D0982429

Microbial
Diseases

Microbial Diseases

A VETERINARIAN'S GUIDE TO LABORATORY DIAGNOSIS

G.R. Carter,
D.V.M., M.S, D.V.Sc., Diplomate ACVM

M.M. Chengappa,
B.V.Sc., M.S., Ph.D., Diplomate ACVM

 Iowa State University Press / Ames

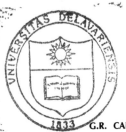

G.R. CARTER received his D.V.M. degree from Ontario Veterinary College, University of Toronto, his M.S. degree from Iowa State University, and his D.V.Sc. degree from the University of Toronto. He formerly held professorships at Ontario Veterinary College, Michigan State University, and Virginia-Maryland Regional College of Veterinary Medicine, Virginia Tech. Dr. Carter is presently professor emeritus, Virginia-Maryland Regional College of Veterinary Medicine, Blacksburg, Virginia.

M.M. CHENGAPPA received his B.V.Sc. and M.V.Sc. degrees in Bangalore, India, and his M.S. and Ph.D. degrees from Michigan State University. He has held positions at Murray State University, University of Kentucky, and Kansas State University. Dr. Chengappa is presently professor and director of clinical microbiology, Department of Pathology and Microbiology, College of Veterinary Medicine, Kansas State University, Manhattan.

© 1993 Iowa State University Press, Ames, Iowa 50010
All rights reserved

Authorization to photocopy items for internal or personal use, or the internal or personal use of specific clients, is granted by Iowa State University Press, provided that the base fee of $.10 per copy is paid directly to the Copyright Clearance Center, 27 Congress Street, Salem, MA 01970. For those organizations that have been granted a photocopy license by CCC, a separate system of payments has been arranged. The fee code for users of the Transactional Reporting Service is 0-8138-0671-2/93 $.10.

♾ Printed on acid-free paper in the United States of America

Microbial Diseases: A Veterinarian's Guide to Laboratory Diagnosis replaces *Veterinarian's Guide to the Laboratory Diagnosis of Infectious Diseases* (© Veterinary Medicine Publishing Company, Lenexa, Kan., 1986).

First edition, 1993

Library of Congress Cataloging-in-Publication Data

Carter, G. R. (Gordon R.)
    Microbial diseases : a veterinarian's guide to laboratory diagnosis / G.R. Carter, M.M. Chengappa. — 1st ed.
        p.   cm.
    Includes index.
    ISBN 0-8138-0671-2 (acid-free paper)
    1. Communicable diseases in animals — Diagnosis. 2. Communicable diseases in animals — North America — Diagnosis. 3. Veterinary clinical pathology.   I. Chengappa, M. M.   II. Title.
SF781.C365   1993
636.089'6904756 — dc20   92-35999

CONTENTS

v

SECTION **2** Microbial Diseases in North America

SECTION **3** **Microbial Diseases Foreign
to North America**

APPENDICES, 291

INDEX, 295

PREFACE

This book replaces *Veterinarian's Guide to the Laboratory Diagnosis of Infectious Diseases* (© 1986 Veterinary Medicine Publishing Co.) and has been updated to include the many changes in the names of important bacteria and fungi. The lists of bacteria and fungi have been expanded to assist veterinarians in the interpretation of reports from the diagnostic laboratory. A number of relatively new diseases have been added and newer diagnostic procedures are referred to where appropriate.

The primary purpose of this book is to provide veterinarians, mainly practitioners, with a summary of important facts of microbial diseases of farm and companion animals in North America; instructions on the use of the diagnostic microbiology laboratory, including, where appropriate, the interpretation of results are also included. The material is organized and presented for quick and ready reference and therefore is also useful to laboratory technicians, as well as students studying for board examinations. For presentation of clinical laboratory data and gross and microscopic pathologic examinations, users should refer to any number of books and manuals that provide in-depth studies (see Appendix B).

The main emphasis is on diseases that occur in North America. Diseases that are foreign to North America are listed separately. Ordinarily the laboratory diagnosis of foreign diseases is the responsibility of federal officials and laboratories; thus, it is not always dealt with in detail in the foreign diseases mentioned. This group of diseases has been included mainly for review purposes because the practitioner should be aware of their principal characteristics and the possibility of their occurrence.

Diseases are listed alphabetically by the currently most acceptable name; synonyms of many of the names used will be found in the index. The diseases are usually discussed, after an introductory definition, under the following headings: Differential Diagnosis, Laboratory Diagnosis, Treatment, and Control. The main emphasis is on Laboratory Diagnosis. Differential Diagnosis, Treatment, and Control are mentioned only briefly in the interest of reviewing salient points.

Not all of the potentially pathogenic bacteria cause important microbial diseases. A considerable number cause or are associated with a variety of usually sporadic and opportunistic infections involving individual or small numbers of animals. These bacteria have been listed under their genus names along with the animals and infections with which they are associated. Each bacterium and fungus has been listed in the index.

The introductory chapter deals in some detail with the selection and submission of specimens. Many diagnostic laboratories provide their own detailed instructions on the selection and submission of specimens.

Appendices include sources of commercially available diagnostic materials and kits that may be useful to the veterinary practitioner, as well as sources for further information.

We wish to thank Dr. John R. Cole, Jr., Mr. A. Wayne Roberts, and Dr. Robert M. Phillips for their many helpful comments and suggestions. We would also like to acknowledge the fine efforts and cooperation of Mrs. Lori Page-Willyard in typing the manuscript and Ms. Sandy Brown in editing the manuscript and preparing the index. The cordial and thoughtful cooperation of Mr. Richard R. Kinney, former director of Iowa State University Press, and his staff is gratefully acknowledged.

Microbial
Diseases

SECTION 1

General Recommendations: Specimens and Interpretation of Reports

Selection and Submission of Specimens

Specific recommendations are given in connection with each disease.

It is of paramount importance to provide an adequate history and to indicate which disease or diseases you suspect. Also advise the laboratory if any antimicrobial (antibiotic) treatment has been given.

Just prior to death, and shortly thereafter, a number of intestinal bacteria may invade host tissues. The significance of these organisms, some of which may be potential pathogens, is difficult to assess when tissue samples have been taken several hours after death, particularly in hot weather. Live, acutely sick animals that can be sacrificed and necropsied are usually the best source of specimens. In all instances, the importance of fresh samples taken as soon after death as possible cannot be overemphasized.

SPECIMENS FOR BACTERIAL AND FUNGOUS EXAMINATIONS
Tissues and Organs

If there are obvious lesions, samples containing these lesions should be included. If there are no apparent lesions and an infectious disease is suspected, samples (about ½ ounce or at least 1 × 2 inches if possible) should be submitted from liver, lung, kidney, spleen, intestine, and lymph nodes. A specimen taken at the margin of diseased and normal tissue is preferred. A rib should also be included.

3

Place tissues in individual plastic bags or leak-proof jars. Twirl plastic bags are convenient and double-bagging is recommended for shipping. Portions of intestines should be packed separately. Specimens can be conveniently shipped in a styrofoam box or picnic-type chest containing a generous amount of ice. Dry ice with plenty of insulation is preferred for prolonged preservation.

Brains sent for examination should be halved longitudinally. One half is refrigerated or frozen over dry ice and the other half is divided into several portions and placed in 10% buffered formalized saline for histopathologic examination. Do not freeze tissues in formalin.

Swabs

Swabs are of value in many instances for the transportation of infectious material to the laboratory. However, because many bacteria are susceptible to desiccation during shipment, it is advisable to place the swab in a nonnutritional transport medium. Swabs referred to as Culturettes and other comparable swab systems that utilize a transport medium are available commercially (see 2,5,10,14, Appendix A).

Equine Cervical Swabs

Special swabs are required for swabbing the cervices of mares and other large animals. These can be prepared by attaching absorbent cotton to the end of an 18- to 24-inch length of wire with a rubber band. Then approximately 1 foot of the portion containing the cotton is enclosed with paper or a pipette paper cover and autoclaved. Sterile swabs with long handles are available commercially (see 2,5,10,14, Appendix A).

Anaerobes

Anaerobes are sensitive to oxygen. Special commercial transport systems are available for transporting materials suspected of containing anaerobes (see 5,10, Appendix A). Some laboratories provide screw-cap tubes containing oxygen-free gas for the submission of swabs. Liquid material can be submitted in a syringe devoid of air.

Dermatophytes (Ringworm)

After first cleaning the area with 70% alcohol, scrapings should be made at the edge of active lesions. Submit samples in a cotton-plugged test tube or paper envelope. Saprophytic fungi will often proliferate rapidly in a sealed tube because of the moisture.

Milk

Collect 5–10 ml in a sterile narrow-necked bottle or Whirl-Pak. For aseptic collection wipe the teat orifice with methylated spirits (not water), discard the milk in the teat cistern, then collect the sample.

Milk samples are of no use for bacteriology if antibiotics have been used in the previous 7 days. Samples must be refrigerated before shipping and packed with coolant packs or ice in insulated boxes for submission to the laboratory.

Urine

Urine is collected in various ways from the domestic animals: bladder tap, particularly in dogs and cats; sterile catheter; midstream catch. In collecting urine for bacteriologic examination, the goal should be to minimize normal flora and environmental bacteria. Strict asepsis should be practiced and urine should be collected in a sterile, sealed container. Because urine can support the growth of bacteria, it should be refrigerated immediately or certainly within 1 hour. It should be cultured as soon as possible after collection. The actual number of bacteria present in the urine sample at the time of collection will indicate whether or not there is a urinary tract infection. The bacteriologist will not be able to reliably estimate the number if multiplication has taken place.

Urine samples must be refrigerated in transit. Urine should not be submitted on a swab.

If the urine is to be examined for leptospira by dark-field microscopy, 1.5 ml of 10% formalin should be added to 20 ml of urine. Leptospira disintegrate shortly after collection unless fixed by formalin.

Abortion Specimens

A complete history of the aborting animals and the herd is particularly important.

For serology: 10 ml of maternal blood for serum must be

submitted. Standard brucella tubes or red-top Vacutainer tubes are convenient. Another blood sample should be collected 2 or 3 weeks postabortion. It may also be helpful to submit blood samples from presuckle calves at birth.

For bacteriology and virology: Fresh placenta; wash if contaminated with dirt and feces.

Uterine discharge is collected on swabs and placed in transport media.

Fresh whole fetus is preferred. If the whole fetus is not submitted, send fresh fetal stomach contents, fetal fluid (heart blood and cavity fluid); and fetal lung, kidney, liver, and thymus. Fresh specimens should be collected, packed, and shipped as described above (SPECIMENS FOR BACTERIAL AND FUNGOUS EXAMINATIONS: Tissues and Organs; Swabs).

For histopathology: Small pieces (see SPECIMENS FOR HISTOPATHOLOGY) of lung, liver, adrenal, kidney, spleen, small intestine, cotyledon, caruncle, and brain should be placed in 10% buffered formalized saline.

Respiratory Tract Infections

Nasal swabs are useful for upper respiratory tract infections. However, nasal swabs have limited value for the recovery of pathogenic bacteria in pneumonias because potential pathogens may be part of the normal flora of the nasopharynx. Nasal swabs are of value for the isolation of viruses in upper and lower respiratory tract infections.

Transtracheal aspiration and the bronchial brush are useful for obtaining materials for culture. The bronchial brush has the advantage that it can sometimes be directed to the lesion fluoroscopically.

SPECIMENS FOR VIRAL EXAMINATION

Specimens are selected and handled as described above for bacterial and fungal diseases. Swabs and transport media specially formulated for the protection and maintenance of viruses are available commercially (see 5,10,14, Appendix A).

Paired serum samples (see SERUM SAMPLES below) are particularly important in the diagnosis of viral infections in that only an appreciable increase (usually at least fourfold) in antibody titer between acute and convalescent sera is significant. The interval between these two samples should be about 3 weeks. To avoid confusion, it is best to submit both samples at the same time.

For electron microscopy: Many laboratories now use the electron microscope to examine for enteric viruses. Feces should be collected directly from the animal within 6 hours of the onset of diarrhea; 5–20 ml are collected, preferably in small wide-mouth containers with secure lids, and promptly shipped under refrigeration.

SERUM SAMPLES

No anticoagulant should be used. Standard brucella tubes or red-top Vacutainer tubes are convenient. Five ml of blood or 2 ml of clear serum is sufficient for most serologic tests. Wet needles, syringes, and tubes and excessive heat will cause hemolysis, which may interfere with such tests as complement fixation.

For clotted blood: Samples are allowed to clot (leave several hours at room temperature) and shipped preferably in wet ice or with coolant but not frozen. Pouring off the serum from a clotted sample will prevent hemolysis. The remaining clotted sample can be kept in the refrigerator for later submission in case anything happens to the submitted serum. Serum can be frozen and shipped on dry ice as an alternative to shipping with wet ice or coolant. Corvac-type separator tubes are useful if it is important to separate serum; centrifuge these separator tubes prior to shipping.

Swine blood is especially susceptible to hemolysis, thus serum should be poured off into clean, dry tubes.

For unclotted blood: This can be conveniently submitted in 5-ml amounts in EDTA Vacutainer tubes (lavender stopper).

SPECIMENS FOR HISTOPATHOLOGY

Slices of tissue, about 5 mm thick, should be fixed as soon after collection as possible. Sections thicker than 5 mm will not fix reliably; very thin sections may twist, making the preparation of sections difficult. Several blocks of tissue from the boundary zone between normal and abnormal tissue should be included so that the most suitable sample can be selected.

Use sharp instruments in preparing tissue samples, and take care that tissue is not crushed with forceps or fingers. Containers should hold about 10 times as much fixative as tissues. Small brains should be fixed whole. Large brains should be divided into several portions to facilitate fixing.

The most common and useful fixative for tissue is 10% formalin, made by diluting 1 volume of commercial formalin with 9 volumes of water or normal saline. Commercial formalin is about 40% formaldehyde gas in water. Never use undiluted commercial formalin. Phosphate-buffered formalin, if available, is preferred. The formalin solution should be free of precipitate.

Specimens for histopathology should never be frozen.

SPECIMENS FOR PARASITOLOGY

Each sample should be carefully identified, including the date taken. Do not submit open containers or containers contaminated on the outside. Do not preserve external parasites in alcohol or other fixative.

Send skin scrapings in a sterile bottle. Samples of hair and wool may be submitted in a plastic container. Send live ectoparasites, larvae, or snails in a jar with moist cotton wool, gauze, or blotting paper to prevent desiccation.

Collect fecal samples from the rectum, not from the ground. Submit individual fecal samples in a separate impervious container such as a small plastic or glass bottle or vial. Eliminate as much air as possible from the container. Eggs may hatch in fecal samples kept for longer than 2 days at room temperature. Keep samples at 4°C.

For diagnosis of abomasal worms, send 10–20 ml of clotted blood or the serum from such samples for a serum pepsinogen determination.

For diagnosis of blood parasites, send a blood sample in EDTA anticoagulant together with a blood smear.

For determination of herbal larval contamination, send 400–600 g of herbage randomly sampled from the pasture; avoid dung pads.

When cestodes, trematodes, or nematodes are to be identified, preserve in 5% formalin. For cestodes, ensure that the scolex is included as well as mature and gravid segments. Specimens should be fully labelled with regard to their source, i.e., animal species and organ or tissue.

SPECIMENS FOR TOXICOLOGY

1. Contents of stomach or abomasum (500 ml).
2. Contents of rumen (500 ml).
3. Perirenal fat (particularly when insecticide examination is required).
4. Liver (about 500 g).
5. Vomitus.
6. Heparinized blood (10 ml) (when nitrate, chlorate, or lead poisoning is suspected).
7. Feces (5–10 g) and urine (60 ml) from a live, affected animal.
8. Stem, leaves, flower, fruit, and root (if plant is suspected to be toxic).
9. Formalin-fixed sections of organs showing gross change; always send sections of liver and kidney.
10. Brain, half fresh and half fixed in formalin (when salt poisoning is suspected in pigs).

Always request a specific analysis. The laboratory cannot check each specimen for the whole range of heavy metals and organic plant poisons.

For mycotoxins, stored grain, feed, or hay may be sent in a closed (not airtight) container, plastic bag (for moist feed sample), or paper bag soon after collection. If delay is anticipated, the specimen should be refrigerated to prevent the overgrowth of some bacteria and fungi.

SUBMISSION KITS

Some diagnostic laboratories provide special submission kits for particular infectious diseases.

Interpretation of Clinical Microbiology Reports

Many bacteria, fungi, and some viruses are found in and on animals. Some knowledge of the normal flora is essential for the interpretation and understanding of reports. When specimens are taken from sites with a normal flora, bacterial cultures will often yield a variety of organisms. For example, the skin may yield *Staphylococcus intermedius, S. epidermidis,* a "viridans" streptococcus, and *Clostridium perfringens.* In selecting the bacterium for an antimicrobial susceptibility test, the experienced microbiologist will usually take into consideration such factors as the potential pathogenicity of the organism, the number of colonies, the condition of the clinical specimen, and the history supplied. Occasionally, susceptibility tests will be performed on more than one bacterium. If the microbial examination is carried out by an inexperienced microbiologist or technologist, the clinician may have to decide which bacterium or bacteria should be susceptibility tested.

The following should be kept in mind when interpreting reports:

1. The sources and condition of the specimens. Unsatisfactory specimens are the principal reason for an unproductive microbial examination.
2. A negative microbial examination does not necessarily rule out an infection. Some organisms are shed intermittently. Another specimen may be indicated.
3. Were antimicrobial drugs used prior to collecting specimens?
4. Because fungi are so prevalent in nature, repeated isolation with histopathologic evidence of infection may be required for confirmation of causality.

2 | Microbial Diseases in North America

ACINETOBACTER

Although only one species, *Acinetobacter calcoaceticus,* is officially recognized, six species have been described. *A. calcoaceticus* and *A. lwoffii* are of greatest veterinary significance. They are gram-negative rods or diplococci that occur frequently in soil, water, sewage, and occasionally as part of the normal flora of animals and humans.

They have been isolated from a variety of opportunistic, usually low-grade, infections of animals. Their occurrence in clinical specimens is not necessarily significant.

ACTINOBACILLOSIS / WOODEN TONGUE

Actinobacillosis is a noncontagious disease, principally of cattle, caused by *Actinobacillus lignieresii* and characterized by the formation of granulomatous abscesses involving the lymph nodes and soft tissues (frequently the tongue), particularly of the head and neck.

Actinobacillus lignieresii is a small, gram-negative aerobic rod that occurs as a commensal in the alimentary tract.

The organism usually enters via small wounds and infects the mucous membrane of the upper digestive tract. Spread is via the lymphatics; those of the head and neck are usually involved; it can spread to other tissues and organs.

Occurrence is worldwide, usually sporadic, and sometimes involves a number of animals in a herd. The disease occurs infrequently in sheep.

Differential Diagnosis

This disease is most easily confused with actinomycosis. The latter usually involves the jawbone and spreads by contiguity.

The granules found in the pus in actinobacillosis are gray-white and smaller (less than 1 mm) than the sulfur granules of actinomycosis.

Abscesses caused by other bacteria are uncommon in this region. When they occur, they are not usually extensive or progressive.

Laboratory Diagnosis

SPECIMENS. Pus is taken from fresh, preferably nondischarging abscesses.

PROCEDURE. Pus is examined for granules and cultured.

Granules are crushed on a slide and Gram stained to identify the bacteria.

A definitive diagnosis is based on the isolation and identification of *A. lignieresii.*

Treatment

1. Surgical drainage.
2. Potassium iodide administered orally.
3. Tetracyclines, streptomycin, erythromycin given systemically and locally are useful.

Control

1. Prevent injuries to the mucosa of the upper digestive tract.
2. Avoid forage and coarse feed that may be injurious.

ACTINOBACILLUS

Members of this genus are small, gram-negative rods that occur as commensals. The following species are recognized:

A. lignieresii: See ACTINOBACILLOSIS.

A. pleuropneumoniae (formerly *Haemophilus pleuropneumoniae*): See CONTAGIOUS PLEUROPNEUMONIA OF SWINE.

A. equuli: See NONENTERIC INFECTIONS OF NEONATAL FOALS.

A. suis: Causes septicemia, arthritis, pneumonia, and other infections in young pigs.

A. capsulatus: Has been recovered from rabbits with septic arthritis.

A. actinomycetemcomitans: Has been isolated frequently

from humans. It has been infrequently associated with epididymitis in rams.

A. actinoides: Not a valid species. It is now thought that isolates given this name are probably *Haemophilus somnus.*

A. seminis: Not considered a valid species within the genus *Actinobacillus.* It is important as a cause of epididymitis of young rams (see OVINE EPIDIDIMYTIS: General), and purulent polyarthritis and gangrenous mastitis of sheep.

ACTINOMYCES

Actinomyces are gram-positive, non-acid-fast rods that frequently display filamentation and branching, and may occur as commensals. The following species are recognized:

Actinomyces bovis: See ACTINOMYCOSIS.

A. pyogenes (formerly *Corynebacterium pyogenes*): See *ACTINOMYCES PYOGENES* INFECTION.

A. viscosus: See CANINE ACTINOMYCOSIS. It occurs as a commensal in the canine mouth. Infections occur infrequently in animals other than the dog.

A. hordeovulneris: See CANINE ACTINOMYCOSIS.

A. suis: See ACTINOMYCOSIS. This name has been proposed for strains of *Actinomyces* recovered from actinomycosis involving the mammary gland of sows.

A. naeslundii: Has been isolated from aborted porcine fetuses.

ACTINOMYCES PYOGENES INFECTION /
PYOBACILLOSIS

Actinomyces pyogenes (formerly *Corynebacterium pyogenes*) causes chronic disease principally in cattle, swine, and sheep. It is characterized most commonly by the formation of abscesses in the lungs (suppurative pneumonia, usually with other agents including nonsporeforming anaerobes). The organism is a frequent commensal in the upper respiratory and digestive tracts. It is involved less frequently in other locations such as the skin (wounds), mammary gland (mastitis), uterus (pyometritis), and joints (suppurative arthritis, joint ill). *A. pyogenes* is frequently recovered along with *Fusobacterium necrophorum* from bovine liver abscesses.

Laboratory Diagnosis

SPECIMENS. Laboratory diagnosis is dealt with under general discussions of RESPIRATORY DISEASE of the various animal species. Fresh material is taken from the abscesses or suppurative lesions and submitted on a swab or in a syringe or other sterile container.

Treatment

Surgical drainage when feasible. *A. pyogenes* is susceptible to many antimicrobial drugs in vitro, but the suppurative nature of the disease process prevents effective antimicrobial action.

ACTINOMYCOSIS / LUMPY JAW

Actinomycosis is a sporadic, chronic progressive disease, principally of cattle, caused by *Actinomyces bovis* and characterized by indurated, granulomatous, suppurative abscesses that most frequently involve the mandible bone and contiguous tissues.

Actinomyces bovis is a gram-positive, filamentous, and branching rod. It is preferentially anaerobic and 10% CO_2 is required for maximum growth. The organism is a commensal in the mouth and usually gains entry to the oral mucosa via wounds. It spreads in tissues by contiguity.

Infections have been reported worldwide in horses, sheep, swine, dogs, and other animals, but they are rare. Infection of the mammary gland of the sow is sometimes seen. Strains that infect the mammary gland of sows differ in several characteristics from *A. bovis* recovered from cattle. They have been given the name *A. suis*.

Differential Diagnosis

In contrast to actinobacillosis, actinomycosis most frequently affects bone, is not spread by lymphatics, and has relatively larger sulfur-colored granules. Abscesses in the head and neck region due to other agents (*A. pyogenes, Fusobacterium necrophorum* or *Bacteriodes* spp.) should be considered.

Laboratory Diagnosis

SPECIMENS. Fresh pus preferably in a sterile container. It is advisable to open an abscess. Draining abscesses are frequently contaminated with extraneous organisms.

PROCEDURES. Pus is examined for sulfur granules and cultured. Granules are crushed and stained to demonstrate the characteristic morphology of the granules and *A. bovis.*

COMMENTS. The characteristic gross pathologic changes along with the finding of typical sulfur granules in pus make possible a highly presumptive diagnosis of actinomycosis. The diagnosis is strengthened by finding the typical gram-positive, filamentous organisms in stained, crushed sulfur granules. The latter are 1–3 mm in diameter while those of actinobacillosis are less than 1 mm.

Treatment
Early cases: Surgery; packing with gauze soaked in Lugol's iodine or other antimicrobials. Potassium iodide orally. Sulfonamides and penicillin. Advanced cases: Do not respond satisfactorily to treatment.

Control
None.

ADENOVIRUS INFECTIONS
Adenoviruses cause a number of infections:
Canine adenovirus 1: See INFECTIOUS CANINE HEPATITIS.
Canine adenovirus 2: See CANINE INFECTIOUS TRACHEOBRONCHITIS, CANINE RESPIRATORY DISEASE.
Bovine adenoviruses: Nine serotypes have been identified thus far. They have been isolated from cattle with subclinical to mild respiratory infections, and from calves and lambs with diarrhea.
Equine adenoviruses: See EQUINE RESPIRATORY DISEASE.

ADIASPIROMYCOSIS / HAPLOMYCOSIS
This disease is caused by the soil-borne fungi *Chrysosporium parvum* and *C. crescens.* The conidia are inhaled resulting in a respiratory infection that has been reported in many species of rodents and other wild animals. There are reports of several canine cases. The conidia do not replicate in the lungs but develop into spherules without endospores. Lesions result

from the granulomatous inflammation.

Diagnosis is based on demonstration of conidia and spherules in tissue sections and isolation and identification of the fungi. The fungi are dimorphic with a yeast-like phase growing at 37°C and a mycelial phase at 25°C on appropriate media.

AEROMONAS

Species of this genus are gram-negative rods that occur widely in freshwater, soil, sewage, and on fish.

Aeromonas hydrophila: The principal species that causes furunculosis in salmonid fish. It is occasionally isolated from cattle, swine, horses, and dogs but is rarely considered pathogenic.

A. salmonicida: A pathogen of fish.

A. media and other species have been implicated in a variety of human infections.

ANAEROBIC BACTERIA (NONSPOREFORMING)

The nonsporeforming anaerobic bacteria comprise a large group that occurs in nature, on mucous membranes, and in the intestinal tract of animals. They are frequently found in association with aerobic pathogens such as streptococci, staphylococci, and corynebacteria in purulent and suppurative infections. Their presence in these mixed infections does not necessarily indicate significance.

The two most common and important species are *Bacteroides nodosus,* the primary cause of contagious foot rot of sheep (discussed separately), and *Fusobacterium necrophorum,* which is involved in a variety of important infections. The most commonly isolated nonsporeforming anaerobic bacteria that have pathogenic significance are listed below:

Bacteroides nodosus: Primary cause of contagious foot rot of sheep (discussed separately).

B. melaninogenicus: Suppurative infections in cattle, sheep, dogs, and cats. It is often found with *F. necrophorum* in foot rot of cattle.

B. fragilis: Recovered occasionally from animal infections.

B. corrodens (B. ureolyticus): Causes infections in humans and animals.

B. asaccharolyticus: Causes osteomyelitis in cats, dogs, cattle, and horses.

B. salivosus: Has been associated with subcutaneous abscesses and empyema in cats.

B. levii: Has been associated with summer mastitis of cattle.

B. heparinolyticus: Has been recovered from oral lesions in cats and horses.

Fusobacterium necrophorum: Cause of bovine liver abscesses, often in association with *Actinomyces pyogenes* (see BOVINE LIVER ABSCESS). Other infections include thrush, a necrotic infection involving the frog of the horse; secondary invader in calf diphtheria (q.v.) and necrotic laryngitis; foot rot in cattle (discussed separately); secondary invader in lip and leg ulceration of sheep (see ULCERATIVE DERMATOSIS); foot abscess in sheep (discussed separately); "bullnose" in swine; and a secondary invader in swine dysentery (discussed separately) and necrotic enteritis of swine. *F. necrophorum* infections are also discussed under NECROBACILLOSIS.

F. nucleatum: Has been recovered from infections in animals.

Three genera of gram-positive anaerobic cocci are recognized: *Peptococcus, Peptostreptococcus,* and *Streptococcus.*

Peptococcus niger: The only species recognized in the genus; it is rarely isolated from animals.

Peptostreptococcus anaerobius: Has been isolated occasionally from veterinary clinical specimens.

P. indolicus: Has been implicated as an infrequent cause of bovine mastitis.

None of the strictly anaerobic streptococci has been implicated as animal pathogens, but some streptococci that are only anaerobic on initial isolation are occasionally recovered from infections in animals. Among the nonsporeforming anaerobic gram-positive rods, *Eubacterium suis* (formerly *Corynebacterium suis*) is the most important pathogen (see PORCINE PYELONEPHRITIS).

Propionibacterium spp.: Are associated with dairy products and the skin. They are occasionally recovered from clinical specimens but their significance in animal disease is not known.

Lactobacilli: Are frequently isolated from animals, but they are not considered to be pathogenic.

Laboratory Diagnosis

SPECIMENS. Some of the nonsporeforming anaerobes are sensitive to oxygen and for this reason, a special effort should be made to exclude oxygen when submitting specimens. Biopsies and exudate or pus submitted in a syringe (needle plugged into a stopper) are satisfactory.

Swabs should be submitted in special tubes from which oxygen has been excluded or a commercially available anaerobic specimen collector should be used (see 5,10, Appendix A).

PROCEDURES/COMMENTS. Gram-stained smears may provide some indication of the probable organisms involved. Isolation and identification procedures are carried out both for aerobic and anaerobic bacteria. Precise identification of some nonsporeforming anaerobes may be rather involved.

Treatment

Among the most useful drugs for empirical treatment are penicillin, clindamycin, and chloramphenicol. When information is available, treatment should be based on the results of antimicrobial susceptibility tests.

ANAPLASMOSIS OF CATTLE / GALLSICKNESS

Anaplasmosis is an arthropod-borne disease of cattle and some other ruminants caused by *Anaplasma marginale* and manifested in acute, subacute, and chronic forms with fever and varying degrees of anemia and icterus.

Anaplasma marginale is a blood-borne rickettsia that parasitizes erythrocytes. *A. centrale* is a relatively avirulent species that sometimes occurs with *A. marginale* in Africa.

The disease occurs widely in tropical and subtropical countries, principally in cattle and water buffaloes. Calves under 6 months of age are relatively resistant to clinical disease but may become carriers.

The principal vectors are ticks, but other biting arthropods may also transmit the disease. The source of infection is always blood, and the disease can be spread by contaminated needles, syringes, and surgical instruments.

Differential Diagnosis

Hemoglobinuria is seen in piroplasmosis but not in anaplasmosis. Salmonellosis, pasteurellosis, and other febrile microbial diseases should be considered. When previously unexposed animals are introduced to infected herds, acute anaplasmosis frequently develops.

Laboratory Diagnosis

1. Unclotted blood for smears.
2. Serum and fresh plasma for serologic tests.

PROCEDURES/COMMENTS

1. Examination of blood smears for characteristic forms of *A. marginale.*
2. Rapid card agglutination test can be carried out with serum or plasma. If plasma is used, the test must be run shortly (2 hours) after bleeding. The rapid card agglutination test is reported as positive or negative.
3. Other tests that are sometimes carried out are complement fixation, capillary tube agglutination, the indirect fluorescent antibody test, and the enzyme-linked immunosorbent assay.

Treatment

Tetracyclines are effective if given early. Long-acting formulations are effective in eliminating the carrier states when administered for prolonged periods.

Control

1. Reduction of arthropod vector population. Eradication can be accomplished by eliminating infected animals.
2. Premunition of young animals with virulent and attenuated *A. marginale* is widely practiced in endemic regions. In adult animals, premunition should include tetracycline administration.
3. A killed vaccine is available that offers some protection.
4. A sheep-adapted strain of *A. marginale* is used as a vaccine in a number of countries but is not approved for use in the United States.

ANAPLASMOSIS OF SHEEP AND GOATS

Anaplasma ovis, a rickettsia, is usually avirulent but, under certain circumstances, it can cause a mild anaplasmosis in sheep and goats that is similar to the mild disease in cattle. It has been reported in the United States and other countries.

A laboratory diagnosis is made by the examination of stained blood smears for *A. ovis* in the same manner as for *A. marginale* in bovine anaplasmosis.

ANTHRAX

Anthrax is most often an acute, toxemic disease caused by *Bacillus anthracis* in animals and humans, and usually characterized by septicemia, sudden death, exudation of tarry blood from body orifices, splenomegaly, and absence of rigor mortis.

Bacillus anthracis is a large gram-positive, sporeforming bacillus. Virulence of strains depends on possession of a capsule and the capacity to produce toxin.

Occurrence is worldwide wherever the spores are present. Spores can survive for years in the soil; flooding may disseminate them. Contaminated oil-cake, tankage, and bone meal are other possible sources of spores.

The disease in swine may be less severe and characterized by acute pharyngitis with extensive swelling and hemorrhage of the pharyngeal region. The disease is rare in dogs and cats.

Differential Diagnosis

Acute infectious diseases such as salmonellosis, leptospirosis, and bacillary hemoglobinuria; acute poisonings such as arsenic, bracken fern, sweet clover, and lead; and other causes of sudden death such as lightning and sunstroke should be considered.

Laboratory Diagnosis

SPECIMENS. To prevent sporulation, the carcass should not be opened.

1. Two swabs and two smears of peripheral blood from an ear vein or other vein.
2. In swine, it may be advisable to remove material from swollen submaxillary or cervical lymph nodes with a syringe in addition to taking swabs and smears from peripheral blood.

PROCEDURES. Isolation and identification of *B. anthracis.*
    With experience, a diagnosis of anthrax can be made on the basis of finding typical large, capsulated rods in smears stained by Giemsa, Wright's, or Loeffler's methylene blue. However, it is advisable when possible to isolate and identify *B. anthracis.*

Treatment
1. Treatment of sick animals with penicillin, tetracyclines, chloramphenicol, sulfonamides.
2. Vaccination of well animals.

Control
Vaccination with Sterne's spore vaccine. Anthrax is a reportable disease in many countries requiring the application of strict regulatory measures.

ASPERGILLOSIS
Aspergillosis is a noncontagious disease of a number of animal species caused by fungi of the genus *Aspergillus* (usually *A. fumigatus*). Other potentially pathogenic species are *A. flavus* and *A. nidulans. A. niger* and *A. terreus* are rarely involved in animal infections. These fungi occur widely in nature, and the usual mode of infection is by inhalation with the production of granulomatous lesions and nodules in the respiratory tract from which there may be dissemination to other tissues and organs. Infections may also begin in the alimentary tract.

The principal forms of aspergillosis are as follows:

Nasal or paranasal aspergillosis: Seen most commonly in the dog (see NASAL ASPERGILLOSIS).

Equine guttural pouch mycosis: Discussed separately.

Bovine and equine abortion: See Index.

Pneumonic and intestinal aspergillosis: Have been reported in many animal species. It is an infrequent disease most often diagnosed following necropsy.

Disseminated aspergillosis: Has been described in dogs.

Aspergillosis: Of poultry (brooder pneumonia).

Laboratory Diagnosis
This will be discussed under specific diseases (except aspergillosis of poultry).

Diagnosis is usually based on the isolation and identification of the *Aspergillus* sp. and the demonstration of septate hyphae in tissue sections. Because this fungus is very widespread in nature, mere isolation may not indicate significance.

ATROPHIC RHINITIS OF SWINE

Atrophic rhinitis of swine (ARS) is a disease of young pigs now considered to be due to combined infection with *Bordetella bronchiseptica* and toxin-producing strains of *Pasteurella multocida*. *B. bronchiseptica* infection is thought to be primary to colonization with toxin-producing *P. multocida*. *B. bronchiseptica* by itself causes a mild transient infection. ARS is characterized by an inflammation of the nasal mucosa, leading often to atrophy of the turbinate bones and distortion of the nasal septum that sometimes results in shortening or twisting of the upper jaw. Prognathism (jutting of the lower jaw) is a common clinical sign.

Occurrence is probably worldwide. *B. bronchiseptica,* a small gram-negative rod, occurs as a commensal in the nasopharynx of some swine, cattle, sheep, dogs, cats, horses, rabbits, and no doubt other animals.

Pasteurella multocida, which is also a small, gram-negative rod or coccobacillus, occurs commonly as a commensal in the nasopharynx of farm animals. Most of the toxin-producing strains associated with ARS belong to serogroup D and occur mainly in swine. Other bacteria may be present but their role in the disease, if any, would seem to be minor.

Differential Diagnosis

Inclusion body rhinitis (discussed separately) and necrotic rhinitis ("bullnose"), a disease of young pigs resulting from wounds to the nasal or oral mucosa. When ARS is well established in a herd, it is usually clinically obvious.

Laboratory Diagnosis

When the disease is well established it is usually clinically obvious. Culturing is carried out mainly to determine the extent of the disease.

SPECIMENS. The external nares should be thoroughly cleaned with either sterile cotton or well-expressed,

70% ethanol-soaked, cotton pledgets. Cotton-tipped applicator sticks are inserted approximately one-half the distance into the nasal cavity, taking care to use a gentle, rotating motion to reduce the chance of trauma to the delicate turbinates. Submit swabs to the laboratory as soon as possible for culturing.

If delivery of the swabs is not immediate, a transport medium or system, e.g., Culturette (see 2,5,10,14, Appendix A), should be used.

PROCEDURES. Swabs are plated on media selective for *B. bronchiseptica* and *P. multocida*.

COMMENTS. The efficiency of culturing for *B. bronchiseptica* has been improved recently by the use of the selective medium of Smith and Baskerville.

An animal is not usually considered free of *B. bronchiseptica* until there have been three successive, negative bilateral swabs.

Treatment

Isolates of *B. bronchiseptica* and *P. multocida* should be tested for antimicrobial susceptibility.

Sulfonamides, tetracyclines, tylosin, and trimethoprim are used for chemoprophylaxis and therapy in sows before farrowing, in newborn piglets, and in newly weaned pigs. Drugs are usually administered in the feed. Bacterins may be used at the same time.

Control

1. Bacterins: Some contain only *B. bronchiseptica*, while others contain both *B. bronchiseptica* and *P. multocida*. They are used to vaccinate baby pigs, sows, and gilts.
2. Live vaccine: A live avirulent culture (*B. bronchiseptica*) vaccine is available. It is administered to baby pigs intranasally and to sows and gilts intramuscularly.
3. Eradication: Eradication is attempted by maintaining a closed herd with segregation, isolation, and eventual marketing of infected animals. The remainder are treated and vaccinated. Culturing and surveillance are continued until no infected animals are found. However, it is very difficult to completely eliminate the disease.

BACILLARY HEMOGLOBINURIA / REDWATER

Bacillary hemoglobinuria is an acute toxemic disease primarily of cattle. It is caused by *Clostridium haemolyticum* and characterized by high fever, hemoglobinuria, and jaundice.

Clostridium haemolyticum is a large, gram-positive, anaerobic, sporeforming rod that produces a potent exotoxin, a lecithinase, within hepatic infarcts resulting from liver fluke infestation.

The disease occurs in many countries in areas where the spores and liver flukes occur. In the United States, it occurs most frequently in western states and around the Gulf of Mexico.

Differential Diagnosis

The hemoglobinuria is particularly significant. Piroplasmosis, anthrax, leptospirosis, bracken fern, and ragwort poisoning are among the diseases that should be considered.

Laboratory Diagnosis

SPECIMENS. Portion of liver with infarct; fresh and in formalin solution.

PROCEDURES. Isolation and identification of *C. haemolyticum* is definitive. The finding of large, gram-positive rods in smears from an infarct and the characteristic gross and microscopic pathologic changes in the liver are supportive. Identification by fluorescent antibody (FA) staining of smears is rapid and reliable.

COMMENTS. The presence of typical liver infarcts, liver flukes, and characteristic clinical signs including hemoglobinuria are highly suggestive of bacillary hemoglobinuria. The organism is fastidious to cultivate and identification by cultural methods is slow. By contrast, FA staining is a rapid and reliable means of identifying *C. haemolyticum.*

Clostridium novyi type B causes a somewhat similar disease in sheep (INFECTIOUS NECROTIC HEPATITIS or Black Disease) but rarely in cattle.

Treatment

1. Early treatment with penicillin, tetracyclines, and chloramphenicol.

2. Whole blood and fluids may be helpful in early cases.

Control

Liver fluke control. Use bacterins annually or semiannually.

BACILLUS

Members of this genus are large, gram-positive, sporeforming rods. Many species occur as saprophytes in soil and water. They are common contaminants in clinical specimens. Several species have been implicated in infections:

Bacillus anthracis: See ANTHRAX.

B. cereus: Can cause gangrenous bovine mastitis and abortion in cows and ewes. It may occasionally have a role in infertility in mares.

B. licheniformis: has been implicated in bovine, ovine, and porcine abortion.

BLACKLEG / BLACK QUARTER

Blackleg is an acute febrile disease, usually of young cattle (occasionally of sheep). It is caused by *Clostridium chauvoei* (*C. feseri*) and characterized by emphysematous gangrene, usually involving large skeletal muscles.

Clostridium chauvoei is a large, gram-positive, anaerobic rod. It is found in the intestine of animals, and spores are widespread in the soil.

The mode of infection in cattle is thought to be by ingestion, although endogenous infections may occur. Sheep are infected via wounds.

Occurrence is worldwide; spores appear to be more common in the soil of certain geographic regions. Young cattle, not more than 2 years of age, are usually affected.

Differential Diagnosis

Malignant edema (usually a sporadic disease initiated from a wound), anthrax, and bracken fern poisoning should be considered.

Laboratory Diagnosis

SPECIMENS. Portions of gangrenous muscle and/or smears from such lesions, which are usually dark red to black, dry, gas bubbles, rancid odor. Lesions may be located in a skeletal muscle, myocardium, or myometrium. Skeletal muscle is most commonly involved.

PROCEDURES. Fluorescent antibody (FA) staining of smears
for *C. chauvoei, C. septicum,* and *C. novyi* type A.
Positive staining of *C. chauvoei* is definitive for blackleg.
Sometimes other clostridia are present. Isolation and identification by cultural methods are slow.

COMMENTS. FA staining has greatly facilitated the laboratory diagnosis of blackleg by the rapid identification of
C. chauvoei. It is important that specimens be taken shortly
after death, for other clostridia, particularly *C. septicum,*
invade the carcass postmortem.

Occasionally blackleg is complicated by the presence of
C. novyi type A, *C. septicum,* or *C. sordellii.* All can be
identified by FA staining.

Treatment
Penicillin may be used for both sick and exposed, healthy
cattle.

Control
Bacterins containing *C. chauvoei, C. septicum* and sometimes *C. novyi* type A, and other bacteria are widely used.

BLASTOMYCOSIS / NORTH AMERICAN BLASTOMYCOSIS
Blastomycosis is usually a severe disease, principally of the
dog and human (rarely the horse, cat, or other animal). It is
caused by the fungus *Blastomyces dermatitidis* and characterized by an infection that usually starts in the lungs and results
in the formation of granulomatous nodules with frequent
metastases to the skin, bone, and other tissues and organs.
Although there are usually numerous nodules in the lungs, in
some instances metastases may come from very limited pulmonary involvement. Occasionally the infection is confined
to lesions involving the skin and subcutis.

Blastomyces dermatitidis is a dimorphic fungus that is
presumed to be soil-borne, although it has only been recovered from soil on a few occasions. It is probably worldwide in
distribution, although the number of cases reported outside
of North America is relatively small. The endemic area in the
United States includes the middle western, southeastern, and
Appalachian states.

Although single cases are most frequent, multiple cases
have been reported in hunting dogs.

Differential Diagnosis

Cryptococcosis, nocardiosis, canine actinomycosis, coccidioidomycosis, histoplasmosis, tuberculosis, chronic granulomatous infections of the skin due to other agents, and pneumonia due to other agents should be considered.

Laboratory Diagnosis

Chest radiographs may suggest blastomycosis.

SPECIMENS

1. Material is taken by transtracheal aspiration, transthoracic biopsy, and from granulomatous nodules or abscesses involving the skin. An ocular tap is used if the eye is thought to be involved.
2. Serum. Paired samples preferable.

PROCEDURES

1. Examination of materials in wet mounts for the characteristic thick-walled, single-budding yeasts. Gram-stained smears. Culture at room and incubator temperature (37°C) on appropriate media.
2. Complement fixation and the immunodiffusion test for antibody.

COMMENTS. Results of the complement fixation test should be considered with other evidence, for some infected dogs may be negative and cross-reactions are encountered with *Histoplasma capsulatum*. Titers usually reflect the status of the disease. Rising titers indicate greater involvement; falling titers indicate improvement.

A positive immunodiffusion test indicates a current or recent infection. This test is relatively sensitive and specific.

Skin-testing is not considered to be of value. Definitive diagnosis depends on the isolation and identification of *B. dermatitidis*.

The finding of the typical organisms in sections of biopsies or affected lung is highly diagnostic.

Treatment

1. Amphotericin B is the treatment of choice.
2. Stilbamidine and dihydroxystilbamidine are also used.
3. Imidazole derivatives: miconazole, ketoconazole are used but relapses have been reported.

Control

There are no practicable preventive measures.

BLUETONGUE / OVINE CATARRHAL FEVER, SORE MOUTH

Bluetongue is an acute, noncontagious, arthropod-borne disease of sheep, goats, cattle, and wild ruminants caused by an orbivirus and characterized by fever; leukopenia; erosive inflammation of the mouth, tongue, and lips; coronitis; and myositis.

The disease in cattle is usually inapparent, but abortion and clinical signs similar to those seen in sheep occur occasionally. The disease in white-tailed deer is particularly severe.

There are at least 24 serotypes of the virus, 5 of which occur in the United States. The virus is transmitted by biting insects of the *Culicoides* genus.

Occurrence is probably worldwide. Cattle and goats with inapparent infections are important reservoirs of the virus. The virus is endemic in certain areas of the United States (e.g., southeast).

Differential Diagnosis

Foot-and-mouth disease, vesicular stomatitis, contagious ecthyma, and ulcerative dermatosis should be considered.

Laboratory Diagnosis

SPECIMENS

1. Unclotted blood samples (25 ml) from several animals with fever (viremia).

    Portions of spleen and mesenteric nodes from dead animals and deformed lambs, calves, and aborted fetuses. In some circumstances it may be advisable to submit the whole animal.
2. Paired serum samples for the complement fixation test and agar gel immunodiffusion test.

PROCEDURES/COMMENTS

1. The virus is present in the blood of febrile sheep but its isolation and identification is cumbersome and time consuming. Immune and nonimmune sheep are sometimes inoculated with suspected blood, spleen, and lymph nodes.

2. The results of the complement fixation test are interpreted as follows:
    Suspect: 1:5–1:10
    Positive: ≥ 1:20
A positive test indicates infection or exposure.

An immunodiffusion test is used in most laboratories for detecting antibodies. The result is reported as positive or negative. Other procedures are virus neutralization, enzyme-linked immunosorbent assay, and indirect fluorescent antibody. An increase in titer in paired sera is especially significant. USDA-licensed test kits are available to detect antibodies in cattle and sheep (see 21, Appendix A).

Treatment
None.

Control
A monovalent (serotype 10) live attenuated vaccine is available for use in sheep in the United States. This vaccine should not be used in areas where the disease does not occur because of the danger of reversion to virulence. Some states have attenuated vaccines for other serotypes.

BORDER DISEASE / HAIRY SHAKER DISEASE OF LAMBS, HAIRY SHAKERS, HYPOMYELINOGENESIS CONGENITA

Border disease is a congenital disease of lambs caused by a togavirus (pestivirus) and characterized by an excessively hairy coat, marked tremors of skeletal muscles, defective myelinization of the central nervous system resulting in retarded growth and varying degrees of skeletal deformity.

Not all lambs in a flock are affected. Those showing clinical signs, including the hairy coat, have a poor survival rate although some will survive and overcome the neurologic involvement. Other features of the disease are infertility in ewes, abortions with some fetuses mummified, and weak lambs. Congenital infection has also been reported in cattle and goats resulting in similar fetal disease.

The disease has been reported from many countries, including the United States, New Zealand, Australia, Britain, and some other European countries. The virus is closely related if not identical antigenically to the agent of bovine virus diarrhea (BVD). Natural spread is both vertical and horizontal. The incidence of the disease in some regions, based on serologic evidence, may be as high as 10%.

Differential Diagnosis

The disease is singular in its clinical manifestations and cannot be confused with other diseases.

Laboratory Diagnosis

The disease can be diagnosed on the basis of the characteristic clinical and epidemiologic features; however, it is advisable to seek laboratory confirmation. Not all diagnostic laboratories have the capability of carrying out all of the procedures described below.

SPECIMENS. Ordinarily an affected lamb (or lambs) is submitted.
1. For histopathology, fluorescent antibody staining, and virus isolation: Brain and spinal cord, fresh and fixed portions.
2. For serology: Clotted blood.

PROCEDURES
1. For histopathology: Sections of the brain and cord disclose characteristic changes, including dysmyelinogenesis. For FA staining: The virus present in the brain and cord fluoresces with BVD conjugate. For virus isolation: The virus can be isolated from the brain and cord using fetal-cell cultures.
2. For serology: Among the tests used to detect and measure antibodies are complement fixation, immunodiffusion, and virus neutralization. The closely related bovine virus diarrhea or hog cholera virus can be used as antigens in the serologic tests.

Treatment

None.

Control

Sheep known to be affected, including ewes, should be segregated and eventually sacrificed.

BORDETELLA

Species of this genus are small, gram-negative rods or cocco-bacilli. Only two species are of veterinary significance:

Bordetella bronchiseptica: See ATROPHIC RHINITIS OF SWINE, CANINE RESPIRATORY DISEASE, EQUINE RESPIRATORY DISEASE. This species, which is found as a commensal in a number of animal species, can also cause a severe bronchopneumonia in young pigs.

B. avium: Causes a rhinotracheitis of turkeys often referred to as turkey coryza.

BOTULISM / LAMZIEKTE, LOIN DISEASE

Botulism is a noncontagious, intoxicative disease of animals caused by the neurotoxins of *Clostridium botulinum,* which are produced in food, decomposing animals (carrion), and plant materials (rarely in the alimentary tract and wounds). The disease is characterized by progressive motor paralysis due to the effect of the neurotoxin blocking the release of acetylcholine at motor end-plates.

Clostridium botulinum is a large, gram-positive, spore-forming, anaerobic rod.

Occurrence is worldwide; the highly resistant spores occur widely in nature.

Pigs, dogs, and cats are relatively resistant to botulism.

Clostridium botulinum multiplies in the anaerobic milieu provided by spoiled or decaying organic material, including necrotic tissue. Botulism resulting from toxin produced in tissues is called toxicoinfectious botulism. Examples are wound botulism, infant botulism (gastrointestinal), and possibly shaker foal syndrome (q.v.). In toxicoinfectious botulism the toxin may be produced in gastric lesions (e.g., ulcers), liver necrosis, septic wounds, and navel and pulmonary abscesses.

The disease, lamziekte, occurs in South Africa but probably also in other countries including the United States (loin disease — rare) and South America. Phosphorus-deficient cattle (pica) acquire toxin from chewing bones with remnants of meat containing toxin; cadavers are not uncommon on large ranges.

Types A, B, C, D, E, F, and G of *C. botulinum* have

been identified on the basis of immunologic differences in neurotoxins (Table 2.1).

Table 2.1. Types of *C. botulinum*

Type	Animals Involved
A,B,E,F,G	Humans
B	Horses, foals, cattle
C-alpha	Wild ducks, pheasants, and chickens
C-beta	Cattle, horses, mink, dogs
D	Cattle, sheep

Differential Diagnosis

Rabies, equine encephalomyelitis, ragwort poisoning, postparturient paresis in cattle, hypocalcemia in sheep, and many other diseases affecting the nervous system should be considered.

Laboratory Diagnosis

SPECIMENS

1. Food including carrion suspected of harboring botulinus toxin (handle with care).
2. Serum; at least 5 ml, preferably more.
3. Tied-off stomach and a portion of small intestine if gastrointestinal botulism (rare) is suspected. In suspected lamziekte, submit gastrointestinal content as well as serum.
4. Liver or a large portion thereof.

PROCEDURES. The specimens, except serum, are processed in order to obtain toxin. The filtrate obtained or serum is used in animal tests to demonstrate toxicity.

Suspected food is sometimes fed to laboratory animals or animals of the same species as those that are affected.

COMMENTS. If botulinus toxin is demonstrated in the serum, liver extract, or food by animal inoculation, a strongly presumptive diagnosis of botulism can be made. A definitive diagnosis depends on the identification of the type of *C. botulinum* involved by toxin neutralization tests in animals.

Recovery of *C. botulinum* alone from food is not sufficient for a diagnosis, for the organism is ubiquitous in its occurrence. An animal may die of botulism and not have a demonstrable level of toxin in its serum.

Treatment

Botulinum antitoxin (type C) has been used effectively in mink and ducks; however, once signs have developed, the efficacy of antitoxins is questionable.

Control

1. Avoid feeding spoiled feed; prevent exposure to decomposing animal and plant materials.
2. Cattle (lamziekte): Types C and D toxoid.
3. Mink: Type C toxoid.
4. Provide adequate mineral supplement to prevent the phosphorus deficiency that contributes to lamziekte.
5. Bury or burn dead animals.

BOVINE BRUCELLOSIS / BANG'S DISEASE

Bovine brucellosis is a contagious disease caused, almost always, by *Brucella abortus* and characterized by abortion and infection of the testicles and accessory sex glands of the male, leading to varying degrees of infertility in both sexes.

Brucella abortus is a small, gram-negative rod that requires CO_2 for primary isolation. It is a facultative intracellular parasite.

The disease occurs in most countries where cattle and water buffalo are raised. *B. abortus* readily infects humans, but rarely domestic animals other than cattle and buffaloes.

Brucellosis is highly infectious. Infection may be by ingestion, coitus, and direct or indirect contact (fomites).

Differential Diagnosis

Abortion usually at 7–9 months; metritis and retained placenta. Occasional infertility in cows; orchitis with occasional sterility in the male.

Leptospirosis; bovine genital campylobacteriosis (vibriosis); trichomoniasis; mycotic abortion; sporadic abortions caused by various bacteria, infectious bovine rhinotracheitis virus, and bovine virus diarrhea virus should be considered.

Laboratory Diagnosis

SPECIMENS

1. Serum.
2. Placenta and aborted fetus.
3. Milk.
4. Semen and testes.

PROCEDURES

1. One of the agglutination procedures—plate, tube, or card test—may be carried out.
2. Cultural procedures are carried out on fetal cotyledons and the aborted fetus. The stomach contents of the aborted fetus is especially useful.
3. Milk may be cultured or subjected to the brucella ring test (BRT).
4. Semen and testes are cultured.

COMMENTS. The mercaptoethanol and rivenol agglutination tests, and the complement fixation procedure detect mainly IgG antibodies specific for *Brucella*. These tests reduce nonspecific reactions and aid in differentiating chronic infection and vaccination responses. These tests are used to confirm positive reactors identified in one of the agglutination tests.

The BRT is mainly used on bulk milk, although it can be used to aid in detecting chronic udder infections.

Guinea pig inoculation is used to recover *B. abortus* from infectious materials.

Brucella abortus antibody test kits are available commercially (see 12, Appendix A).

Treatment

None.

Control

1. Blood testing with removal of reactors.
2. Calfhood vaccination with *B. abortus* strain 19 vaccine.
3. Adult vaccination with strain 19 or strain 45/20 (killed oil-adjuvant) in heavily infected areas.
4. Periodic ring tests are used for surveillance of herds.

BOVINE GENITAL CAMPYLOBACTERIOSIS / BOVINE
VIBRIOSIS, EPIZOOTIC BOVINE INFERTILITY

Bovine genital campylobacteriosis is a venereal infection acquired from the bull, caused by *Campylobacter fetus* ssp. *venerealis* and characterized by metritis, leading to infertility with frequent resorption of embryos and occasional abortions.

Campylobacter fetus ssp. venerealis is a small, gram-negative, microaerophilic rod.

Distribution is probably worldwide. The disease is widespread in both dairy and beef herds. Transmission is by coitus. Bulls may be carriers and the disease is often introduced to a herd by a carrier bull.

Differential Diagnosis

There is often a herd history of repeated returns to service with irregular estrous cycles, especially in young cows and heifers. Occasionally there are early abortions.

Consider particularly trichomoniasis, leptospirosis, and brucellosis. The history and clinical manifestations are usually sufficiently characteristic to differentiate bovine genital campylobacteriosis from other infections that result in abortions.

Laboratory Diagnosis
SPECIMENS

1. Fetus, cervical mucus, preputial washings. Methods for the collection of cervical mucus and preputial washings are described in clinical and diagnostic texts. Transport media are made available by some laboratories for submitting preputial washings; they are available commercially (see 2, Appendix A). *C. fetus* ssp. *venerealis* will survive at room temperature for 2–3 days in suitable transport media.

   Fetuses should be refrigerated and sent to the laboratory as soon as possible. Unless cervical mucus can be delivered to the laboratory within 4 hours, it should be kept on dry ice.

2. Cervical mucous samples (do not collect at estrus).

PROCEDURES/COMMENTS

1. Fluorescent antibody staining of fetal stomach contents,

cervical mucus, and preputial washings are useful in the identification of *C. fetus.* It does not distinguish between *C. fetus* ssp. *venerealis* and *C. fetus* ssp. *fetus.*

Isolation and identification of *C. fetus* ssp. *venerealis* from the fetus, cervical mucus, and preputial washings is definitive.

2. The cervical mucus agglutination test (CMAT) is a reliable procedure that requires collection of cervical mucus from each animal. CMAT is interpreted as follows:

   Suspect: any agglutination
   Positive: 75% agglutination at titers between 1:25
             and 1:50

   An enzyme-linked immunosorbent assay has been used to detect and measure antibodies in cervical mucus.

Treatment

1. Intra-uterine infusion of streptomycin, or streptomycin and penicillin.
2. In bulls, the same antibiotics may be administered systemically or locally into the preputial sac.

Control

1. Artificial insemination. The herd frees itself of the disease if infection is not reintroduced.
2. Bacterins are used particularly in bulls and replacement heifers.

BOVINE LEPTOSPIROSIS

Bovine leptospirosis is caused by various *Leptospira* serovars and is often characterized by an asymptomatic course, but also on occasions by multiple infections with such manifestations as fever, icterus, hemoglobinuria, nephritis, uremia, infertility, abortion, atypical mastitis, and death. Abortion occurring in late pregnancy is the principal manifestation.

The leptospira pathogenic for animals are serovars of the species *L. interrogans.* The serovars that cause most cases of bovine leptospirosis in order of their frequency of occurrence are *L. pomona* (most frequent), *L. hardjo, L. grippotyphosa, L. canicola,* and *L. icterohaemorrhagiae.*

The generic name and the serovar name are usually employed as above. The species name *interrogans* is not always included.

Both *L. pomona* and *L. hardjo* can cause infertility but the former causes more abortions.

There is a wild animal reservoir of leptospira species, and other sources of infection are asymptomatic domestic animals shedding leptospira in urine.

The disease is endemic in cattle populations worldwide. Its occurrence depends largely upon the wild and domestic animal reservoir, environmental stresses, and the immune status of animals.

Differential Diagnosis

Clinical diagnosis is difficult. Abortions: 6 months or later.

Brucellosis, bovine genital campylobacteriosis, trichomoniasis, bacillary hemoglobinuria, and other diseases resulting in abortions should be considered.

Laboratory Diagnosis

Laboratory diagnosis in cattle is usually based on serologic tests.

SPECIMENS

1. Paired serum samples or multiple samples from animals with no evidence of the disease and cattle that have aborted or have had other signs suggesting leptospirosis.
2. Urine, portions of kidney and liver. Because of the fragility of leptospira and the time and effort involved, culture is not usually practicable.
3. Portions of liver and kidney, both fresh and fixed.
4. Fresh urine or urine containing formalin. Add 1.5 ml of 10% formalin to 20 ml of urine. The latter will keep leptospira intact for days or weeks.
5. Bovine fetus for fetal serology, fluorescent antibody (FA), and culture.

PROCEDURES/COMMENTS

1. Serologic tests: Microscopic agglutination (MA).
   Single or individual samples: These are not recommended. A titer of 1:100 or greater generally indicates that the animal has sustained a leptospira infection at some time. Titers less than 1:100 are considered negative.
   Multiple herd samples: A diagnosis of probable leptospirosis can be made if MA titers are below 1:100 in animals with no evidence of clinical disease, while samples

from animals that have aborted or have had other signs of leptospirosis are high, i.e., ranging from 1:100 to 1:800 and greater.

Acute and convalescent sera:

> Positive: Fourfold or greater increase in titer, e.g., acute sample 1:50 and convalescent sample 1:200. Conclusion: Animal has probably sustained an infection.
>
> Negative: None or less than a fourfold increase in titer of the paired sera. Conclusion: Animal has probably not sustained an infection.
>
> Vaccinal titers: These are usually less than 1:100 after 2–3 months postvaccination.
>
> It should be kept in mind, however, that an animal can have leptospirosis without developing a significant titer.

2. Isolation, cultivation, and identification: Because of the fragility of leptospires and the time and effort involved, isolation is not usually practicable.
3. FA and silver-impregnation staining: Microscopic lesions are usually absent, although leptospira can be seen.
4. Dark-field examination: Demonstration of leptospira in formalized urine along with typical clinical signs is significant. Without clinical signs, it simply means the animal is a shedder. Considerable experience is needed to identify leptospira by dark-field examination; they disintegrate soon after collection if not preserved with formalin.
5. MA test using fetal serum. FA identification of leptospires in fetal liver and kidney smears. Leptospires can frequently be isolated from the fetal kidney, liver, and eye.

    Leptospira antigens are available commercially for macroscopic agglutination procedures (see 11, Appendix A).

Treatment

Streptomycin and tetracyclines. Treatment must be early to be effective. A single large, intramuscular dose of dihydro-streptomycin (25 mg/kg) will cure the carrier state.

Control

1. Effective rat control: Fence off ponds and streams; screen replacement stock.
2. Bacterins: These may contain as many as five serovars.

BOVINE LEUKOSIS / BOVINE LYMPHOSARCOMA, BOVINE LEUKEMIA, MALIGNANT LYMPHOMA

Bovine leukosis is an insidious but highly fatal disease caused by a retrovirus and characterized by the development of aggregations of immature lymphoblastic cells in many organs with a resulting variety of clinical signs. Only a small percentage of seropositive animals develop the progressive, fatal disease.

A number of forms of the disease are recognized: the adult or enzootic form (most common); the thymic form (rare); the juvenile or calf form with multiple lymph node enlargement; the cutaneous form (rare); and persistent lymphocytosis (benign). Bovine leukosis virus is associated with the adult or enzootic form and the persistent lymphocytosis form.

Bovine leukosis is worldwide in distribution and widespread in occurrence. It is estimated that 10–20% of dairy herds in the United States are infected. Losses in individual heavily infected herds may be as great as 5% per year. It is less frequent in beef cattle.

Transmission of the virus between cattle is mainly by blood (horizontal transmission). Blood on instruments and needles and such procedures as dehorning, ear-tagging, and castration involving interchange of blood are considered important means of transmission. Bloodsucking insects may be mechanical vectors. Prenatal vertical transmission occurs in utero to the fetus and to the newborn calf via milk. The virus in milk is destroyed by pasteurization.

The virus has been propagated in a variety of cells.

Differential Diagnosis

Because of its variable manifestations, depending upon the organs involved and rate of tumor growth, this disease can mimic many other diseases. When superficial lymph nodes are involved, they are swollen and can be seen as lumps beneath the skin, usually in the neck and rear flank regions. If suspected, a serologic test should be carried out.

Laboratory Diagnosis
SPECIMENS
1. Serum sample.
2. Affected tissues (lymphoid and bone marrow): Take at necropsy, formalized and fresh.

3. Blood: Buffy coat.

PROCEDURES
1. An agar gel immunodiffusion (AGID) test is performed. It is reported as positive (infected) or negative (not infected).
2. The characteristic gross and microscopic changes of tissues are supportive.
3. Virus may be isolated from the buffy coat.

COMMENTS. Less than 10% of the cattle that are found to be infected (positive AGID test) go on to develop lymphoid neoplasms.

It is thought that when a case (or cases) with lesions is diagnosed as bovine leukosis in a herd, 80% or more of the herd can be considered infected or will give a positive AGID test.

Antibodies can be detected by other procedures, but the AGID test is the most practical procedure.

Bovine leukemia antibody test kits are available commercially (see 16,18, Appendix A). They employ the AGID procedure.

A persistent lymphocytosis occurs in many infected animals prior to the development of lesions.

Treatment
None.

Control
Control programs that eliminate infected animals and establish leukosis-free herds are carried out in some countries. If herds are heavily infected, it may be advisable to slaughter and reestablish with seronegative animals.

The disease can be eliminated by testing at 2- to 3-month intervals and removing the seropositive animals.

No vaccine is available.

BOVINE LIVER ABSCESS /
BOVINE HEPATIC NECROBACILLOSIS
Bovine liver abscess is a widespread disease mainly of feeder cattle caused by *Fusobacterium necrophorum* (sometimes with *Actinomyces pyogenes, Streptococcus* spp., and *Staphylococcus* spp.). *F. necrophorum* gains entrance to the liver via

lesions of the mucosa of the rumen.

The disease is recognized at slaughter and results in the condemnation of a large percentage of livers.

Control

Tylosin is the most commonly used feed additive in the feed-lot industry for the control of liver abscesses.

BOVINE MASTITIS

Several microbial agents cause most cases of bovine mastitis. They are listed below along with the considerable number of other agents that cause fewer and usually sporadic cases of mastitis.

Streptococcus agalactiae: Mastitis is widespread, contagious, but eradicable; it usually runs a chronic course but also has intermittent phases of acute reaction. There is a reduced milk yield and the chronic disease leads to progressive parenchymatous fibrosis.

Staphylococcus aureus: Mastitis is widespread, contagious, and noneradicable; it is usually of a mild and chronic nature. *S. aureus* occurs as a harmless commensal on the skin of the udder and teat. When the usually mild disease flares up and becomes acute, the secretion is purulent and yellow. Abscessation, usually microabscesses, is characteristic of staphylococcal mastitis and is responsible in part for the often poor response to therapy. This form of mastitis is most prevalent when the milking system and practices are faulty. *S. aureus* can, on occasion, cause gangrenous mastitis.

Streptococcus dysgalactiae and *S. uberis:* These are responsible for roughly 15% of mastitis while *S. agalactiae* causes about 50% or more and *S. aureus* causes roughly 30%. These four gram-positive organisms account for about 95% of bovine mastitis.

Actinomyces pyogenes: This organism alone or with one of the streptococci listed above, causes a suppurative mastitis sometimes called "summer mastitis," which is usually seen in dry cows and in recently calved or lactating cows. If not treated early, there are often multiple abscesses leading to total loss of function of a quarter or quarters. Anaerobic bacteria may be associated with *A. pyogenes.*

Escherichia coli, Enterobacter, or *Klebsiella:* These organisms cause coliform mastitis. The endotoxin released during infection may result in a peracute mastitis with a systemic toxemia, which can be fatal.

Nocardia asteroides: This soil-borne organism, which is usually introduced to the udder by a lack of asepsis during treatment, can cause an acute destructive mastitis.

Mycoplasma spp. (e.g., *M. bovis, M. californicum,* etc.): These organisms cause mycoplasmal mastitis that is characterized by the following: rapid onset and spread, usually all quarters affected, udder swollen but not hot and painful, serous exudate followed by purulent exudate, rapid drop in milk production, no systemic involvement, and no response to treatment. Asymptomatic carriers occur.

Among the agents that can cause mastitis are:

Streptococcus agalactiae	*Pasteurella haemolytica*
S. dysgalactiae	*P. multocida*
S. uberis	*Bacillus* spp.
Fecal streptococci	*B. anthracis*
Group G streptococci	*Bacteroides* spp.
Staphylococcus aureus	*Mycoplasma* spp.
S. epidermidis	*Nocardia* spp.
Micrococci	*Trichosporon* spp.
Escherichia coli	*Candida* spp.
Klebsiella spp.	*Cryptococcus neoformans*
Enterobacter spp.	*Saccharomyces* spp.
Actinomyces pyogenes	*Torulopsis* spp.
Corynebacterium bovis	*Mycobacterium* spp.
C. ulcerans	*Fusobacterium necrophorum*
Pseudomonas spp.	*Leptospira* serovars
Serratia marcescens	*Brucella* spp.
Clostridium perfringens	*Prototheca* spp.
(gangrenous mastitis)	Various anaerobic bacteria, usually in mixed infections

Laboratory Diagnosis

To exclude extraneous contaminating bacteria, it is imperative that milk samples be taken aseptically into sterile vials. If mycoplasmal mastitis is suspected, the clinician should so inform the laboratory, for special media are required. Milk samples should be refrigerated as soon as possible and kept in this state until they reach the laboratory. To isolate some of the potential causes of mastitis, blood agar plates may have to be incubated for at least 5 days.

The clinician should base the diagnosis on results obtained from the laboratory. An antimicrobial susceptibility test should be carried out routinely.

There is an enzyme-linked immunosorbent assay diagnostic kit available commercially for the detection of *Staphylococcus aureus* antibody in milk (see 13,17, Appendix A). Good correlation of test results with culture is claimed.

Treatment

Treatment will be based on the kind of mastitis and the results of the antimicrobial susceptibility tests.

Control

The control and prevention of mastitis depends upon good milking practices and appropriate antimicrobial therapy.

BOVINE PAPULAR STOMATITIS / INFECTIOUS BOVINE ULCERATIVE STOMATITIS, STOMATITIS PAPULOSA OF CATTLE

Bovine papular stomatitis is usually a mild contagious disease of young cattle (<2 years) caused by a parapoxvirus and manifested by papules leading in some animals to erosions and ulcers of the buccal and nasal mucosa and muzzle. Esophageal and rumen lesions may also be seen.

The course is usually about 7 days and suckling calves may be infected from teat lesions. Occasionally there are secondary bacterial invaders.

The disease is probably worldwide in distribution and seen fairly frequently in cattle in North America, particularly in feedlots.

The virus is closely related or identical to that causing pseudocowpox and milker's nodules.

Differential Diagnosis

Bovine virus diarrhea, infectious bovine rhinotracheitis, endemic erosive stomatitis (Africa), necrotic stomatitis, and mycotic stomatitis should be considered. Uncomplicated bovine papular stomatitis is distinguishable clinically from the latter two diseases.

Laboratory Diagnosis

SPECIMENS. Material from papules; scrapings from erosions and ulcers; biopsies or portions of lesions (fixed).

PROCEDURES/COMMENTS. The most convenient procedure is the demonstration of the parapoxvirus in clinical material by means of electron microscopy.

The characteristic intracytoplasmic inclusions seen in tissue sections are diagnostic. The virus can be cultivated in bovine and ovine cell cultures in which characteristic plaques are produced. A fluorescent antibody test is useful to confirm the results of isolation or to identify virus in infected cells in diseased tissue.

Treatment

Not usually necessary.

Control

The generally mild character of the disease does not require preventive measures.

BOVINE PARVOVIRAL INFECTION

The bovine parvovirus causes mainly subclinical infections in calves. Fetal infections and reproductive failure in cows appear to be infrequent.

Diagnosis is based on isolation and identification of bovine parvovirus and/or seroconversion. The fastest method of identification of parvovirus in calves is by examination of the feces by electron microscopy (see SPECIMENS FOR VIRAL EXAMINATION, Section 1).

BOVINE PNEUMONIC PASTEURELLOSIS / SHIPPING FEVER

Bovine pneumonic pasteurellosis is a contagious disease thought to be initiated by various stresses, such as those incidental to transport, and probably caused initially by various viruses or mycoplasmas (see BOVINE RESPIRATORY DISEASE), followed by the invasion of *Pasteurella haemolytica* (most frequently) and/or *P. multocida*. The disease varies in severity from a mild pneumonia involving mainly anterior lobes to a fulminating fibrinous bronchopneumonia affecting large portions of the diaphragmatic lobes.

Clinical signs include depression, anorexia, fever (104–108°F), serous nasal discharge, rapid shallow respirations, and a diminution of lung sounds as consolidation develops. The morbidity is high and the disease spreads readily to unstressed native cattle.

Abscesses due to *Actinomyces pyogenes* are frequently found complicating pneumonic pasteurellosis, particularly in young cattle. Such cases respond poorly to treatment. *Haemophilus somnus* infection may also complicate pneumonic pasteurellosis.

Differential Diagnosis

A clinical diagnosis is usually based on the history and clinical signs; however, in appreciable outbreaks, a laboratory diagnosis should be sought.

Some of the other agents that cause bovine respiratory infections are listed under the discussion of BOVINE RESPIRATORY DISEASE.

Laboratory Diagnosis

See BOVINE RESPIRATORY DISEASE.

Treatment

Pasteurella haemolytica and *P. multocida* should, if isolated, be subjected to routine antimicrobial susceptibility tests, for multiple drug resistance occurs in these species. Broad-spectrum antibiotics, combined penicillin and streptomycin, and sulfonamides such as sulfamethazine have been effective if given early.

Control

Good management practices with a view to reducing stresses are of paramount importance. Vaccination with bacterins and live *P. haemolytica* vaccines is practiced prior to shipment.

BOVINE PYELONEPHRITIS

Bovine pyelonephritis is a chronic, sporadic disease, principally of cows and heifers (infrequently the bitch, ewe, sow, and mare), caused by *Corynebacterium renale, C. cystitidis* or *C. pilosum* (rare), and characterized by purulent inflammation of the urethra, bladder, ureters, and kidney, resulting in fibrotic thickening of these structures.

These closely related *Corynebacterium* spp. are small, gram-positive, pleomorphic rods. *C. renale* causes most bovine pyelonephritis. It occurs as a commensal in the male and female genital tract. *C. cystitidis* is found on the prepuce of many bulls and can cause severe hemorrhagic cystitis and pyelonephritis. *C. pilosum,* which also occurs as a commensal, is an infrequent cause of cystitis and pyelonephritis.

Distribution is worldwide. Transmission is venereal and by indirect contact.

Differential Diagnosis

Leptospirosis, postparturient hemoglobinuria, bacillary hemoglobinuria. Other urinary tract infections, most frequently due to *E. coli.*

History of previous cases is suggestive. Rectal examination is helpful.

Laboratory Diagnosis
SPECIMENS
1. A midstream sample of urine in a sterile container should be refrigerated immediately after collection and kept at that temperature until it reaches the laboratory.
2. Necropsy: Fixed and fresh portions of affected kidney, ureter, bladder, and urethra.

PROCEDURES
1. The urinary sediment is cultured.
2. Fresh tissues are cultured. A fibrinonecrotic inflammation with pseudomembrane formation in the bladder and urethra is highly suggestive of the disease.

COMMENTS. Definitive diagnosis depends on the isolation and identification of *C. renale, C. cystitidis,* or *C. pilosum* in conjunction with clinical signs or gross pathologic lesions.

Treatment

Penicillin (preferred) or sulfonamides for at least a week. Efficacy of treatment should be checked by urine culture 1 month after treatment.

Control

If feasible, infected cows should be isolated until cured.

BOVINE RESPIRATORY DISEASE

A number of microbial agents have the capacity to infect the bovine respiratory tract. One or more agents may be recovered from the lungs of cattle with bovine respiratory disease (BRD). It is widely thought that viruses and mycoplasmas are the most frequent primary agents, while bacteria such as *Pasteurella haemolytica* (most frequently) and *P. multocida* are secondary invaders. Fungi cause infrequent sporadic respiratory infections.

Some of the microbial agents that are involved in BRD are listed in Table 2.2. The more important agents and the disease manifestations they produce will be dealt with separately. In the investigation of BRD it is incumbent upon the clinician to indicate to the laboratory what particular agents are suspected.

Table 2.2. Microbial agents associated with bovine respiratory disease

Viruses	Bacteria
Parainfluenza-3 virus	*Pasteurella haemolytica*
Infectious bovine rhinotracheitis virus	*Pasteurella multocida*
(bovine herpesvirus-1, BHV-1)	*Haemophilus somnus*
Bovine virus diarrhea virus	*Actinomyces pyogenes*
Bovine respiratory syncytial virus	*Chlamydia psittaci*
	Mycoplasma spp.

Laboratory Diagnosis

The laboratory diagnosis of some of the diseases caused by agents referred to above is dealt with separately. The characteristic gross pathologic finding in BRD is bilateral consolidation of the ventral anterior lobes of the lungs.

SPECIMENS

1. Nasal swabs in viral transport media. Swab-transport systems are available commercially for viruses (see 5,10,14, Appendix A).
2. Sample taken by transtracheal aspiration (tracheal wash). The latter is preferred for the isolation of bacteria (including mycoplasmas and chlamydia) from the trachea and lung. Viruses can also be isolated from the aspirate.
3. Portions of affected lung including margin of the lesion; fresh and fixed.
4. Paired sera.

PROCEDURES/COMMENTS
1. Isolation and identification of viruses: Because commensal bacteria are frequently present in the normal upper respiratory tract, their isolation from nasal swabs is not necessarily significant.
2. Isolation and identification of bacteria and viruses: Fluorescent antibody staining of smears or sections is often useful for the identification of viruses although in advanced BRD, viruses may not be demonstrable.
3. Serologic tests are available in many laboratories for antibodies to the most important viruses.
4. Characteristic gross and microscopic change involving the lung are supportive in a diagnosis of BRD.

BOVINE RESPIRATORY SYNCYTIAL VIRUS INFECTION

Bovine respiratory syncytial virus infection occurs widely in cattle. The most severe disease is seen in calves and is characterized by an acute pneumonia with fever, anorexia, nasal discharge, and respiratory distress. There is a bronchitis, interstitial pneumonia, and alveolitis with alveolar hyperplasia and characteristic multinucleted syncytia. The causal agent, a paramyxovirus, may be involved as a primary agent in bovine pneumonia (see BOVINE RESPIRATORY DISEASE).

The laboratory diagnosis is essentially the same as that described under BOVINE RESPIRATORY DISEASE.

Antimicrobial drugs are used to control secondary bacteria; inactivated and modified live virus vaccines are available for prevention.

BOVINE TUBERCULOSIS

Bovine tuberculosis is a chronic, contagious disease almost always caused by the acid-fast organism *Mycobacterium bovis* and characterized by the formation of granulomatous nodules called tubercles whose location depends largely on the route of infection.

The distribution is worldwide although the incidence in some countries is very low as a result of eradication programs. In the absence of control programs, the incidence may reach 75%. Dairy and other confined cattle have a higher incidence than range animals.

In calves the mode of infection is usually by ingestion,

and lesions involve the mesenteric lymph nodes with possible spread to other organs. In older cattle, infection is usually by the respiratory tract with lesions in the lungs and dependent lymph nodes.

Cattle are refractory to members of the *M. avium* complex and *M. tuberculosis,* but they are rendered sensitive to tuberculin. Some of the so-called atypical mycobacteria, including members of Runyon Group IV, may sensitize cattle to tuberculin. The latter organisms may be soil-borne.

Skin tuberculosis or mycobacterial ulcerative lymphangitis is characterized by nodulo-ulcerative lesions on the ventral body and legs. These tubercle-like lesions yield noncultivable acid-fast bacteria, which may sensitize cattle to tuberculin.

Mycobacterium bovis is a small, gram-positive, aerobic, acid-fast rod. It is a facultative intracellular parasite, which elicits a predominantly cell-mediated immune response.

Differential Diagnosis

Bovine tuberculosis is usually diagnosed either by tuberculin tests or at slaughter on the basis of stained smears and gross pathology.

Given the usually chronic nature of tuberculosis and the great difference in its severity and consequent clinical signs, differential diagnosis is difficult. It can mimic many diseases.

Laboratory Diagnosis

SPECIMENS. For culture and histopathology, use affected tissues, fresh and formalized. Great care should be exercised in handling suspected tubercular tissue because of the danger of human infection.

PROCEDURES. Because culture takes several weeks, bovine tuberculosis is often diagnosed on the basis of finding typical acid-fast organisms in smears from characteristic granulomatous lesions in lymph nodes and organs.

A highly presumptive diagnosis can also be based on the recognition of characteristic tubercles by gross and microscopic examination.

Treatment

Ordinarily cattle are not treated.

Control

Test and slaughter programs are carried out to eliminate the disease. Tuberculin for intradermal testing of animals is available commercially (see 8, Appendix A).

BCG (Bacille Calmette-Guerin) vaccine is used in calves in some countries where the incidence of the disease is high.

BOVINE ULCERATIVE MAMMILLITIS / BOVINE HERPES DERMOPATHIC DISEASE, PSEUDO–LUMPY SKIN DISEASE

Bovine ulcerative mammillitis is a severe disease of the teats of principally dairy cattle, caused by a herpesvirus, and characterized by edema of the teats, followed by vesicle production and subsequent erosion, ulceration, and scab formation.

There may be a marked loss in milk production due to secondary mastitis. Recovery usually takes place in 3–4 weeks. Lesions may be seen on the face and muzzle of nursing calves.

Probably worldwide in distribution, affecting mainly dairy cows.

This herpesvirus (bovine herpesvirus-2) is indistinguishable from the Allerton virus, the cause of pseudo–lumpy skin disease. The latter disease is now considered to be a manifestation of bovine ulcerative mammillitis.

Differential Diagnosis

Cowpox (infrequent), pseudocowpox, staphylococcal infections (impetigo) involving the udder, and black pox involving the teats should be considered.

Laboratory Diagnosis

SPECIMENS

1. Vesicular fluid and scrapings from fresh lesions.
2. Biopsies.

PROCEDURES

1. Isolation and identification of the virus using cell cultures.
2. Electron microscopic examinations of scrapings for herpesviruses to distinguish from the viruses of pseudocowpox and cowpox. Intranuclear inclusion bodies are seen in epithelial and giant cells of biopsy sections.

Treatment

1. Emollient ointments.
2. Udder disinfectants and treatment for mastitis if the latter is a complication.

Control

1. Isolate infected cows.
2. Employ strict sanitary measures and separate milking utensils.

BOVINE VIRUS DIARRHEA / MUCOSAL DISEASE

Bovine virus diarrhea (BVD) is a contagious disease of cattle caused by a togavirus (pestivirus) and characterized by inflammation and erosions of the mucous membrane of the alimentary tract and manifested in two principal forms: a diarrhea with a low mortality rate and a high morbidity rate; "mucosal disease" also with diarrhea but having a high mortality rate and a low morbidity rate. Infection of the pregnant cow may lead to abortion, congenital deformities, and birth of normal and/or weak calves. Surviving infected calves may harbor the virus for life. These persistently infected calves are often "poor doers" and will develop mucosal disease when superinfected with cytopathic strains of BVD.

Although only one serotype of the virus has been found, strains may vary antigenically and in virulence.

The disease occurs worldwide and the virus is endemic in many cattle populations. Many cattle are consequently exposed but only a small number develop clinical disease. Current research indicates that "typical" BVD signs are seen only in animals that are persistently infected with a noncytopathic strain of BVD, which they acquired in utero. The disease occurs most frequently in the age range of 6–18 months.

Differential Diagnosis

Salmonellosis, malignant catarrhal fever, rinderpest, bracken poisoning, coccidiosis, infectious bovine rhinotracheitis (IBR), and parainfluenza-3 infection.

Laboratory Diagnosis

Laboratory confirmation is required for definitive diagnosis.

SPECIMENS

1. For virus isolation: Swabs of nasal discharge; feces; blood (unclotted); portions of spleen, intestine, turbinates, and lymph nodes; fetal liver and kidney.
2. For fluorescent antibody (FA) staining: Portions of spleen, kidney, trachea, intestine, and lymph nodes; fetus; liver and kidney; nasopharyngeal brush swabbings.
3. Paired serum samples.
4. For histopathology: Formalized portions of the tissues referred to above.

PROCEDURES/COMMENTS

1. For virus isolation and identification: Some strains of BVD virus do not produce a cytopathogenic effect and are thus difficult to identify by virus neutralization.
2. For FA staining: This procedure can be used to identify the virus in cell cultures, nasopharyngeal brush swabbings, and in sections of the tissues referred to above.
3. For serology: Many normal cattle have antibody to BVD virus. The virus neutralization titers will usually range from 1:32 to 1:512. To make a serologic diagnosis of BVD, paired sera should show at least a fourfold increase in titer between the acute and convalescent samples.
4. For histopathology: Finding of the typical histopathologic changes, mainly lymphoid necrosis of gut-associated lymphoid tissue, is strongly suggestive and helps distinguish BVD from malignant catarrhal fever.

Treatment

None.

Control

Live modified virus and inactivated virus vaccines provide significant protection. Persistently infected animals may develop typical mucosal disease following vaccination with modified live vaccines.

Simultaneous vaccination with IBR and PI-3 vaccines is practiced.

BRAXY / BRADSOT, CLOSTRIDIAL ABOMASITIS

Braxy is an uncommon disease, mainly in sheep, generally conceded to be caused by *Clostridium septicum* and characterized by a severe abomasitis with toxemia and a high mortality rate.

Braxy occurs most commonly in England, Australia, Scotland, Ireland, Iceland, and Scandinavia. The incidence of the disease is highest in yearlings and weaner sheep wintered on mountainous and hill pastures. Based on reports, braxy would seem to be an infrequent disease in North America.

The precise conditions that give rise to braxy are not known. The causal organism, *C. septicum,* which multiplies in the wall of the stomach, is a normal inhabitant of the intestine.

The clinical diagnosis of braxy is difficult. A history of previous occurrence of the disease in yearling sheep wintered on frozen and snowy pastures would be suggestive.

Laboratory Diagnosis

Definitive diagnosis depends upon the isolation and/or identification of *C. septicum* from characteristic abomasal lesions.

SPECIMENS
1. After necropsy, affected abomasal wall is submitted.
2. Smears or films are made on microscope slides from incised abomasal lesions. These should be spread in the manner of blood smears. The smears can be prepared in the diagnostic laboratory from the tissue submitted if this is preferred by the veterinarian.

PROCEDURES/COMMENTS
1. Attempts are made to isolate and identify *C. septicum.* The finding of abomasal lesions with edema and emphysema will strongly suggest braxy. Isolation and identification procedures are time consuming and laborious.
2. Smears are stained by a fluorescent antibody (FA) specific for *C. septicum.* Identification by FA staining is accurate and rapid.

Treatment

Treatment has not been effective.

Control
1. Avoidance of frozen forage.
2. Vaccination with a *C. septicum* bacterin has been effective.

CALF DIPHTHERIA

Calf diphtheria is mainly an endogenous infection of the larynx (necrotic laryngitis), oral cavity (necrotic stomatitis), or pharynx and characterized by fever, ulceration and swelling of affected tissues, often rapid respiration, and profuse salivation. The principal bacterium involved is the gram-negative anaerobe, *Fusobacterium necrophorum,* which invades tissues as a result of trauma, including coarse feed, eruption of teeth, and various primary infections. The principal lesions are necrotic ulcers involving the mucous membranes of the mouth, larynx, or pharynx. In some severe cases the lesions may extend to involve the nose, trachea, and lungs. Necrotic stomatitis is usually seen in calves less than 3 months of age; necrotic laryngitis is usually seen in older calves.

The disease is readily diagnosed clinically. Although *F. necrophorum* is the most important microbial agent, infections are usually mixed. Isolation of *F. necrophorum* is not usually attempted.

Treatment/Control

Affected animals should be isolated and treated with such antimicrobials as sulfamethazine, sulfamerazine, penicillin, and streptomycin and broad-spectrum antibiotics. Conditions contributing to trauma should be eliminated, and feeding and drinking facilities should be cleaned and disinfected.

CAMPYLOBACTER

This genus contains a number of species of small, gram-negative, spirally curved, motile rods. They are found on the mucous membranes of the reproductive and alimentary tracts of animals and humans.

Campylobacter fetus ssp. *fetus:* See BOVINE GENITAL
    CAMPYLOBACTERIOSIS and OVINE GENITAL
    CAMPYLOBACTERIOSIS.

C. fetus ssp. *venerealis:* See BOVINE GENITAL CAMPY-
    LOBACTERIOSIS.

C. jejuni: See CANINE CAMPYLOBACTERIOSIS, FE-

LINE CAMPYLOBACTERIOSIS. A frequent commensal in the intestinal tract of many domestic and wild animals, including birds and poultry. It is an important cause of enteritis in humans.

C. mucosalis (formerly *C. sputorum* ssp. *mucosalis*): See SWINE PROLIFERATIVE ENTERITIS COMPLEX.

C. hyointestinalis: See SWINE PROLIFERATIVE ENTERITIS COMPLEX. Has been recovered from the intestine of cattle, foals, hamsters, and humans. In humans it has been associated with gastrointestinal disease.

C. coli: Occurs as a commensal in the intestinal tract of pigs, poultry, and humans. It can cause diarrhea in humans and probably, on occasion, in animals, but it is not considered a significant pathogen in the latter.

C. laridis: Has been recovered from birds, dogs, horses, and humans but its role in disease is not clear.

C. upsaliensis: Has been recovered from the feces of normal and diarrheic dogs, cats, and children. Its role, if any, in disease has not yet been established.

C. sputorum ssp. *bubulus:* A commensal found in healthy cattle and sheep.

C. fecalis: Has been recovered from ovine feces and from bovine semen and vaginas. Pathogenic significance, if any, is not known.

C. butzleri: A recently described species that has been isolated from humans with diarrhea and from swine and cattle. The sources from swine: aqueous humor, stillborn piglet, thoracic fluid; from a bovine: stomach contents.

C. cryaerophila: A recently described species that has been isolated from humans, swine, sheep, and cattle. Sources were bovine: brain, amniotic fluid; swine: aqueous humor, kidney, placenta, and stillborn piglet; sheep: placenta and blood.

CANDIDIASIS / CANDIDOSIS, MONILIASIS, THRUSH

Candidiasis is an infrequent disease of domestic animals (except poultry), most commonly caused by the yeast-like fungus *Candida albicans* and characterized by infection of the mucous membrane of the alimentary tract (occasionally the genital tract) with infrequent spread to lungs, heart, kidneys, placenta, and other tissues. The organism may also cause mastitis and, rarely, dermatitis.

Candida albicans is a commensal in the alimentary tract and the disease is worldwide in occurrence. Young and debilitated animals are most often affected. Prolonged antibiotic treatment and immunodeficiency may predispose animals to candidiasis.

The oral form of the disease is seen most commonly in puppies and kittens. Genital candidiasis has been described in cows, mares, bulls, and stallions, but it appears to be uncommon. Systemic infections have been described in calves, pigs, and horses that have been on prolonged antibiotic treatment. Crop mycosis is an important disease of poultry.

Candida albicans and other species of *Candida* can cause bovine mastitis. These organisms are usually introduced during treatment.

Differential Diagnosis

Candidiasis has to be distinguished from a number of other diseases affecting mainly the mucous membranes of the alimentary and genital tracts. White to gray patches of pseudomembranous inflammation are characteristic.

Laboratory Diagnosis

SPECIMENS. Collect material by deeply scraping the surface of affected tissue below the pseudomembrane or other extraneous material.

PROCEDURES. Smears and wet mounts are examined for the characteristic yeast-like cells and pseudohyphae. Definitive diagnosis requires the isolation and identification of *C. albicans*.

COMMENTS. Systemic infections are usually only diagnosed after necropsy by culture and histopathologic examination of tissues. Serologic procedures (immunodiffusion, latex agglutination, and counterimmunoelectrophoresis) are used to aid in the diagnosis of human infections.

Candida candidum, C. tropicalis, and other species can be readily isolated from milk samples in the case of mastitis due to these organisms.

Treatment
1. Nystatin may be administered topically or orally.
2. Clotrimazole topically to treat chronic candidiasis.
3. Amphotericin B and fluorocytosine are used in systemic candidiasis.
4. The less toxic antifungal agents such as the imidazoles are preferred for mastitis.

Prolonged treatment is usually required; however, mycotic mastitis may clear up spontaneously.

CANINE ACTINOMYCOSIS
Canine actinomycosis is a chronic, sporadic disease most commonly caused by *Actinomyces viscosus* and/or *A. hordeovulneris* (rarely by *A. bovis*), and occasionally by unnamed *Actinomyces*. Two principal forms are recognized: a localized granulomatous abscess(es) involving the skin and subcutis; a pyothorax with granulomatous, suppurative lesions involving the lungs, pericardium, and pleura and extending in some cases to involve the peritoneal cavity.

Occurrence is probably worldwide. These actinomycetes occur as commensals in the oral cavity of dogs. Infection is via wounds, occasionally due to gunshot or grass awns, and also by inhalation.

Differential Diagnosis
The disease resembles nocardiosis clinically. The latter disease is also seen in the two forms mentioned above. Other diseases to be considered are blastomycosis, cryptococcosis, other fungous infections, abscesses due to other causes, and various pulmonary infections.

Because the treatment of actinomycosis and nocardiosis is different, it is advisable to seek a definitive diagnosis by the isolation and identification of the causative organism.

Laboratory Diagnosis
SPECIMENS
1. Fresh material from the localized form (skin, subcutis); the granulomatous abscess may have to be opened surgically.
2. A tracheal wash and/or fluid obtained by thoracocentesis should be submitted in the thoracic form.

PROCEDURE/COMMENTS
1. Demonstration of the organism in Gram-stained smears.
2. Isolation and identification of *A. viscosus* or *A. hordeovulneris* from characteristic lesions are definitive.

   Actinomyces viscosus, A. hordeovulneris, and *Nocardia asteroides* resemble one another morphologically; however, the latter organism can be distinguished from the other two in that it is partially acid-fast. A highly presumptive diagnosis of these diseases can be made on the basis of the Gram and acid-fast staining of smears from typical lesions.

Treatment
1. Surgical debridement and drainage.
2. Prolonged treatment with penicillin, sulfonamides, tetracyclines, or chloramphenicol is usually effective; however, because there may be a difference between the antimicrobial susceptibility of *A. viscosus* and *A. hordeovulneris,* all significant isolates should be subjected to drug susceptibility tests.
3. Penicillin is not effective in the treatment of nocardiosis.

CANINE BRUCELLOSIS
Canine brucellosis is a contagious disease of dogs caused by *Brucella canis* and characterized in the bitch by metritis, abortion, prolonged bacteremia, and vaginal discharge; in the male, disease is characterized by infection of the testicles and accessory sex glands, leading occasionally to irreversible sterility. Sequellae include infections of bones, particularly the intervertebral disks.

Canine brucellosis is probably widely distributed in North and South America and Europe, but it has not been reported from Australia. The incidence of the disease is not high except in some kennels and colonies.

Differential Diagnosis
Abortion during the last trimester of pregnancy is the cardinal sign. Stillbirths and failure to conceive also suggest canine brucellosis. Infectious abortion due to other agents is infrequent.

Laboratory Diagnosis
SPECIMENS
1. Females: Blood (heparinized), fetus (lung and liver preferred), placenta.
   Males: Semen, testes, epididymis, prostatic fluid. *B. canis* has been recovered from urine.
2. Serum.

PROCEDURES
1. Isolation and identification of *B. canis:* Blood cultures are particularly useful.
2. The mercaptoethanol tube agglutination test (TAT) is widely used and usually read as follows:
   Negative: titer 1:50 or less
   Suspicious: 1:50 and 1:100
   Positive: 1:200
   The agar gel immunodiffusion test (AGID): A reliable procedure carried out in some laboratories.
   Canine brucellosis screening test: The specificity of this commercial slide agglutination procedure (see 16,18, Appendix A) has been improved with the use of mercaptoethanol. This test is usually performed by practitioners.

COMMENTS. Dogs positive to the canine brucellosis screening test should be retested with the TAT or AGID test. Positive reactions to the latter tests are particularly significant when there are clinical signs of the disease. Dogs may be bacteremic for long periods and confirmation of brucellosis can sometimes be conveniently obtained with a positive blood culture.

Treatment
Treatment is not usually attempted; however, it may be attempted in order to save valuable bloodlines. The human regimen of combined tetracycline and streptomycin has been used.

Control
Elimination of infected animals after serologic testing and cultural examinations.

CANINE CALICIVIRUS INFECTION

There have been a small number of caliciviruses isolated from cases of glossitis and enteritis in dogs. Their significance in these diseases is not yet clear.

Laboratory diagnosis involves isolation and identification of the canine calicivirus.

CANINE CAMPYLOBACTERIOSIS

Canine campylobacteriosis is a contagious disease caused by *Campylobacter jejuni* and characterized by a diarrhea that has been described as lasting from 1 to 2 weeks and also as being chronic. Other clinical signs that may be observed are anorexia, vomiting, and a low fever. Dogs less than 6 months of age are more severely affected. The organism has been reported to cause abortion in bitches.

Distribution of *C. jejuni* is probably worldwide in dogs, cats, and other animals. A considerable percentage of dogs carry and shed *C. jejuni* (up to 10% or more) but not all of them develop enteritis and diarrhea.

Campylobacter jejuni is an important cause of gastroenteritis in infants, children, and adults. Potential sources of this organism for humans include carrier poultry and a number of animals, in addition to dogs and cats.

Differential Diagnosis

Among the diseases and agents that should be considered are salmonellosis, canine parvovirus infection, pancreatitis, intestinal parasites, and poisons.

Laboratory Diagnosis

SPECIMENS. For culture: Rectal/fecal swabs in transport media (Cary and Blair medium preferred; see 2, Appendix A) or feces in sealed containers. Specimens should be refrigerated and delivered to the laboratory so that they can be cultured within 48 hours of collection. Failing this, feces should be frozen on dry ice.

PROCEDURES/COMMENTS. Special media must be used to isolate this fragile and fastidious organism. Without special selective media the organism is rapidly overgrown by other enteric bacteria.

Antimicrobial susceptibility tests should be performed.

Isolation of the organism in itself does not necessarily mean the dog has campylobacteriosis. Such an isolation should be considered along with the clinical picture, the results of other diagnostic tests, and the results of antimicrobial therapy.

Treatment

It would seem that most cases of canine campylobacteriosis recover without treatment, although the course is probably shortened by the administration of erythromycin, chloramphenicol, tetracyclines, or other drugs shown to be effective in susceptibility tests.

Control

There are reports that shedding of the organisms can be reduced and possibly eliminated by erythromycin administration. Several negative cultures are required before the dog is no longer considered a carrier.

Owners of dogs with diarrhea should be advised to exercise appropriate hygienic measures to prevent possible exposure to *C. jejuni*.

CANINE CORONAVIRUS GASTROENTERITIS

Canine coronavirus gastroenteritis is a relatively mild disease of neonatal and older dogs. Clinical signs are anorexia, depression, and loose stools. Occasionally, sudden onset with vomiting and diarrhea occurs. Mucus is usually present in the feces, which have a foul-smelling odor.

Occurrence is probably worldwide. It appears to be more common where numbers of dogs are raised in kennels and colonies. Virus is shed in the feces and the mode of infection is by ingestion. The coronavirus is carried by many dogs. Disease is thought to occur in the absence of protection acquired from the bitch.

Differential Diagnosis

This disease is most likely to be confused with canine parvovirus infection. Other enteric infections such as coccidiosis, salmonellosis, campylobacteriosis, hookworm infection, acute pancreatitis, and renal or hepatic failure should be considered (see ENTERIC INFECTIONS OF PUPPIES).

Laboratory Diagnosis

SPECIMENS. Fresh feces and/or fresh and fixed portions of small intestine.

PROCEDURES. The virus is difficult to isolate. A diagnosis is most readily made by the demonstration of coronavirus in fecal lysates with the electron microscope.

A fluorescent antibody conjugate can be used to identify coronavirus in frozen sections of small intestine and in feces.

Finding the characteristic histopathologic changes (particularly villous atrophy) in the small intestine is supportive.

Treatment

Supportive. Fluid therapy.

Control

An inactivated virus vaccine is available. The virus retains its infectivity for considerable time under cool conditions.

CANINE DISTEMPER

Canine distemper is a highly contagious disease usually of young dogs caused by a paramyxovirus and characterized by a diphasic fever, leukopenia, acute coryza, later bronchitis and catarrhal pneumonia, gastroenteritis, and neurologic signs and complications.

The mode of infection is inhalation, and transmission is by direct contact and fomites. Large numbers of viruses are shed in secretions and excretions during the active stage of the disease. Because of maternal antibody many infections are subclinical.

This important disease of dogs occurs worldwide and is endemic in urban areas.

Differential Diagnosis

Infectious canine hepatitis, leptospirosis, lead poisoning, and granulomatous meningoencephalomyelitis are among the diseases that should be considered. A number of viral, bacterial, and parasitic infections may flare up during the course of distemper, complicating the clinical diagnosis.

The disease is usually diagnosed clinically or after necropsy examinations.

Laboratory Diagnosis
SPECIMENS
1. Live animals: Conjunctival, tracheal, vaginal scrapings, and buffy coat are taken early in the course of the disease.
2. Necropsy: Fixed and fresh portions of intestine, pancreas, stomach, bladder, brain, and lung.
3. Paired sera or plasma.

PROCEDURES
1. Fluorescent antibody (FA) staining to identify the distemper virus. Inclusion bodies can sometimes be demonstrated in scrapings with appropriate stains. The later the course, the more difficult it is to demonstrate virus by the FA procedure because of antibody production.
2. Histopathologic examination of tissues for the characteristic cytoplasmic inclusion bodies in the bladder, lung, stomach, and pancreas. In the neurologic form the microscopic lesions located in the white matter near the ventricular and meningeal surface are diagnostic. They involve demyelination with inclusions in glial cells and neurons.

    FA test is extremely reliable on frozen sections of tissues taken at necropsy.
3. An enzyme-linked immunosorbent assay (ELISA) is performed in some diagnostic laboratories. An indirect immunofluorescence test kit is available to detect antibodies in serum or plasma (see 15, Appendix A).

COMMENTS. The virus is not readily cultivated in cell cultures or embryonated eggs. Ferrets are excellent laboratory animals and are occasionally used for virus isolation.

Rising IgG titers in the ELISA are significant.

Treatment
Supportive. Antimicrobial drugs for secondary bacteria.

Control
Vaccination is effective after loss of maternal immunity, which is usually by 12 weeks of age. Measles virus vaccine is sometimes administered before 12 weeks of age and prior to canine distemper vaccination.

CANINE EHRLICHIOSIS /
TROPICAL CANINE PANCYTOPENIA

Canine ehrlichiosis is an acute to chronic disease caused by the rickettsia (bacterium) *Ehrlichia canis* and is transmitted by the dog tick *Rhipicephalus sanguineus*. Disease is characterized by infection of monocytes and neutrophils, resulting in various clinical signs including recurrent fever, epistaxis, mucopurulent nasal discharge, vomiting, subcutaneous hemorrhages and edema, emaciation, splenomegaly, meningoencephalitis, convulsions, and paralysis.

Epistaxis may follow bone marrow hypoplasia a number of weeks after initial infection. Without antibiotic therapy, dogs may remain carriers for many months.

Occurrence is worldwide, with puppies and German Shepherds seeming to be particularly susceptible. Ehrlichiosis may be complicated by concurrent infections with babesia and haemobartonella. A small number of human infections have been reported.

Differential Diagnosis

Babesiosis and other infectious diseases produce some clinical signs similar to those of ehrlichiosis. Rocky Mountain spotted fever, a relatively uncommon disease of dogs, is also clinically similar to ehrlichiosis. A clinical diagnosis should be confirmed by laboratory means.

Laboratory Diagnosis
SPECIMENS
1. Unclotted blood for buffy coat and regular smears. In necropsied dogs, smears should be made from the lungs and other organs.
2. Serum.

PROCEDURES
1. Smears stained by Giemsa and fluorescent antibody procedures.
2. Serum is tested by the indirect fluorescent antibody procedure. A titer of 1:10 or greater with the indirect fluorescent antibody test is considered positive. The test may be negative early in the disease.

COMMENTS. The characteristic morulae of *E. canis* are not always present in Giemsa-stained smears. The optimum time for their demonstration is about 13 days postinfection.

A thrombocytopenia along with other clinical signs is suggestive.

Treatment

Tetracyclines are effective if the disease is diagnosed early; treatment should be given for at least 2 weeks. Additional treatment may be necessary, particularly in the chronic disease.

Control

1. Isolation, treatment, or elimination of seropositive animals.
2. Spraying and dipping to eradicate ticks.

CANINE EXTERNAL EAR INFECTIONS /
CANINE OTITIS EXTERNA

Among the factors predisposing dogs to external ear infections are accumulation of excessive amounts of hair, wax, dirt, and other extraneous matter; anatomic characteristics (certain breeds); trauma sometimes as a result of careless cleaning; and allergic dermatitis. The principal organisms involved are listed in Table 2.3.

Table 2.3. Organisms implicated in causing canine external ear infections

Bacteria	Fungi	Parasites
Pseudomonas aeruginosa	*Pityrosporum canis*	*Otodectes cynotis*
Proteus spp.	(*Malassezia pachydermatis*)	(ear mite)
Staphylococci	*Candida* spp.	
Streptococci	*Aspergillus* spp.	
Escherichia coli	*Geotrichum candidum*	
Enterobacter	*Penicillum* spp.	
Klebsiella	Occasionally other fungi	
Occasionally other bacteria		

Almost all of the above listed organisms can be recovered on occasion, usually in small numbers, from healthy ears. Rather characteristic exudates are attributed to some of the more common causative agents; however, microbial examination is recommended.

Laboratory Diagnosis

SPECIMENS. Two swabs are taken, preferably through a sterile otoscope canula, before cleaning or medicating the ears.

PROCEDURES. Appropriate media (bacterial and fungal) are inoculated from one swab, while a smear is made from the second for Gram staining.

COMMENTS. Cultures are frequently mixed. An antimicrobial susceptibility test should be conducted if the cultures indicate a probable pathogen. Occasionally, it may be advisable to perform susceptibility tests on more than one organism.

Treatment

Treatment can be rather involved and clinical texts should be consulted. If bacteria are involved, the susceptibility test will indicate what drugs may be effective.

CANINE HERPESVIRUS INFECTION

Canine herpesvirus infection is a contagious, often fatal disease of puppies (3 weeks of age or less) characterized by a viremia with disseminated necrosis and hemorrhage involving the kidney, liver, lungs, and other organs.

Among the clinical signs are a soft, yellowish green stool, anorexia, labored breathing, abdominal pain, and finally death or recovery.

Occurrence is probably worldwide. The disease in previously unexposed adults is characterized by mild rhinitis and vaginitis. The virus can cause abortion and infertility.

The virus is carried by many adult dogs, and puppies are usually protected by maternal antibody. Infection of puppies is considered to take place transplacentally or by contact during or shortly after parturition. The virus is a cause of vesicular vaginitis in adult females.

Differential Diagnosis

Distemper, canine hepatitis, toxoplasmosis should be considered.

Canine herpesvirus infection should be suspected in an acute, frequently fatal, febrile disease of young puppies (3 weeks of age or less) that does not respond to antibiotics.

Laboratory Diagnosis

SPECIMENS. Portions of lung and kidney, fixed and fresh, are submitted for virus isolation and histopathology.

PROCEDURES. The disease is diagnosed by one or both of the following along with a typical history: isolation and identification of the virus in canine cell cultures; the finding of the characteristic inclusion bodies in the lung, liver, and kidney.

Treatment

None.

Control

No practicable measures are available for prevention.

CANINE LEPTOSPIROSIS

Canine leptospirosis is a disease of varying severity, from latent to acute, caused by the spirochete *Leptospira interrogans* serovar *canicola* (*L. canicola*) and less frequently by serovar *icterohaemorrhagiae* (*L. icterohaemorrhagiae*).

In the acute disease, a bacteremia follows introduction of the leptospira with later localization in various tissues and organs, including the liver, kidney, and lymph nodes. Among the clinical signs are anorexia, vomiting, and fever; followed by depression, reluctance to move, labored breathing, sometimes icterus, hemorrhages and necrotic patches involving the oral mucosa, muscular tremors, bloody feces, and vomitus resulting from a severe gastroenteritis. Frequent urination results from acute nephritis. Uremia may also develop. The mortality rate is approximately 10%.

Epidemics of the hemorrhagic type of leptospirosis are considered to be due to *L. canicola,* while the disease in which icterus more often occurs is thought to be caused by *L. icterohaemorrhagiae.*

The disease is worldwide in distribution and common in occurrence. The reservoir for *L. canicola* is mainly carrier dogs and for *L. icterohaemorrhagiae,* rats and mice. The organism may be shed in the urine for months from dogs and other animals with asymptomatic kidney infections. Infection occurs by direct or indirect contact via the skin, conjunctiva, or oral mucous membrane.

Differential Diagnosis

Canine hepatitis, distemper, ehrlichiosis, babesiosis, and sporadic febrile diseases caused by various bacteria and viruses should be considered.

Laboratory Diagnosis

The diagnosis of canine leptospirosis is essentially the same as for bovine leptospirosis. In brief, it involves the following:

1. Dark-field examination of urine to which formalin has been added at the rate of 0.75 ml of 10% formalin to 10 ml of urine.
2. Serologic tests, preferably the microscopic agglutination, on paired sera. A fourfold increase in titer is significant. *Leptospira* antigens are available commercially for this procedure (see 11, Appendix A).
3. Culture of fresh urine and heparinized blood. Not all diagnostic laboratories are prepared to do this.
4. Histopathologic examination of sections of liver and kidney for leptospiras (silver impregnation staining). Microscopic tissue changes alone are not usually characteristic.
5. Fluorescent antibody staining of tissues, particularly the kidney, and urine.

Treatment

1. Penicillin, streptomycin, chloramphenicol, and erythromycin given early.
2. Dihydrostreptomycin in large doses along with vaccination is used to eliminate the latent kidney infections and urine shedding.
3. General supportive treatment.

Control

1. Exposure can be reduced by leashing and restricting access to other dogs.
2. Bacterins prepared from *L. canicola* and *L. icterohaemorrhagiae* are of value, although the duration of immunity is less than 1 year.

CANINE ORAL PAPILLOMATOSIS / CANINE WARTS

Canine oral papillomatosis is an often highly contagious disease, primarily of young dogs caused by a papovavirus (papillomavirus) and characterized by multiple papillomas or warts on the mucous membrane of the mouth, lips, and pharynx.

Laboratory Diagnosis

A laboratory diagnosis is not ordinarily carried out, for the lesions are sufficiently characteristic to warrant a clinical diagnosis; however, histopathologic examination of tissue biopsies may be helpful.

Treatment

1. Surgical.
2. Application of various chemicals.
3. Autogenous wart vaccines. The value of the latter is questionable; warts frequently disappear spontaneously within a few weeks.

Control

Autogenous wart vaccines are sometimes used.

CANINE PARVOVIRUS INFECTION /
CANINE PARVOVIRUS ENTERITIS

Canine parvovirus infection is a contagious disease that affects dogs of all ages and is characterized by vomiting, diarrhea (may be hemorrhagic), fever, weakness, dehydration, and marked leukopenia. The disease is most often seen in the age range of 6–16 weeks. Myocarditis may occur in puppies less than 6 weeks of age.

Although first recognized in 1978, canine parvovirus would appear to be worldwide in distribution. The disease is seen in household dogs and may involve whole litters and kennels. Young and aged dogs are most susceptible. The virus is shed in the feces and the mode of infection is by ingestion.

The virus is closely related to the parvovirus causing feline panleukopenia.

Differential Diagnosis

Canine parvovirus can only be diagnosed with certainty by laboratory procedures. Among other causes of diarrhea in dogs are canine coronavirus, hookworm infection, *Salmonella* spp., and *Campylobacter jejuni*.

Laboratory Diagnosis
SPECIMENS
1. Feces and portions of fresh intestine and heart.
2. Unclotted blood samples.
3. Formalin-fixed portions of intestine and heart.

PROCEDURES
1. Virus identification is accomplished by electron microscopic (EM) examination of feces or fluorescent antibody staining sections of intestine or heart. The characteristic morphology of the parvovirus allows it to be readily recognized by EM examination.
   Viral hemagglutination (HA): Canine parvovirus agglutinates certain species of red blood cells. A HA titer of 1:64 (dilution of feces) provides presumptive evidence of infection. The higher the titer the more virus present.
   The enzyme-linked immunosorbent assay (ELISA) is also used to detect parvovirus in feces and commercial kits for this purpose are available to practitioners (see 9, Appendix A).
2. For hematology: A leukopenia is suggestive.
3. For histopathology: Crypt necrosis with collapse of mucosal architecture and villus loss is diagnostic. Intranuclear inclusion bodies are infrequent to rare in the gut and myocardium.

   COMMENTS. Because the virus presents some difficulties in cultivation, virus isolation and identification is not generally carried out.
   False negative results are common with both the HA test and ELISA in the later stages of the illness, for developing antibodies interfere with the tests.

Treatment
Fluid therapy; antimicrobials; intensive care.

Control
Isolation of infected animals.
Killed virus vaccines and modified live virus vaccines are

used. Modified live and inactivated feline panleukopenia vaccines have been found to protect dogs. Maternal antibody interferes with vaccination.

The virus can persist for long periods on the premises.

CANINE RESPIRATORY DISEASE

The principal microbial agents associated with canine respiratory disease are listed in Table 2.4.

Table 2.4. Principal microbial agents associated with canine respiratory disease

Bacteria	Viruses	Fungi
Bordetella bronchiseptica	Canine distemper virus	*Blastomyces*
Actinomyces hordeovulneris	Canine adenovirus 1	*dermatitidis*
A. viscosus	and 2	*Cryptococcus*
Nocardia asteroides	Canine paramyxovirus	*neoformans*
Pasteurella multocida	(parainfluenza type	*Aspergillus*
P. pneumotropica	2 virus)	*fumigatus*
Klebsiella spp.	Canine rotavirus	*Histoplasma*
Escherichia coli	Canine herpesvirus	*capsulatum*
Streptococci		Infrequently
Staphylococci		other fungi
Pseudomonas aeruginosa		
Mycoplasma cynos (see MYCOPLASMA		
INFECTIONS OF DOGS AND CATS)		
Infrequently other bacteria		

Laboratory Diagnosis

This usually involves the isolation and identification of the causative agent from material taken by transtracheal or transthoracic aspiration, or throat swabs. See the specific diseases for further details.

CAPNOCYTOPHAGA

Species of this genus are slender, pleomorphic, gram-negative rods that are found as commensals in the mouth and nasopharynx of dogs and possibly cats. Two species are recognized:

Capnocytophaga canimorsus (formerly designated DF-2): Produces infections following dog bites in humans. Serious and even fatal infections may develop in variously compromised human patients.

C. cynodegmi: Less virulent than the afformentioned species and the cause of localized dog-bite infections and keratitis resulting from cat scratches.

CAPRINE ARTHRITIS AND ENCEPHALITIS

Caprine arthritis and encephalitis is a disease of goats caused by a retrovirus and characterized by a leukoencephalomyelitis in young goats and chronic arthritis in adult goats.

There is serologic evidence that the disease is widespread in the United States. Reports indicate that the disease occurs in many countries.

Dairy goats are more susceptible than the indigenous goats of developing countries. The prevalence in a dairy herd is usually less than 25%. Transmission is mainly by milk and colostrum. Most goats are infected while young but develop the clinical disease months or even years later. The encephalitis results in an ascending paralysis that may terminate with seizures and death.

Differential Diagnosis

Scrapie, rabies, progressive pneumonia, listeriosis, louping ill, and infections of the central nervous system and joints caused by various agents. Chlamydial and mycoplasmal arthritis, and septic arthritis in young goats.

Laboratory Diagnosis
SPECIMENS
1. Usually a moribund or dead goat is preferred, or brain in the encephalitic form and joints in the arthritic form; fresh or fixed tissues.
2. Serum.

PROCEDURES
1. Histopathologic examination.
2. Agar gel immunodiffusion test; enzyme-linked immunosorbent assay.
3. A commercial diagnostic kit that uses the agar gel immunodiffusion procedure is available (see 21, Appendix A).

COMMENTS. A presumptive diagnosis is made on the basis of the gross and microscopic pathologic changes. There is a characteristic lymphocytic encephalomyelitis.

The virus can be isolated and identified by immunodiffusion and immunofluorescence.

The characteristic morphology of the virus can be seen in

cell cultures by electron microscopy.

Goats without clinical disease may have specific antibody by the agar gel immunodiffusion test.

Treatment
None.

Control
Eradication of the disease is not widely practiced. Testing and removal of reactors. Only serologically negative animals should be admitted to the herd.

CAPRINE BRUCELLOSIS
Brucellosis of goats is a generalized infection caused by *Brucella melitensis* and characterized by abortion in the second half of pregnancy, the production of weak kids, and orchitis in the male.

The disease is quite similar to bovine brucellosis. Large numbers of brucellae are shed with the placenta, uterine discharges, urine, and milk; in the latter, for prolonged periods of time. After one or two abortions, the infection becomes quiescent with localization in the udder, lymph nodes, and other tissues.

The disease is widespread, occurring in the Middle East, Asia, the former USSR, Africa, and South America. It appears to be a rare disease in North America. Sheep are susceptible to *B. melitensis* but there is considerable variation in the degree of susceptibility among breeds.

Brucella melitensis causes undulant fever or human brucellosis and great care should be exercised in handling suspect goats and specimens, for the organism is highly infectious.

Differential Diagnosis
If testing discloses reactors to *B. melitensis,* brucellosis would be a prime suspect. Other diseases that should be considered are *Chlamydia psittaci* abortion (enzootic abortion), ovine genital campylobacteriosis, listeriosis, and toxoplasmosis.

Laboratory Diagnosis
SPECIMENS
1. For serology: Serum samples, preferably from all of the goats in the herd.

2. For culture: Fresh placenta(s) and fetus(es).

PROCEDURES/COMMENTS
1. A special tube agglutination test is used for suspected *B. melitensis* infections.

   The Rose Bengal plate agglutination test and the card test are also useful.

   The most reliable test is complement fixation.

   The Brucella ring test is useful if conducted on individual samples rather than on bulk samples.
2. The isolation and identification of *B. melitensis* provides a definitive diagnosis.

   A presumptive diagnosis can be made on the basis of demonstrating typical bacteria in stained smears from fetal stomach contents and cotyledons.

   A skin test is used to detect animals that have been infected.

Treatment

None.

Control

Eradication involves skin testing and repeated serologic testing with removal of reactors. All replacement or additions must be brucellosis negative. If the flock is heavily infected it may be advisable to depopulate and begin with negative stock.

A live attenuated vaccine strain of *B. melitensis* called Rev 1 has been used successfully to protect sheep and goats in a number of countries. A killed adjuvant vaccine has also been used.

CASEOUS LYMPHADENITIS / PSEUDOTUBERCULOSIS

Caseous lymphadenitis is a chronic, slowly progressive disease of adult (primarily) sheep and goats, caused by *Corynebacterium pseudotuberculosis* (*C. ovis*) and characterized by extensive caseous necrosis and abscessation, most commonly and initially of the precrural and prescapular lymph nodes. Later, the mediastinal, bronchial, and sublumbar lymph nodes may be involved and, on occasion, abscesses are found in vital organs and their dependent lymph nodes. The disease is not usually fatal.

The disease occurs worldwide and is widespread. The mode of infection is by wounds and ingestion. Discharging abscesses are the principal source of the infection. The disease may be introduced to small flocks by an infected sheep or goat.

Differential Diagnosis

Although other bacteria (streptococci, *Actinomyces pyogenes,* staphylococci) can cause superficial abscesses in sheep and goats, if there are multiple superficial abscesses, the most likely cause is *C. pseudotuberculosis.* Definitive diagnosis by cultural means is advisable if control measures are planned.

Laboratory Diagnosis

SPECIMENS. Fresh pus is collected on a swab from several excised abscesses.

PROCEDURES. The isolation and identification of *C. pseudotuberculosis* does not ordinarily present any difficulty.

Treatment

Excision of affected nodes.

Control

Avoid shearing injuries; shear young sheep first. Culling of sheep with abscesses.

CAT SCRATCH DISEASE /
CAT SCRATCH FEVER, BENIGN LYMPHORETICULOSIS

Although cat scratch disease (CSD) is not an animal disease, it is of interest because the cat is the source of this not infrequent zoonosis.

This is a noncontagious disease of humans resulting from contact with cats. The cause is now thought to be a small, non-acid-fast, pleomorphic, coccoid, gram-negative bacterium. The disease is most often acquired from cats less than 1 year old, due to a scratch or a puncture wound. Some infections have been initiated via the conjunctiva. Multiple cases have been reported in families and attributed to the same cat. The causal bacterium is thought to be a commensal in the mouth or on the skin of cats. The latter show no evidence of infection.

The incubation period may range from 3 to 90 days, and the course usually ranges from 2 to 4 months. The principal sign is regional lymphadenopathy, usually accompanied by a low-grade fever and mild, systemic symptoms. The disease is usually self-limiting and complications are rare.

Laboratory Diagnosis

This is carried out in medical diagnostic laboratories. It involves a skin test, using an antigen consisting of heated pus from a patient with CSD, and demonstration of characteristic bacteria in sections of biopsies with the Warthin-Starry stain.

Treatment

Most cases of CSD recover without treatment. Inflamed, fluctuant abscesses may be aspirated or excised for the relief of symptoms.

Control

Disposal of the suspected cat is not usually indicated.

CHLAMYDIAL POLYARTHRITIS /
TRANSMISSIBLE SEROSITIS

Chlamydial polyarthritis is a disease of calves, sheep, and pigs, caused by *Chlamydia psittaci* and characterized by some of the following signs: stiffness, lameness, conjunctivitis, fever, diarrhea, swollen and painful joints and tendons.

The disease, which probably occurs worldwide, is seen most frequently in lambs and calves 1–4 weeks of age. In pigs, the disease occurs in both piglets and feeder pigs. It is thought that the infection begins in the intestines, with subsequent spread and localization in joints and synovial sacs. There have been several reports of chlamydial polyarthritis in horses.

Differential Diagnosis

Because a variety of organisms can cause arthritis in these animals, chlamydial polyarthritis can only be diagnosed with certainty by the isolation of the agent from the synovia of affected joints and sacs.

Laboratory Diagnosis
SPECIMENS
1. For complement fixation test: Serum samples from normal and affected sheep; paired samples if possible.
2. For culture: Joints and joint fluids.

PROCEDURES/COMMENTS
1. Significant increases in the complement fixation titer between sera from normal and affected animals and between paired sera strongly suggest a chlamydial infection. Titers of 1:32–1:256 suggest a chlamydial infection.
2. The causal agent can be cultivated in embryonated eggs or cell cultures.
   Smears from joint surfaces and fluids are stained in an attempt to demonstrate the chlamydial organisms.

Treatment
Tetracyclines and tylosin are effective if treatment is early.

Control
It is likely that various stresses contribute to this disease but they may not be apparent. Thus, little can be done in the way of prevention and control.

CHLAMYDIOSIS: GENERAL
Strains of the bacterium *Chlamydia psittaci* cause a number of important diseases in domestic animals. All are listed below and the most important ones will be discussed separately. All strains share a group antigen that is used in the complement fixation test; however, there are some antigenic differences among strains. Chlamydia have a predilection for epithelial cells of mucous membranes, although other tissues in various locations are also infected. Latency is a common feature of chlamydial infections and various stresses can activate this latency resulting in serious disease. They are all obligate intracellular parasites.

The principal chlamydial diseases, discussed separately, are the following:

Feline pneumonitis (see FELINE RESPIRATORY DISEASE)
ENZOOTIC ABORTION OF EWES
SPORADIC BOVINE ENCEPHALOMYELITIS
Polyarthritis of calves, lambs, and swine (see CHLA-

MYDIAL POLYARTHRITIS)
Infectious keratoconjunctivitis of sheep
Feline conjunctivitis
Psittacosis-Ornithosis, a disease primarily of birds and
    poultry

Laboratory Diagnosis

This is discussed under each of the diseases that are listed
separately.

CHROMOBACTERIUM

Chromobacteria are short to medium-sized, pigment-produc-
ing, gram-negative, motile rods that occur in soil and water.
Only the following species has been incriminated in diseases:

Chromobacterium violaceum: Causes suppurative pneumo-
    nia in cattle and swine in tropical and subtropical coun-
    tries including southern United States.

C. fluviatile: May cause human infections but does not ap-
    pear to be pathogenic for animals.

CHROMOBLASTOMYCOSIS

Chromoblastomycosis is an infrequent fungal disease, which
has been reported in horses, dogs, cats, and humans. The
fungi, some of which are listed below, enter via a wound or at
the site of trauma and produce a granulomatous mass at or
near the site of entry. It may spread peripherally and, on
occasion, to the lymphatics and other tissues and organs. The
disease is chronic and if not treated it may persist and progress.

Some of the dematiaceous (dark pigmentation) fungi
that have been involved are *Fonsecaea pedrosoi, F. campacta,
Cladosporium carrionii,* and *Phialophora verrucosa.*

Differential Diagnosis

Chromoblastomycosis should be suspected when chronic
granulomatous lesions resulting from wounds and trauma are
seen involving the skin, lymphatics, and regional lymph
nodes. Blastomycosis, nocardiosis, canine actinomycosis,
and phaeohyphomycosis are among the diseases that should
be considered.

Laboratory Diagnosis

SPECIMENS

1. Material from granulomatous and/or ulcerous lesions.

2. Biopsies or portions of lesions, fixed.

PROCEDURES/COMMENTS. The characteristic brown-pigmented, branching, hyphal elements can be seen in wet
mounts. The same fungal structures are seen in stained sections. Finding the fungal elements in tissue sections is confirmatory.

Definitive diagnosis is based upon the isolation and identification of the fungus, which may take as long as 6 weeks to
grow.

Treatment
1. Surgical excision in some cases.
2. Amphotericin B, locally and systemically.
3. Thiabendazole has been used effectively.
4. 5-fluorocytosine appears to be the treatment of choice.

CLOSTRIDIAL ENTEROTOXEMIA
Clostridial enterotoxemia is an acute, highly fatal intoxication of sheep, especially lambs, calves, piglets, and possibly
horses. It is caused by types of *Clostridium perfringens* (Table
2.5). Types A, B, C, D, E, and F of *C. perfringens* have been
identified on the basis of immunologic differences in their

Table 2.5. Principal clostridial enterotoxemias of animals

Type	Animal Species	Disease
A	Humans	Food poisoning
	Horses	Enterotoxemia (clostridiosis)
	Calves	Enterotoxemia
	Lambs	Yellow lamb disease
	Piglets	Enterotoxemia
	Dogs (rare)	Enterotoxemia
B	Calves (neonates)	Enterotoxemia
	Lambs (neonates)	Lamb dysentery
	Foals (neonates)	Enterotoxemia
C	Calves (neonates)	Enterotoxemia
	Lambs (neonates)	Enterotoxemia
	Piglets (neonates)	Enterotoxemia
	Adult sheep	Struck
	Adult goats	Enterotoxemia
	Adult cattle	Enterotoxemia
	Foals	Enterotoxemia
D	Sheep (2 days to adult)	Enterotoxemia (overeating disease)
	Goats	Enterotoxemia (occasionally)
E	Cattle (rare), sheep	Enterotoxemia

exotoxins, which are produced in the intestine and absorbed, resulting in enteritis and toxemia.

The diseases are worldwide in occurrence. The various types of *C. perfringens* are frequently part of the normal flora of the intestine of animals; type A is the most common. Enterotoxemia is thought to result when toxin-producing strains of *C. perfringens* grow excessively, usually as a result of some disturbance in digestion, e.g., overeating.

Differential Diagnosis

This will vary with the different animal species. Salmonellosis, *E. coli* infection, viral (rota- and coronavirus) diarrheas, coccidiosis, and other infections that give rise to diarrhea or dysentery.

Among the signs are diarrhea, dysentery, convulsions, opisthotonos, ataxia, and coma. Animals are often found dead.

Definitive diagnosis requires laboratory confirmation.

Laboratory Diagnosis

SPECIMENS. At least 20–30 ml of ileal content in a tied-off portion of intestine, including portion of duodenum. The contents should be fresh, immediately refrigerated or frozen, and dispatched to the laboratory.

PROCEDURES. Intestinal content is inoculated into mice to determine if toxin is present. Toxin is identified by neutralization tests in mice or guinea pigs.

Smears from the duodenal mucosa are stained to determine if clostridial organisms are present; their presence in considerable numbers is supportive.

The duodenal mucosa is cultured for *C. perfringens*.

COMMENTS. Neutralization tests to determine the type of *C. perfringens* are laborious and expensive. A laboratory diagnosis is usually based on the demonstration of toxin in the ileal contents by mouse inoculation along with typical clinical signs, lesions, and history.

The probable type of *C. perfringens* can be conjectured fairly reliably on the basis of the history, the animal species, and its age.

Culture of *C. perfringens* in large numbers from the ileal

contents and duodenum is supportive of a diagnosis of enterotoxemia but is not definitive. *C. perfringens* type A occurs frequently in the intestinal tract of farm animals.

CLOSTRIDIAL ENTEROTOXEMIA OF CALVES

Clostridial enterotoxemia of calves is an acute, frequently fatal intoxication caused by the exotoxins of *Clostridium perfringens,* type B or C and occasionally type A, and is manifested by severe diarrhea or dysentery, opisthotonos, and tetany.

Clostridium perfringens type B does not appear to occur in North America. There are some reports of type D enterotoxemia in calves.

See CLOSTRIDIAL ENTEROTOXEMIA for further details and for laboratory diagnosis.

CLOSTRIDIAL ENTEROTOXEMIA OF HORSES /
EQUINE CLOSTRIDIOSIS

Clostridial enterotoxemia of horses is a recently described disease considered to be due to toxigenic strains of *C. perfringens* type A and characterized by sudden onset, fever, anorexia, and diarrhea with copious, watery, foul-smelling, dark feces. The course is short, 24–48 hours, and many cases terminate fatally.

Some workers have equated colitis-X with equine clostridiosis.

Enterotoxemia in foals, which would appear to be rare, has been attributed to *C. perfringens* types B and C.

Laboratory Diagnosis

See CLOSTRIDIAL ENTEROTOXEMIA for specimens and procedures; it may be desirable to examine intestinal contents from the large intestine as well as the small intestine as indicated.

CLOSTRIDIAL ENTEROTOXEMIA OF SHEEP /
LAMB DYSENTERY, ENTEROTOXEMIA, OVEREATING DISEASE

Clostridial enterotoxemia of sheep is an acute, frequently fatal intoxication caused by the exotoxins of *Clostridium perfringens* types B (lamb dysentery), C, or D (enterotoxemia, overeating disease) and is characterized by severe diarrhea or dysentery, opisthotonos, and tetany. Lamb dysentery is not thought to occur in North America. *C. perfringens* type A has been implicated as a cause of enterotoxemia in nursing lambs (yellow lamb disease).

See CLOSTRIDIAL ENTEROTOXEMIA for further details and for laboratory diagnosis.

CLOSTRIDIAL ENTEROTOXEMIA OF SWINE

Clostridial enterotoxemia of pigs (usually piglets) is an acute, usually fatal, intoxication caused by the exotoxins of *Clostridium perfringens* type C and characterized by a severe diarrhea or dysentery, convulsions, opisthotonos, and death. *C. perfringens* type A enterotoxemia has been reported recently in neonatal pigs.

See CLOSTRIDIAL ENTEROTOXEMIA for further details and for laboratory diagnosis.

COCCIDIOIDOMYCOSIS / COCCIDIOIDAL GRANULOMA

Coccidioidomycosis is a noncontagious disease of domestic animals, humans, and various wild animals, caused by the soil- or dustborne dimorphic fungus, *Coccidioides immitis*. It occurs in a benign, subclinical form and infrequently in a progressive, disseminated form, which usually begins with the formation of tuberculosis-like granulomas in the lung.

The disease occurs in the arid, acid-soil regions of the United States (mainly Arizona and California) and South America.

Differential Diagnosis

Blastomycosis, histoplasmosis, nocardiosis (dog), canine actinomycosis. Pneumonic infections caused by other agents should be considered.

Most diagnoses of coccidioidomycosis, with the possible exception of cases in the dog, are made by pathologic examination after necropsy. Pulmonary nodules can be seen in radiographs. The skin test may be of value in areas other than where the organism is widespread in the soil.

Laboratory Diagnosis
SPECIMENS
1. Exudate and biopsies taken from nodules in the disseminated disease.

Biopsies from liver, spleen, and lymph nodes.

Transthoracic aspirates if pulmonary disease is suspected.

For necropsy: Fresh and fixed portions of tissues and organs with granuomatous lesions.
2. Paired sera, or sequentially drawn sera.

PROCEDURES
1. Demonstration of the yeast-like forms in wet mounts and smears using fluorescent antibody and other stains.

    Culture, identification, and histopathologic examination.
2. For serology: Complement fixation (CF) test; the titer usually rises as the disease progresses.

    The precipitin and agar gel immunodiffusion (AGID) tests are useful.

COMMENTS. It should be kept in mind that many animals in areas where the fungus occurs in nature will have antibodies to this fungus and react positively to the skin test.

If the CF and AGID tests are positive, it indicates a recent or active infection.

Treatment
Amphotericin B is the drug of choice. Prolonged treatment is required for disseminated infections. Ketoconazole given over a period of months has been curative.

Control
Cases should be isolated. Although human infections are not ordinarily traced to animals, it is advisable to prevent human exposure to infected animals.

COLIBACILLOSIS OF CALVES
Although *E. coli* is part of the normal flora of calves, certain strains are pathogenic. Colibacillosis includes the disease manifestations caused by these strains of *E. coli*. They are as follows:

Colisepticemia: Occurs during the first week of life and is characterized by depression, fever, and anorexia with recumbency and death. The course may be as short as 48 hours.

Enteric or enterotoxic colibacillosis: Occurs during the first 3 weeks of life and is characterized by diarrhea with marked dehydration, acidosis, and emaciation. Death often ensues in several days if treatment is not initiated. White scours of calves is a manifestation of enteric colibacillosis.

The disease occurs worldwide and is more common in dairy calves than in beef calves.

Those strains responsible for colisepticemia have the capability of invasiveness. This property can be demonstrated in the Sereny test.

Enteric or enterotoxic colibacillosis is usually caused by one of a relatively small number of *E. coli* strains that produce enterotoxins referred to as heat labile (LT) and heat stable (ST). These strains also possess pili that enable them to adhere to epithelial cells. The most common pilus antigens associated with *E. coli* in calves is K99. Strains possessing the 987P or F41 pilus antigen have also been implicated. Some strains of *E. coli* that cause diarrhea in calves also produce a verotoxin, which effaces epithelial cells of the small intestine. It resembles the toxin of *Shigella*.

The development of colibacillosis in calves is dependent upon whether or not they acquire sufficient colostral protection.

Differential Diagnosis

Because there are a number of agents that cause diarrhea and rapid death in young calves, laboratory confirmation is required.

Salmonellosis, rota- and coronavirus infection, and cryptosporidiosis should be considered.

Laboratory Diagnosis
SPECIMENS
1. A sick or recently dead calf. *E. coli* may invade tissues shortly after death, which could confuse a diagnosis of colisepticemia.
2. Portions of small intestine (including duodenum), liver, and spleen.
3. Fecal swabs.

PROCEDURES/COMMENTS

1. In enterotoxic colibacillosis (EC), isolation, except from fresh duodenum, is not necessarily significant. Regardless of the source, all cultures from suspected EC should be examined for K99 and F41 pilus antigens (see 2 below).
2. For K99 and F41 antigens: The identification of the pilus antigens in cultures by an agglutination procedure is highly presumptive, as is the identification of these antigens in fecal smears and cryostat sections by fluorescent antibody (FA) tests. Stained sections will usually disclose gram-negative bacteria adherent to the villi. As pilus antigens are often not expressed when organisms are cultured by routine methods, the FA test on clinical specimens is usually considered more reliable.
3. A commercial serologic test is available to test feces for K99 antigen (see 20,22, Appendix A).
4. The invasive strains causing colisepticemia usually produce alpha hemolysin and are hemolytic on blood agar.
5. A positive Sereny test on *E. coli* recovered from fresh tissues supports a diagnosis of colisepticemia.

The demonstration of enterotoxins is laborious and expensive and thus is not usually carried out.

Rota- and coronaviruses may be involved with *E. coli* in the production of diarrheic disease. Consult the ROTAVIRUS AND CORONAVIRUS INFECTIONS OF CALVES for further information.

Treatment

Treatment of colisepticemia is not usually effective because of the short duration of the disease.

Treatment of enteric colibacillosis usually involves replacement of electrolytes and fluids and/or blood transfusion. Antimicrobial drugs as indicated by in vitro susceptibility tests.

Control

Pilus vaccines administered to the dam.

Good management practices including calving in an isolated area and provision of adequate amounts of colostrum.

COLIBACILLOSIS OF PIGS

Colibacillosis is usually an acute, contagious disease of pigs a few days of age caused by enterotoxigenic strains of *E. coli*. Among the clinical signs are depression; shivering; coma, with or without a yellow, watery diarrhea. Those pigs with diarrhea do not feed adequately, become dehydrated, and usually die.

The major predisposing factor is insufficient immunity through a lack of colostrum. Other contributing factors are poor care and sanitation, and exposure to new virulent varieties of *E. coli*.

The disease is worldwide in distribution, and explosive outbreaks often occur when a new virulent, enterotoxigenic strain is introduced to a herd. Strains of *E. coli* that cause diarrhea in pigs usually have the K88 or 987P pilus antigen and produce enterotoxins. The K88 or 987P pili enable *E. coli* to adhere to the mucosa of the small intestine, where it grows and produces enterotoxin(s) (heat labile and/or heat stable) that result in the diarrhea and dehydration.

Differential Diagnosis

A number of different agents cause clinical disease similar to colibacillosis. The agents and diseases are listed under ENTERIC INFECTIONS OF PIGLETS.

Laboratory Diagnosis

1. Preferably several sick or recently dead pigs.
2. Portions of small intestine, spiral colon, liver, and spleen.
3. Fecal swabs or feces.

PROCEDURES/COMMENTS

1. For culture: In addition to culturing for *E. coli*, it is usually advisable to also examine for rotavirus, coronavirus, and the virus of transmissible gastroenteritis.

   Because *E. coli* is carried in the intestine normally, its isolation alone is not necessarily significant. However, its isolation in pure culture from the small intestine immediately after death suggests significance. Cultures should be examined for pilus antigen (see 2 below).
2. For K88 and 987P antigens: The identification of the K88 and 987P antigens by an agglutination procedure is highly presumptive. Some laboratories have K88– and 987P–flu-

orescent antibody reagents for the identification of these pilus antigens in sections of intestine. It is not usually feasible to demonstrate enterotoxin(s).

Treatment
1. Antibiotics, as indicated by susceptibility tests, may be of some value.
2. Replacement of electrolytes and fluids.

Control
1. Pilus vaccines administered to the sow. Live autogenous oral vaccines have been widely used.
2. Good management practices with attention to comfort and sanitation are important.

CONTAGIOUS ECTHYMA / SORE MOUTH, SCABBY MOUTH, CONTAGIOUS PUSTULAR DERMATITIS, ORF

Contagious ecthyma is an acute, eruptive dermatitis of sheep and goats caused by a parapoxvirus and characterized by the formation of papules, vesicles, pustules, and scabs (in that order) on the lips, mucous membranes of the oral cavity, nostrils, eyelids, teats, udder, and feet. The most prominent lesions are around the nose and mouth. Secondary bacterial infections are frequent.

Occurrence is worldwide. These infections are most common in young, nonimmune sheep. Those recovering are immune. The virus is particularly resistant and thus tends to persist on premises. A carrier state has not been demonstrated.

The disease is transmissible to humans, with lesions occurring most commonly on the hands and face. In humans it is called orf, and those associated with sheep, including slaughterhouse workers and veterinarians, are often infected.

Differential Diagnosis
Ulcerative dermatosis is a relatively minor disease of sheep; the crateriform ulcers are characteristic. Mycotic dermatitis (streptothricosis or dermatophilosis), photosensitization, and scald (interdigital dermatitis) should be considered.

Laboratory Diagnosis
SPECIMENS. Scrapings and/or biopsies from lesions.

PROCEDURES. The characteristic elementary bodies of the parapoxvirus can be seen with the light microscope after suitable staining of smears or sections of biopsies from the lesions. The electron microscope is particularly useful to demonstrate the virus in homogenates prepared from lesions. The virus is difficult to propagate in cell cultures.

Treatment
Antimicrobial drugs are administered to combat secondary bacterial infections.

Control
A live, single-strain virus vaccine is applied to scarified areas of the skin. All unaffected sheep are vaccinated when faced with an outbreak.

CONTAGIOUS EQUINE METRITIS
Contagious equine metritis (CEM) is a highly contagious venereal disease of horses caused by a fastidious, gram-negative rod, *Taylorella equigenitalis,* and characterized by the development of an endometritis, cervicitis, and vaginitis with a copious, mucopurulent vaginal discharge. Although the stallion may carry the causal agent, it does not show clinical signs.

It has been reported from Australia, England, Ireland, a number of European countries, and the United States. It is not thought to be a prevalent disease.

Differential Diagnosis
The copious mucopurulent vaginal discharge occurring after breeding or during the breeding season is highly suspicious. All suspected cases should be reported and subjected to appropriate laboratory procedures.

Bacteria other than *T. equigenitalis* can, on occasion, cause a purulent metritis in mares.

Laboratory Diagnosis
SPECIMENS
1. For culture: Swabs from the cervix, urethra, and clitoral fossa including the clitoral sinuses of the mare and the urethral fossa and penile sheath of the stallion should be refrigerated and sent to the laboratory in a transport me-

dium (preferably Amies) as soon after collection as possible. Regional laboratories may provide suitable swabs and transport media.

2. For serology: Clotted blood samples or serum.

PROCEDURES/COMMENTS
1. For culture: The disease can only be diagnosed definitively by the isolation and identification of the causal agent. Repeated swabbings may be necessary to confirm the carrier state in stallions.
2. For serology: Among the serologic tests used are complement fixation (CF), passive hemagglutination, enzyme-linked immunosorbent assay, and agglutination (plate and tube). Serologic tests may serve as an aid in identifying infected mares. The CF test is not reliable for detection of carriers.

Treatment
Carrier stallions are treated by cleansing the penis and sheath with various antiseptics.

Treatment of mares with antimicrobial drugs is not always effective even though *T. equigenitalis* is broadly susceptible to antibiotics. Many mares remain clitoral carriers after treatment.

Control
This is a reportable disease in North America. Quarantine or isolation with attempts to eliminate actively infected animals and positive carriers by antimicrobial therapy and surgery (clitoral sinusectomy). Antibiotics added to the semen inactivates the organism.

CONTAGIOUS FOOT ROT OF SHEEP /
FOOT ROT OF SHEEP, INFECTIOUS FOOT ROT OF SHEEP,
OVINE DIGITAL DERMATITIS
Contagious foot rot of sheep (CFRS) is an acute or chronic disease caused by *Bacteroides nodosus* (usually in association with *Fusobacterium necrophorum*). It commences as an interdigital dermatitis and extends to large areas of the sensitive laminae of the hoof. It results in varying degrees of lameness and frequently detachment of the hoof.

The disease affects goats but is less severe. Less virulent strains of *B. nodosus* have been recovered from cattle and swine.

Bacteroides nodosus is an obligate parasite that can be eliminated from a flock because it does not survive longer than 2 weeks on pasture.

Differential Diagnosis

Foot abscess, "scald" (interdigital dermatitis of unknown origin), contagious ecthyma, injuries to the foot.

The disease affects a number of sheep and it is characteristic clinically.

Laboratory Diagnosis

SPECIMENS. Smears are made on microscope slides with the aid of a scalpel from material taken well down in the lesion after the horn and necrotic material have been pared away.

PROCEDURES. The organisms associated with CFRS are sufficiently characteristic in Gram-stained smears to warrant a diagnosis.

COMMENTS. This anaerobic organism is difficult to isolate and identify, thus, culture, which is not necessary for diagnosis, is seldom attempted.

Treatment

Affected and lame sheep should be isolated, then treated. Two procedures are used, topical or systemic.

Topical: Pare diseased feet and apply daily 5% formalin, 10% copper sulfate, 10% tincture of tetracycline or chloramphenicol. It is claimed that a 10% solution of zinc sulfate as a footbath is superior to 10% formalin or 10% copper sulfate.

Systemic: Penicillin and streptomycin; extensive paring not required. Foot rot vaccine may increase the cure rate.

Control

Nonaffected sheep should be put through a 10% formalin footbath, then put on a pasture that has been free of sheep for at least 2 weeks.

Isolate additions before introducing to flock.

Foot rot vaccines containing the appropriate serotype have been of value.

CONTAGIOUS OPHTHALMIA OF SHEEP AND GOATS

Contagious ophthalmia is a disease of sheep and goats caused by *Rickettsia* (*Colesiota*) *conjunctivae* and possibly, on occasion, by or in association with other bacteria, chlamydia, and mycoplasmas. The disease is widespread and is characterized by a conjunctivitis and keratitis affecting, most commonly, weanling rather than neonatal lambs and kids.

The disease is most common during the hot summer months when the pastures are dry and dusty. Transmission is by direct contact and mechanically by insects. The morbidity may be as high as 50%. Host specific strains of *R. conjunctivae* may produce conjunctivitis in cattle and swine.

Other associated agents:

Branhamella catarrhalis (Neisseria catarrhalis): Carried on the conjunctiva of sheep, but of questionable significance.

Mycoplasma oculi: Also present in the eyes of sheep with ophthalmia, but of doubtful significance.

Mycoplasma conjunctivae: Reports support the claim that this organism can cause ophthalmia in sheep.

Various other *Mycoplasma* spp.: Have been recovered.

Chlamydia psittaci: Is frequently recovered along with other bacteria from cases of ophthalmia in sheep.

Differential Diagnosis

The disease, which usually runs its course in less than 10 days, is most often diagnosed clinically. Among the clinical signs are excessive lacrimation, blepharospasm, vascularization, mucopurulent discharge, cloudiness of the cornea, and ulceration in some cases.

Laboratory Diagnosis

This is not commonly carried out.

SPECIMENS/PROCEDURES. Swabs are taken for culture of bacteria and mycoplasmas. These should be plated as soon as possible. Similar swabs can be used to isolate and cultivate rickettsia and chlamydia.

Conjuctival scrapings should be taken for smears for rickettsia and chlamydia and also for the cultivation of these organisms.

Treatment
Local irrigation with various collyria. Tetracycline and chloramphenicol collyria have reduced the severity of lesions.

Control
Isolation of infected animals. Insect control and removal to less dusty pastures.

CONTAGIOUS PLEUROPNEUMONIA OF SWINE
Contagious pleuropneumonia of swine is an acute, subacute, or chronic respiratory infection affecting principally, but not exclusively, pigs up to 5 months of age. It is caused by *Actinobacillus pleuropneumoniae* (*Haemophilus pleuropneumoniae*) and is characterized by an acute fibrinous pneumonia or a chronic form with pleuritis and pulmonary abscessation. The mortality rate in the acute disease may exceed 10%.

The disease is probably worldwide in distribution and occurs sporadically as well as in herd outbreaks. The infection is most severe in stressed pigs or in those that have not been previously exposed. Meningitis and arthritis may be seen in nursing pigs. At least 12 capsular serotypes have been identified; types 1 and 5 are the most frequent.

The infection usually results from the introduction to a herd of a carrier or subclinically infected pig. The disease may be chronic in feeder pigs and result in delayed weight gains and condemnations at slaughter.

Differential Diagnosis
Swine influenza, enzootic pneumonia of swine, Glasser's disease, mycoplasma polyserositis, and *Streptococcus suis* polyserositis are among the diseases that should be considered.

Definitive diagnosis is dependent upon laboratory confirmation.

Laboratory Diagnosis
SPECIMENS. Portions of lungs with lesions.

PROCEDURES/COMMENTS. Isolation and identification of *A. pleuropneumoniae*. *A. pleuropneumoniae* is a fastidious bacterium and provision must be made for the V factor in the blood agar plates used.

A number of serologic tests including complement fixation, agglutination, and enzyme-linked immunosorbent assay are available to confirm infection or exposure.

Treatment

Although penicillin and broad-spectrum antibiotics have been successful, it is advisable to carry out antimicrobial susceptibility tests on isolates. Pigs with the chronic form do not respond well to antimicrobial therapy. Some practitioners employ simultaneous treatment and vaccination.

Control

Because survivors are frequently carriers, control of the disease is difficult. Serologic tests have been used to screen pigs and to detect carriers in infected herds.

Various vaccines are available containing the appropriate serotypes. They reduce the severity and mortality of the disease.

CORYNEBACTERIUM

Several important species of this genus have been moved to new genera. The corynebacteria are small, gram-positive, pleomorphic rods with club-shaped swellings at one or both ends. The animal corynebacteria are nonmotile, nonspore-forming, aerobic or facultatively anaerobic, and frequent commensals on the skin and mucous membranes. Corynebacteria, also called diphtheroids, are frequently recovered from clinical specimens where they are usually considered nonpathogenic.

Some of the following species of the genus have been reclassified:

Corynebacterium pyogenes to *Actinomyces pyogenes*.

C. equi to *Rhodococcus equi*.

C. suis to *Eubacterium suis*.

C. renale: See BOVINE PYELONEPHRITIS, ENZOOTIC BALANOPOSTHITIS AND VULVITIS.

C. pilosum: See BOVINE PYELONEPHRITIS.

C. cystitidis: See BOVINE PYELONEPHRITIS.

C. pseudotuberculosis: See CASEOUS LYMPHADENITIS, ULCERATIVE LYMPHANGITIS. One biotype of *C. pseudotuberculosis* causes caseous lymphadenitis in sheep and goats. Another biotype is responsible for pectoral abscesses in horses and infrequent skin abscesses in cattle.

C. ulcerans: Has been recovered infrequently from bovine mastitis.

C. minutissimum: Has been isolated from docking wounds in lambs and from "scald" (inflammation of the interdigital spaces) and scabs on the brisket.

C. bovis: A nonpathogenic diphtheroid frequently recovered from bovine milk. It is a commensal that occurs normally in the region of the teat orifice.

COWPOX

Cowpox is a benign, contagious disease involving the skin of the teats and udder caused by an orthopoxvirus and characterized by the formation of papules, which become vesicles that rupture leaving scabs. There is a loss of milk production, but without secondary bacteria, the disease usually runs its course in 2 weeks.

Cowpox is potentially transmissible to humans.

Differential Diagnosis

Pseudocowpox is a milder disease that occurs much more commonly than cowpox. It is now thought that cowpox no longer occurs in North America. There are reports of its occurrence in Western Europe.

Bovine ulcerative mammillitis and various bacterial and fungal infections of the teat and udder should be considered.

Cowpox, like pseudocowpox, is usually diagnosed clinically. Laboratory confirmation should be sought if the more serious disease, bovine ulcerative mammillitis, is suspected.

Laboratory Diagnosis

SPECIMENS. Vesicular fluid and tissue from lesions are collected as aseptically as possible.

PROCEDURES. Vesicular fluid and tissue are examined by electron microscopy.

The virus can be cultivated in cell cultures and identified

by the cytopathic effect and the character of the inclusion bodies. It also grows in a characteristic way on the chorioallantoic membrane of the embryonated chicken egg.

Treatment
None, except in some instances, antiseptic ointments to control secondary infection.

Control
1. Isolation of affected animals.
2. Affected cows are milked last.
3. Disinfection of teat cups between cows.

CRYPTOCOCCOSIS / TORULOSIS
Cryptococcosis is a subacute to chronic, frequently fatal disease of dogs, cats, horses, cattle, sheep, goats, and other animals. Disease is caused by the yeast-like fungus, *Cryptococcus neoformans,* and is manifested most commonly as a paranasal infection that often extends to the meninges, brain (particularly in cats), and lungs. The characteristic tumor-like granulomatous lesions may also involve the skin and subcutis. When the infection is well established, metastases may develop in various tissues and organs.

In veterinary practice, most cases of cryptococcosis are seen in dogs, cats, horses, and cows (mastitis). In the latter disease, which can be severe, the fungi are thought to be introduced during udder treatment.

The organism is soil-borne and multiplies to large numbers in the feces of pigeons; however, it is not found in the intestinal tract of live pigeons.

Differential Diagnosis
Paranasal cryptococcosis must be distinguished from other respiratory diseases in the various species. The subcutaneous form must be distinguished from a number of diseases such as blastomycosis, nasal aspergillosis (dogs), nocardiosis, and canine actinomycosis that may produce discharging, granulomatous lesions.

Laboratory Diagnosis
The paranasal and subcutaneous forms of the disease can be presumptively diagnosed on the basis of clinical signs and the

demonstration of yeast-like cells (different from those of blastomycosis and coccidioidomycosis) in wet mounts and Gram-stained smears of material taken from lesions.

SPECIMENS. Material is collected aseptically from the nasal passages in the paranasal form, and from the granulomatous lesions in the subcutaneous form.

It may be advisable in certain cases to take biopsies. If there is evidence of involvement of the brain and meninges, cerebrospinal fluid (CSF) should be collected.

Milk in suspected cryptococcal mastitis.

Necropsy: Portions of affected tissues, fresh and fixed, are submitted.

PROCEDURES. All materials collected, including CSF, are examined by stains and wet mounts, then cultured for *C. neoformans.*

Fixed tissues are examined for the typical lesions containing the yeast-like organisms.

COMMENTS. Although *C. neoformans* is not the only capsulated cryptococcus, the association of a capsulated yeast-like organism with the morphology of cryptococci from an animal with typical clinical signs or lesions is considered sufficient for a firm diagnosis.

Sensitive serologic tests, e.g., the tube agglutination and latex agglutination tests, are available for the detection of *C. neoformans* antibody and antigen, respectively, in humans but they have seldom been employed in the animal disease. An indirect fluorescent antibody test has also been used although a negative test does not exclude cryptococcosis.

Treatment

Amphotericin B and flucytosine are used, alone or in combination. Resistance may develop to either drug. Miconazole and ketoconazole have shown some promise.

Control

Cases should be isolated. Because humans contract this disease, human exposure to infected animals should be avoided. However, human cases ordinarily are not thought to be acquired from animals.

DERMATOPHILOSIS /
STREPTOTHRICOSIS, MYCOTIC DERMATITIS (SHEEP), LUMPY WOOL

Dermatophilosis is a contagious disease of horses, cattle, goats, sheep, and other animals caused by the actinomycete, *Dermatophilus congolensis,* and is characterized by dermatitis of the superficial layers of the skin resulting in the formation of crusts or scabs. Initial lesions may be circumscribed but later they may coalesce resulting in extensive encrustation.

The disease in sheep is referred to as mycotic dermatitis and is seen in the following forms:

Dermatitis of wool-covered areas or "lumpy wool."

Dermatitis of face and scrotum.

Dermatitis of the lower leg and foot, which may result in an ulcerative dermatitis called "strawberry foot rot."

Although the disease has been diagnosed in swine, dogs, cats, primates, and humans, its occurrence is infrequent to rare in these species.

The disease occurs worldwide but it is probably more common in tropical and subtropical countries. Moist and wet conditions contribute to its spread. Biting arthropods and trauma may initiate infections.

Differential Diagnosis

Ringworm, scabies, contagious ecthyma (sheep).

Although the encrustations and scabs are characteristic, allowing for a highly presumptive clinical diagnosis, laboratory confirmation should be sought.

Laboratory Diagnosis
SPECIMENS

1. Scabs, crusts, and plucked hair are collected.
2. Skin biopsies taken after removal of scabs.

PROCEDURES

1. A diagnosis can usually be made by demonstrating *D. congolensis* in Gram- or Giemsa-stained smears.
2. Isolation, culture, and identification of *D. congolensis.*
3. The characteristic morphologic elements can be seen in Gram-stained sections of skin.

COMMENTS. The finding of the characteristic morphologic elements of *D. congolensis* in Giemsa- or Gram-stained smears is sufficient to make a definitive diagnosis of dermatophilosis. Although culture is not usually difficult, it is not required for diagnosis. There is a good correlation between the results of the examination of smears and of culture.

Treatment

Cases should be isolated. Acute cases are often of short duration and clear up without treatment.

Single large doses of penicillin-streptomycin and long-acting tetracyclines given intramuscularly have been found effective. Washing and using disinfectant solutions may reduce spread, although topical treatment is not effective. Mild cases may respond to good, regular grooming.

Control

Isolation of infected animals.

DERMATOPHYTOSIS / RINGWORM

Dermatophytosis is a contagious disease caused by fungi of the genera *Microsporum* and *Trichophyton* that infect the keratin-containing tissues (skin, nails, and hair) of domestic animals, humans, and other animals. The infections are superficial, starting in the stratum corneum and invading hair follicles and hair, with the production of hyphae and spores within (endothrix) and/or on (ectothrix) hairs. The lesions spread out from a central locus resulting in circular and patchy lesions.

The dermatophytoses are of worldwide occurrence. Among the domestic animals, ringworm is found less frequently in sheep, goats, and swine. *Microsporum gypseum* occurs naturally in soil and *M. nanum* will survive in soil and pig yards for long periods. Infected animals and fomites are the usual source of the dermatophytes (Table 2.6). Inapparent infections are common in kittens.

Differential Diagnosis

The circular or roughly circular lesions of ringworm are variable in size and develop from raised plaques on the skin. The hair becomes thin, broken, and finally there is bareness that may become scaly and scabby. Most lesions occur on the head and neck.

Table 2.6. Principal dermatophytes of domestic animals

	Organism
Dog	*Microsporum canis*
	M. gypseum
	Trichophyton mentagrophytes
	M. distortum
Cat	*M. canis*
	M. gypseum
	T. mentagrophytes
	M. distortum
Horse	*T. equinum*
	M. canis
	M. gypseum
	T. mentagrophytes
	M. distortum
Cattle	*T. verrucosum*
	M. canis
	M. gypseum
Swine	*M. nanum*
	M. distortum
	M. canis
Sheep	*T. verrucosum*
	T. mentagrophytes (uncommon)
Goats	*T. verrucosum* (rare)

Eczema, dermatitis, pyoderma, dermatophilosis, and mange should be considered.

Laboratory Diagnosis

If feasible, examine lesions with a Wood's lamp; *M. canis* and *M. distortum* may fluoresce (greenish color). Negative fluorescence does not exclude ringworm.

SPECIMENS. Plucked hair (especially those that fluoresce) and skin scrapings from the edge of lesions. These are sent to the laboratory in a paper envelope (to prevent moisture and the growth of saprophytic fungi).

Some veterinarians inoculate one of the several commercial media (Dermatophyte Test Media, Fungassay, etc.) that are available for the selective growth of dermatophytes. If the results are equivocal, the media may be submitted to a diagnostic laboratory for interpretation.

PROCEDURES. The specimen is first examined microscopically in wet mounts for the presence of spores and other fungal elements.

Appropriate media are inoculated. Isolation and identification may take several weeks.

Treatment

Isolation of infected animals if feasible. These fungi are often zoonotic so contact with humans should be prevented. It is often a self-limiting disease.

Treatment will depend to some extent on the animal species and economic considerations.

Local: clipping, dipping, and thorough washing with mild soap; Lugol's iodine; equal parts tincture of iodine and glycerine; sprays for large animals, such as 75% thiabendazole, detergent, and other disinfectant solutions; natamycin. An aqueous solution of lime-sulfur (2%) is used in dogs. Zinc and sodium salts of fatty acids such as propionic, undecylenic, and caprylic acids are useful.

Systemic: griseofulvin; iodides for cattle and horses; various imidazoles (e.g., ketoconzaole, miconazole, clotrimazole).

EDEMA DISEASE / GUT EDEMA

Edema disease is an acute disease usually occurring in pigs from 1 month to 14 weeks of age and characterized by sudden onset, incoordination, and edematous swelling, particularly of the cardiac region of the stomach, mesenteric folds, and coils of the colon. The disease is thought to be due to a toxic factor (verotoxin) of certain strains of *Escherichia coli.*

Distribution is probably worldwide; it occurs periodically in weaned pigs following sudden changes in feed presumably resulting in excessive multiplication of certain strains of *E. coli.*

Acute postweaning enteritis, thought to be due to the same *E. coli* that causes edema disease, sometimes occurs with the latter disease.

Differential Diagnosis

Distinguish from salt poisoning, mulberry heart disease, stomach ulcers, Teschen and Teschen-like diseases, arsenic poisoning, and pseudorabies.

Laboratory Diagnosis

The disease can be diagnosed clinically on the basis of the gross changes, viz., edema (clear, gelatinous fluid) involving the stomach wall, mesenteric folds, coils of the colon, and subcutaneous tissues of the forehead and eyelids.

SPECIMENS. A sick or recently dead pig should be submitted or necropsied on the premises. A portion of the anterior part of the small intestine is submitted in the latter instance.

PROCEDURES/COMMENTS. Cultural procedures are carried out for *E. coli* or other enterobacteria.

A diagnosis of edema disease is usually made on the basis of finding the characteristic gross pathologic changes, viz., edema in various locations.

Supportive of this diagnosis is the recovery of a heavy culture of *E. coli* from the duodenum. Certain serotypes of *E. coli* have been found in edema disease although very few laboratories carry out serotyping. It is ordinarily not practicable to test for verotoxin.

Treatment

Usually impracticable. Antimicrobial drugs may reduce the number of cases.

Control

Reduction of predisposing factors such as sudden changes in feed.

EHRLICHIA

Species of this genus are rickettsial parasites of white blood cells. The following are significant species:

Ehrlichia canis: See CANINE EHRLICHIOSIS.

E. platys: Parasitizes canine thrombocytes causing a nonclinical thrombocytopenia.

E. risticii: See POTOMAC HORSE FEVER.

E. equi: See EQUINE EHRLICHIOSIS.

E. phagocytophilia: See Microbial Diseases Foreign to North America, TICK-BORNE FEVER.

E. ondiri: See Microbial Diseases Foreign to North America, BOVINE PETECHIAL FEVER.

E. bovis and *E. ovina:* Parasitize bovine and ovine mononuclear cells respectively. Clinical disease is not apparent in these infections.

ENCEPHALOMYOCARDITIS VIRUS DISEASE OF PIGS

Encephalomyocarditis virus disease of pigs (EVDP) is usually a sporadic disease of young pigs caused by a cardiovirus (picornavirus) and characterized by depression, inappetence, difficult breathing, and incoordination. One or more litters may be infected and mortality, after a short course, may reach 50%; adults are resistant. Reproductive failure and transplacental infection have been reported.

The virus is thought to be contracted from infected rodents. The porcine disease has been reported in Australia and North and South America, and given the wide distribution of the virus in rodents, it probably occurs worldwide.

Differential Diagnosis

Mulberry heart disease, edema disease, and various acute viral and bacterial diseases are among the diseases that should be considered. The presence of myocardial lesions with pale longitudinal necrosis, calcifications, and lymphocitic infiltration are indicative of EVDP.

Laboratory Diagnosis

Laboratories should be alerted when the disease is suspected.

SPECIMENS
1. Brain, heart, spleen, liver, and kidney.
2. Paired serum samples preferred.

PROCEDURES/COMMENTS
1. The disease is only diagnosed with certainty by isolation and identification of the virus.
2. Serologic tests, such as virus neutralization for specific antibody on unpaired sera, are of limited value because pigs may die before producing appreciable antibody response and because normal pigs may have antibodies as a result of exposure. A demonstration of increase in titer between acute and convalescent sera would be significant.

Treatment

None.

Control
Rodent eradication if there is a persistent problem.

ENTERIC INFECTIONS OF PIGLETS
The agents commonly associated with enteric disease in young pigs are listed in Table 2.7 with some of their diagnostically significant features. See also ENTEROVIRUS INFECTIONS OF SWINE.

Table 2.7. Agents commonly associated with enteric disease in young pigs

Agent	Age	Features
E. coli	First few days	Yellow to watery feces, dehydration
Clostridium perfringens type C enterotoxemia	First few days	Diarrhea, dysentery
Rotavirus	Usually 1–4 weeks but up to 8 weeks	White scours; milk scours
Enteric coronavirus	Usually prior to weaning	Diarrhea; reported from Europe
Transmissible gastroenteritis	Birth to 10 days usually	Severe diarrhea, dehydration, high mortality
Virus of vomiting and wasting disease	5–21 days	Vomiting; neurologic signs; infrequent
Virus of Teschen and Teschen-like disease	All ages; most common 7–12 weeks	Varying degrees of paralysis
Salmonella spp.	All ages	Signs depend on form; septicemia more common in piglets
Serpulina hyodysenteriae	All ages	Bloody diarrhea
Coccidiosis (*Eimeria, Isospora*)	5–15 days	Enteritis and diarrhea
Cryptosporidiosis	5–15 days	Diarrhea; extent not known

Laboratory Diagnosis
Because the clinical signs of these various enteric diseases are often similar, a laboratory diagnosis is important. Refer to specific diseases for details (see Table 2.7).

ENTERIC INFECTIONS OF PUPPIES
The principal microbial enteric infections of the dog are listed below. Readers are referred to the separate discussions as indicated for details.

SALMONELLOSIS: Dogs frequently carry salmonellas and

shed them intermittently in their feces but, except for puppies and dogs under severe stress (e.g., racing grey-hounds), the acute, septicemic form of the disease is rarely seen. As in other domestic animals, the serotypes or species vary considerably.

CANINE PARVOVIRUS INFECTIONS.
CANINE CAMPYLOBACTERIOSIS.
CANINE CORONAVIRUS GASTROENTERITIS.
COLIBACILLOSIS.

Other diseases that may result in diarrhea and enteritis are canine rotavirus infection, histoplasmosis, canine hemor-rhagic enteritis (cause unknown), intestinal parasites, poi-sons, pancreatitis, chronic bacterial enteritis (cause un-known), and infection due to *Clostridium difficile.*

ENTERIC INFECTIONS OF YOUNG CALVES /

NEONATAL CALF DIARRHEA

The agents commonly associated with enteric disease in young calves are listed in Table 2.8 along with some of their significant features.

Table 2.8. Agents commonly associated with enteric disease in young calve

Agent	Age	Features
E. coli (colibacillosis)		
Enterotoxic colibacillosis		
(white scours)	1st 2 weeks	Dehydration, diarrhea
Colisepticemia	1st week	Sudden death
Clostridium perfringens		
Type C enterotoxemia	up to 1 month	Dysentery, opisthotonos, convulsions
Type D enterotoxemia	uncommon	Dysentery, opisthotonos, convulsions
Rotavirus	up to 7 days	Profuse watery diarrhea, dehydration
Coronavirus	1–3 weeks	Profuse watery diarrhea
Salmonella spp.	all ages	Signs depend on form; septicemia more common in young

Other agents that may be involved in either a primary or secondary capacity are the protozoans *Cryptosporidium* and *Eimeria* (coccidiosis), and the breda virus, bovine viral diar-rhea virus, and astroviruses. *Chlamydia psittaci* is thought to be an occasional cause of enteritis in calves. Enteroviruses can be isolated from calves, but their significance in disease is questionable.

Laboratory Diagnosis

Consult specific diseases and agents listed in Table 2.8 for details of laboratory diagnosis.

ENTERIC INFECTIONS OF YOUNG FOALS

Neonatal foals are largely dependent upon an adequate supply of colostrum for protection against infectious agents. The foal is most susceptible to enteric infections during the first 10 days of life. The principal enteric infections of young foals are listed below. Readers should consult the separate discussions as indicated for further information, including Laboratory Diagnosis.

Actinobacillus equuli: Causes diarrhea shortly after birth. However, because infections often involve other organs, *A. equuli* is discussed under NONENTERIC INFECTIONS OF NEONATAL FOALS.

COLIBACILLOSIS: *E. coli* infection in foals is similar clinically to that of calves, lambs, and piglets. Septicemia is usually seen early in the first week, while the diarrheic form occurs toward the end of the first week.

Treatment and Laboratory Diagnosis is essentially the same as that for: COLIBACILLOSIS OF CALVES, SALMONELLOSIS, ROTAVIRUS INFECTION OF FOALS, and Sleepy Foal Disease (see NONENTERIC INFECTIONS OF NEONATAL FOALS).

Coronaviruses: There have been several reports of the demonstration and isolation of these organisms associated with diarrhea in foals.

Clostridium difficile: Has been reported as a cause of diarrhea in foals.

ENTERIC INFECTIONS OF YOUNG LAMBS

Enteric infections of neonatal and young lambs are not a major disease problem. Some of the infections that are encountered are listed below:

CLOSTRIDIAL ENTEROTOXEMIA OF SHEEP.

ROTAVIRUS INFECTION OF LAMBS.

Coronaviruses: Have been implicated in diarrhea in lambs.

COLIBACILLOSIS: With diarrhea and/or septicemia, it is seen in lambs occasionally and is essentially the same as colibacillosis in other domestic animals.

Coccidiosis: Is seen in lambs in the age range of 2 weeks to 3 months.

Cryptosporidia: Cause diarrhea in lambs.

ENTEROBACTERIACEAE

Members of this family are frequently called enterobacteria or enteric bacteria because most are part of the normal flora of the intestine of animals; some also occur in nature. They are gram-negative rods and include nonpathogens, opportunists, and frank pathogens. Only those species that are known to cause disease in animals are listed below:

Arizona: This genus is now included in *Salmonella.*

Citrobacter: Members of this genus are isolated from the feces of animals. They are infrequent, opportunistic pathogens in animals.

Edwardsiella: E. tarda and *E. ictaluri* are common pathogens of catfish. A small number of opportunistic infections due to *E. tarda* have been reported in animals.

Enterobacter: A few members of this genus are opportunistic pathogens in animals. *E. aerogenes* and possibly other species cause bovine mastitis and occasionally other infections in animals.

Escherichia coli: See COLIBACILLOSIS. In addition to colibacillosis, this species frequently causes severe bovine mastitis, urinary tract infections in all domestic species, wound infections, and a variety of infections including arthritis, septicemia, metritis, and meningitis. *E. coli* causes edema disease in pigs (discussed separately).

Certain strains of *E. coli* produce enterotoxins, the most important of which are the heat-stable and heat-labile. Not all strains produce both of these plasmid-based enterotoxins. Colonization of intestine by pathogenic strains of *E. coli* depends on certain types of pili. Important pilus antigens of *E. coli* associated with diseases are as follows: in swine, K88 or F4, K99 or F5, 987P or F6; in calves, K99; and in lambs, K99. Certain strains of *E. coli* produce verotoxin (Shiga-like toxin), which is thought to play a role in the pathogenesis of edema disease in pigs, and diarrhea in calves and rabbits.

Klebsiella (most commonly *K. pneumoniae*): It has been implicated in pneumonia and suppurative infections in foals; cervicitis and metritis in mares; mastitis and urinary tract infections in cows; and pneumonia and septicemia in dogs. *Klebsiella* organisms occur in nature and are associated with wood shavings used as bedding for cows. Consequently, *Klebsiella* mastitis is more common when cows are on such bedding.

Morganella: M. morganii is associated with urinary tract and ear infections of dogs and cats.

Proteus (most commonly *P. mirabilis*): A variety of sporadic infections have been reported in cattle, fowl, cats, ponies, and dogs particularly. *P. mirabilis* causes urinary tract infections in dogs and ponies.

Salmonella: Also see SALMONELLOSIS. All *Salmonella* organisms are now considered to belong to one species. However, there are 7 distinct subgroups and more than 2000 serovars in this genus, all of which are potentially pathogenic, causing many sporadic and multiple infections (Table 2.9). *Salmonella arizonae* serovar (formerly known as *Arizona hinshawii*) causes fatal infections in turkey poults and occasionally severe infections in humans, dogs, cats, and other animals.

Table 2.9. Important diseases caused by *Salmonella* serovars

Serovar	Disease
S. typhimurium	Gastroenteritis in humans; most prevalent species causing infection in various animal species
S. agona	Various infections in horses and other animals
S. abortusequi	Abortion in mares and jennets
S. abortusbovis	Abortion in cattle
S. abortusovis	Abortion in sheep
S. choleraesuis	Enteritis in swine; frequent secondary invader in hog cholera
S. typhisuis	Infections in young pigs
S. montevideo	Infections in cattle and swine primarily
S. newport	Infections in various animals, especially cattle
S. enteritidis	Infections in various animals
S. dublin	Severe infections in calves
S. muenster	Infections in cattle primarily

Serratia: Serratia marcescens can cause bovine mastitis, wound infections, and a variety of infrequent sporadic infections in cattle and horses.

Shigella: Members of this genus cause intestinal infections and dysentery in humans and primates.

Yersinia: See *YERSINIA ENTEROCOLITICA* INFECTION, *Y. PSEUDOTUBERCULOSIS* INFECTION, and PLAGUE. The important pathogenic species are those just mentioned, and *Y. pestis,* the cause of plague.

Several other species have been described, but they do not cause significant infections in domestic animals.

Laboratory Diagnosis

See disease or organism of interest. These organisms are relatively hardy and material for culture can be submitted on swabs with a transport medium.

Definitive diagnosis depends on the isolation and identification of the causal bacterium. Because these organisms often possess multiple drug resistance, antimicrobial susceptibility tests should be carried out.

ENTEROVIRUS INFECTIONS OF SWINE / SMEDI VIRUS INFECTION OF SWINE

SMEDI is an acronym for stillbirths, mummification, embryonic death, and infertility. Several picornaviruses have been incriminated as causes of SMEDI. These infections are probably widespread where swine are raised intensively; however, porcine parvovirus is considered to be a much more important cause of reproductive problems. The picornaviruses are distributed widely and probably only cause disease in immunologically susceptible sows and gilts.

Differential Diagnosis

Parvovirus infection, leptospirosis, and brucellosis, should be considered. Similar disease manifestations may result from pseudorabies, hog cholera, and several bacterial pathogens.

Laboratory Diagnosis

SPECIMENS

1. For virus isolation: Fresh fetuses and stillborn pigs.
2. For serology: Paired serum samples or multiple samples from affected and nonaffected pigs.

PROCEDURES/COMMENTS

1. The laboratory diagnosis of enterovirus infection is not very satisfactory. Although the viruses can be cultivated, there have been few isolations. Fetal lesions have been absent or minimal.
2. A laboratory diagnosis has usually been based upon the results of serologic tests. A fourfold increase in the titers

of paired samples or high titers in affected animals strongly supports a diagnosis of enteroviral infection. Unfortunately, few laboratories carry out the serologic tests.

Treatment
None.

Control
1. Isolation of affected swine with appropriate sanitary measures to limit spread.
2. Exposure of breeding gilts to mature sows and boars 3 weeks before breeding appears to be helpful.
3. Isolation of all mature, newly purchased swine is also recommended.

ENZOOTIC ABORTION OF EWES / CHLAMYDIAL AND ENDEMIC ABORTION OF EWES

Enzootic abortion of ewes is caused by the bacterium *Chlamydia psittaci* (*C. ovis*), and is manifested by a placentitis leading to premature lambing, stillbirths, and, more frequently, abortion.

The disease has been reported from Britain, a number of European countries, the United States, and South Africa. Lambs and sheep are thought to be infected by ingestion. Infections appear to be latent until conception occurs.

The disease affects goats similarly.

Differential Diagnosis
This disease should be suspected if there are stillbirths, premature lambing, abortions in late gestation, and retained placentas.

Abortions are also caused by *Campylobacter fetus* ssp. *fetus, Listeria monocytogenes, Toxoplasma gondii, Brucella ovis,* leptospires, *Salmonella* serovars, bluetongue virus, and *Coxiella burnettii.*

A consistent gross lesion seen in chlamydial abortion is placentitis with multifocal cotyledonary necrosis and red-brown intercotyledonary exudate.

Laboratory confirmation should be sought.

Laboratory Diagnosis
SPECIMENS
1. Fresh placenta and fetus.
2. A number of serum samples; paired samples are preferred.

PROCEDURES
1. Examination of stained smears. Flourescent antibody-stained smears have no advantage over regularly stained smears (modified Ziehl-Neelsen or Gimenez).

    Isolation and identification of *C. psittaci* in embryonated chicken eggs or cultures of McCoy cells.
2. Complement fixation test. A number of reactors with titers in the range of 1:32–1:256 suggest a chlamydial infection. A fourfold rise in titer between paired serum samples is significant.

COMMENTS. A strongly presumptive diagnosis can be made on the basis of demonstrating the elementary bodies of *C. psittaci* in stained smears from cotyledons and fetal tissues. A definitive diagnosis is dependent on the isolation and identification of the agent from fetal tissues. It should be kept in mind that chlamydia are frequently shed in the feces and thus clinical specimens may easily be contaminated.

Treatment
Tetracyclines have been used for infected newborn lambs and for ewes that have aborted. Long-acting tetracyclines are administered to pregnant ewes intramuscularly to prevent abortion.

Control
1. Segregation of infected and aborting ewes.
2. Bacterins are available.

ENZOOTIC BALANOPOSTHITIS AND VULVITIS /
PIZZLE ROT, SHEATH ROT
Bacterial balanoposthitis and vulvitis (BBV) is a disease mainly of wethers and rams, less commonly of ewes, and infrequently in goats. It is associated with protein-rich feed, and characterized by necrosis and ulceration involving the prepuce, and sometimes the penis and vulva. Both *Coryne-*

bacterium renale and *C. pilosum* are thought to be causally involved in the ovine disease.

The primary lesion, which begins from an injury of the prepuce, becomes ulcerous and may spread to involve much of the prepuce and even the penis. There is pus, necrosis, and scab formation leading to difficult urination. Much of the inflammatory process is attributed to the ammonia released as a result of the hydrolysis of urea by the organism. Other bacteria, including anaerobes, may be involved.

Differential Diagnosis

The ulcerative dermatosis virus can cause a balanoposthitis in sheep that is clinically indistinguishable from the bacterial disease. In most countries, ulcerative dermatosis is a much less frequent disease than BBV.

Laboratory Diagnosis

SPECIMENS. Pus is collected on swabs from several animals.

Unless they are being cultured within a few hours, the swabs should be placed in a transport medium. See ULCER-ATIVE DERMATOSIS for its laboratory diagnosis.

PROCEDURES. A definitive diagnosis of BBV is based on the isolation of the gram-positive diphtheroid *C. renale* or *C. pilosum* from characteristic lesions.

Treatment

1. Withhold food for 2–3 days, then feed small quantities of low-protein hay.
2. Give ammonium chloride orally for a week.
3. Treat locally with nonirritant antiseptics after removing pus, necrotic debris, and scabs.
4. Use antibiotics systemically.
5. Perform surgery if indicated.

Control

Isolation of affected animals. Chronic cases are usually sacrificed.

ENZOOTIC NASAL ADENOCARCINOMA OF SHEEP /
NASAL ADENOCARCINOMA, OVINE NASAL ADENOPAPILLOMA

Nasal adenocarcinoma of sheep is thought to be an infectious disease most probably caused by a retrovirus. The tumors involve the nasal mucosa and are usually bilateral and located in the ethmoturbinate region. They are classified as papillary adenomas or adenocarcinomas with little tendency to metastasize.

The most apparent clinical sign is a serous, mucous, or mucopurulent nasal discharge with death frequently occurring as a result of inanition and asphyxiation.

Laboratory Diagnosis

This is based on the gross and histopathologic changes. The probable viral cause is supported by demonstration of retroviruses in sections examined by electron microscopy.

ENZOOTIC PNEUMONIA OF SHEEP /
OVINE PNEUMONIC PASTEURELLOSIS

Enzootic pneumonia of sheep (EPS) is a major, widespread, contagious disease caused almost always by *Pasteurella haemolytica* (biotype A) and characterized by a bronchopneumonia, which varies in severity from a mild chronic pneumonia (most common) to an acute fulminating disease.

This disease is worldwide in distribution and can affect sheep of all ages. As in pneumonic pasteurellosis of cattle, factors such as viral and mycoplasmal (*Mycoplasma ovipneumoniae*) infections, and various stresses predispose to the disease. Relatively mild pneumonic lesions may lead to acute bronchopneumonia under particularly stressful conditions.

Differential Diagnosis

Diseases that should be considered are progressive pneumonia of sheep, verminous pneumonia, sporadic infectious pneumonias due to various organisms, and pulmonary adenomatosis.

Enzootic pneumonia of sheep is frequently diagnosed clinically; however, in severe outbreaks, laboratory confirmation should be sought.

Laboratory Diagnosis

A diagnosis of EPS is based on the recovery of *P. haemolytica* from the lungs of one or several sheep with bronchopneumonia. *P. multocida* and *Actinomyces pyogenes* are occasionally recovered with *P. haemolytica* and sometimes by themselves.

Mycoplasma ovipneumoniae and several viruses (parainfluenza-3, adenovirus, reoviruses, etc.) are thought to be primary agents in some outbreaks. The identification of these agents will require special procedures.

Antimicrobial susceptibility tests should be conducted on the bacterial isolates. *P. haemolytica* may show multiple drug resistance.

Treatment

Tetracyclines, sulfonamides, and other drugs selected on the basis of the results of susceptibility tests. The prognosis is poor when abscessation due to *A. pyogenes* is extensive.

Control

Sheep with fever and signs of pneumonia should be isolated.

Viral vaccines (e.g., to prevent PI-3 infection) and bacterins containing *P. haemolytica* and sometimes other bacteria are available for prevention.

ENZOOTIC PNEUMONIA OF SWINE /
VIRUS PNEUMONIA OF PIGS,
MYCOPLASMA PNEUMONIA OF SWINE,
ENDEMIC PNEUMONIA OF SWINE

Enzootic pneumonia of swine is a widespread, chronic, contagious disease caused by *Mycoplasma hyopneumoniae* (*M. suipneumoniae*) and characterized usually, by a chronic, low-grade bronchopneumonia complicated frequently by the secondary invasion of *Pasteurella multocida,* and occasionally other bacteria such as *Haemophilus parasuis.* Under certain circumstances, usually involving stress, an acute, fulminating pneumonia may develop.

The disease is probably widespread in most swine-raising regions of the world. When present in the low-grade form, the principal effect is a moderate to small loss in weight gains. A debilitating pleuritis may be present in older pigs. The only clinical sign observed may be repeated coughing.

Differential Diagnosis

Although the disease is usually diagnosed on the basis of clinical signs and gross and microscopic pathologic changes, it can only be identified with certainty by laboratory procedures. The latter are usually carried out only if this ordinarily mild disease becomes acute or eradication is being attempted.

Laboratory Diagnosis

The causative agent, *M. hyopneumoniae,* is particularly difficult to grow and identify.

SPECIMENS. Portions of affected lungs, fresh and fixed. Sick or recently dead pigs are necropsied.

PROCEDURES. Cultural procedures are not usually available for *M. hyopneumoniae* but should be employed for potential secondary bacteria.

Tissue sections are examined for histopathologic changes.

Mycoplasma hyopneumoniae can be identified in smears and sections with fluorescent antibody staining.

COMMENTS. A presumptive diagnosis of this disease is usually made on the basis of the clinical signs, gross pathology, and the recovery of secondary bacteria such as *Pasteurella multocida.*

A number of serologic procedures including enzyme-linked immunosorbent assay, latex agglutination, and complement fixation are effective in determining the extent of infection in herds; however, they are not routinely employed.

Treatment

Antimicrobial drugs are employed when serious pneumonias develop. These are determined by the results of susceptibility tests on secondary bacteria. Antimicrobial treatment will reduce the severity of the disease but not eliminate it.

Control

The use of specific-pathogen-free (SPF) pigs.

No attempt is made to eliminate the disease in many herds; the consequent economic loss is considered acceptable.

Although vaccines may reduce the severity of the disease, they do not prevent it.

EPERYTHROZOON

Members of this rickettsial genus consist of small, ring- and rod-shaped forms found in and upon erythrocytes and in plasma. They have not been cultivated in cell-free media and some species are transmitted by arthropods. Species of veterinary interest are as follows:

Eperythozoon suis: See PORCINE EPERYTHROZOONO-SIS.

E. ovis: Causes a disease mainly of lambs and is characterized by fever, retarded growth, anemia, hemoglobinuria, and considerable mortality. The agent is carried by ewes and transmission is probably by biting arthropods. The disease occurs in many countries including the United States. Subclinical infections are thought to become clinical as a result of a concomitant disease or various stresses.

Laboratory diagnosis is essentially the same as for porcine eperythrozoonosis.

Neoarsphenamine or antimosan is effective in treatment; however, reinfection usually occurs.

E. wenyoni: Causes bovine eperythrozoonosis, which has been reported from Africa and Europe. The disease resembles porcine eperythrozoonosis.

EPIZOOTIC BOVINE ABORTION / FOOTHILL ABORTION

Epizootic bovine abortion is a disease of beef cattle thought to be tick-transmitted. It occurs on pastures in the foothills of northern California during the summer and also in Italy, Germany, and Spain. There is considerable evidence that the disease is caused by *Chlamydia psittaci.*

Pregnant animals abort only during their first exposure to the foothills and are immune to infection in subsequent pregnancies. Abortions occur in the last trimester, with a peak incidence from July to October.

Diagnosis is usually based on fetal pathology. The consistent lesions in most cases are hemorrhages in multiple organs, particularly the thymus, granulomas in the liver, and occasionally other organs. Attempts should be made to isolate and identify *C. psittaci.*

EQUINE COITAL EXANTHEMA

Equine coital exanthema is a benign, for the most part, venereal disease caused by equine herpesvirus-3. It usually runs an uneventful short course of less than 2 weeks and is characterized by the formation of papules followed by pustules then ulcers about 2 cm in diameter on the mucosa of the vulva, penis, and prepuce. The ulcers heal with the production of scabs. Affected skin may lose pigmentation.

The disease is probably worldwide and is perpetuated by asymptomatic carriers. Although lesions are seen most commonly involving the genital tract, they also occur in the mouth and nostrils.

Differential Diagnosis

The lesions are sufficiently characteristic to allow for a reliable clinical diagnosis.

Laboratory Diagnosis

Laboratory diagnosis is not usually sought.

SPECIMENS/PROCEDURES. Scrapings from the affected mucosa of the vulva and penis. The virus can be cultivated and identified in equine cell cultures.

Treatment

1. Lesions are cleansed. Antibiotics may be used to control secondary bacteria.
2. Sexual rest.

Control

Horses should not be bred if lesions are present.

EQUINE EHRLICHIOSIS

Equine ehrlichiosis is a sporadic, noncontagious disease caused by the rickettsia *Ehrlichia equi* and is characterized by fever, thrombocytopenia, mild anemia, leukopenia, and edema of the limbs.

The mode of transmission is not known although ticks are suspected. In the United States the disease has only been reported from California and Florida. The disease varies in severity from inapparent, very mild to moderately severe with acute manifestations being rare. Old horses are most severely affected.

Differential Diagnosis

Equine infectious anemia, piroplasmosis, purpura hemorrhagica, leptospirosis, Potomac horse fever, and viral arteritis should be considered.

Laboratory Diagnosis

This is essentially the same as for canine erhlichiosis and involves the examination of stained blood and buffy coat smears for the morulae of *E. equi* in neutrophils, and the testing of sera with the indirect fluorescent antibody (FA) procedure. An indirect FA procedure is available for the diagnosis of the other ehrlichiosis of horses, viz., POTOMAC HORSE FEVER.

Treatment

Tetracyclines daily for at least a week.

Control

Isolation of infected animals and arthropod control.

EQUINE ENCEPHALOMYELITIS / EQUINE ENCEPHALITIS, VIRAL EQUINE ENCEPHALOMYELITIS

Viral equine encephalomyelitis is a disease of horses usually caused by one of three alphaviruses. The viruses are transmitted mainly by mosquitoes but also by ticks, lice, and mites, the natural reservoir being in wild birds or forest rodents. Disease is characterized by deranged consciousness, motor irritation, paralysis, and high mortality.

These viruses also infect humans, producing disease of varying serverity that constitutes a serious but sporadic public health problem.

The three most common viral equine encephalitides are as follows:

Western equine encephalomyelitis (WEE): Generally occurs west of the Mississippi; mortality rate is 20–40%.

Eastern equine encephalomyelitis (EEE): Generally occurs east of the Mississippi; mortality rate is 90%.

Venezuelan equine encephalomyelitis (VEE): South and Central America and southwestern United States; mortality rate is 50–80%.

Several other viruses occasionally cause infrequent cases of equine encephalitis.

Differential Diagnosis

Seasonal occurrence and a history of previous outbreaks often suggest viral equine encephalomyelitis.

Rabies, Borna disease, botulism, some plant poisonings, moldy corn poisoning (leukoencephalomalacia), tetanus, listeriosis, and other infections of the central nervous system should be considered.

Laboratory Diagnosis

SPECIMENS

1. Whole brain or head; portions of the brain, fresh and formalized.
2. Serum; paired samples are preferred.

PROCEDURES

1. Isolation, cultivation, and identification of the viruses using chicken embryos or cell cultures. The three viruses can be differentiated by virus neutralization.

   Examination of tissue sections of brain disclose characteristic microscopic changes with EEE, i.e., perivascular cuffing with neutrophilia.
2. Complement fixation, hemagglutination inhibition, and virus neutralization tests.

COMMENTS. Antibodies may develop 2–3 days after clinical signs. A rise in the titer between paired sera is significant. Animals may die before there is an appreciable antibody response.

No gross lesions are seen.

Virus isolation is recommended.

Treatment

Supportive.

Control

1. Mosquito control.
2. Stabling during outbreaks.
3. Inactivated vaccines are available for the prevention of all three encephalitides. They are usually given in the spring, annually, in endemic areas.

   Horses that recover from the disease are immune for life. There is no cross protection between strains.

EQUINE INFECTIOUS ANEMIA / SWAMP FEVER

Equine infectious anemia is usually a chronic disease of Equidae spread mainly by mosquitoes. It is caused by a retrovirus and characterized by intermittent fever, progressive weakness, loss of condition, jaundice, anemia, edema of dependent parts, with widespread petechial hemorrhages. A variety of clinical forms are seen from the rare acute disease to an asymptomatic carrier state. Once infected the animal remains infected indefinitely.

The disease is worldwide in distribution occurring most frequently in swampy, low-lying areas where mosquitoes are prevalent. The virus is spread mainly by mosquitoes, but also by other biting arthropods, hypodermic syringes, and surgical instruments. Infection can also take place by ingestion of contaminated food and water, to the fetus transplacentally, and to the neonate through the first milk.

Differential Diagnosis

Purpura hemorrhagica, ehrlichiosis, influenza, babesiosis, leptospirosis, severe parasitic infections, and anemias due to various causes should be considered.

A definitive diagnosis can most readily be obtained by the agar gel immunodiffusion test.

Laboratory Diagnosis

Serum is required for the agar gel immunodiffusion test (Coggins test). A positive test indicates clinical or subclinical infection. All animals that are positive are potential sources of infection. Positive nursing foals should be retested in 6 months if they have not nursed from an infected mother for 60 days.

The competitive enzyme-linked immunosorbent assay (C-ELISA) has been approved as an alternative official test.

Commercial kits are available for the detection of antibody to equine infectious anemia virus (see 9,16, Appendix A).

Treatment

None.

Control

Eradication has been impeded because positive animals frequently show no evidence of the disease. Control and elimination of the disease can only be achieved by strict isolation or, preferably, by removal of positive horses from the possibility of exposure to uninfected horses.

The spread of infection can be reduced by insect control.

Immunization is not practiced.

EQUINE INFLUENZA

Equine influenza is an acute, highly contagious, rapidly spreading respiratory disease caused by an orthomyxovirus (type A influenza virus) and characterized by fever and persistent cough.

The severity of the infection depends upon the immune state. All gradations in severity occur from asymptomatic infections to severe infections with pneumonia and bacterial complications, particularly in foals.

The disease is caused by one of two antigenically related, but not reciprocally immunogenic, serologic varieties of type A influenza virus designated A/Equi 1 and A/Equi 2.

The disease is probably worldwide in distribution and endemic in many regions. It is frequently associated with movement of horses in connection with shows, sales, and racetracks. The source of the virus is horses with apparent or inapparent infections. There is probably a short-term carrier state. The mode of infection is mainly by droplet inhalation.

Differential Diagnosis

The signs are those of a febrile upper respiratory infection. The dominant sign is a dry, hacking cough. Course: 1–3 weeks. Pneumonic signs are uncommon except in severe cases.

Equine rhinopneumonitis, equine viral arteritis, and strangles are the principal respiratory infections that should be considered. For other viruses and bacteria that cause equine respiratory disease, see EQUINE RESPIRATORY DISEASE.

Laboratory Diagnosis

Laboratory confirmation is required.

SPECIMENS

1. Nasal swabs and tracheal wash.
2. Paired serum samples are preferable.

PROCEDURES/COMMENTS
1. Virus isolation and identification.
2. Hemagglutination inhibition, complement fixation, and virus neutralization are also used. A fourfold rise in titer between paired serum samples indicates recent infection.

A definitive diagnosis is made on the basis of the isolation and identification of the virus in chicken embryos or cell cultures.

Treatment
Antibiotics for secondary bacterial infections.

Control
Vaccination with killed virus vaccine containing the two antigenic types of influenza virus.

EQUINE LEPTOSPIROSIS
Leptospirosis of horses is caused mainly by *Leptospira interrogans* serovar *pomona* and characterized usually by a mild or subacute form with fever, depression, and icterus resulting occasionally in abortion and periodic ophthalmia. Eye lesions may result from clinically mild or inapparent infections.

The disease is probably worldwide. *L. pomona, L. hardjo,* and other serovars have been isolated from normal horses.

Urine of carrier or infected cattle, swine, and horses is the usual source of infection. The organism is also shed in the urine of the skunk, raccoon, wildcat, deer, and opossum. The reservoir of *L. hardjo* is cattle. Other serovars are shed by various wild (particularly the rat and mouse) and domestic animals.

The organism can survive for days in alkaline water, e.g., ponds and streams. Most infections result from direct or indirect exposure to infectious urine. Infection is via nasal, oral or conjunctival mucous membranes, and abraded skin.

Differential Diagnosis
Other febrile diseases and causes of abortion such as equine viral abortion, equine viral arteritis, and various bacteria should be considered.

Laboratory Diagnosis
Laboratory confirmation is required.

SPECIMENS
1. Preferably paired serum samples or multiple samples from the herd.
2. 20 ml of fresh urine.
3. 20 ml of midstream urine to which 1.5 ml of 10% formalin is added immediately after voiding.
4. For necropsy: Kidney and liver; fetus and cotyledons in case of abortion; fresh and formalized.

PROCEDURES/COMMENTS
1. For microscopic agglutination test: A fourfold increase in titer between paired serum samples is considered significant. If titers are greater than 1:100 in a number of serum samples from a herd, they are considered positive or highly suspicious.
2. Leptospirae can be isolated, cultivated, and identified from fresh urine if it is processed and added to media right after voiding. This is seldom practicable.
3. Leptospira can be demonstrated in the sediment of positive urine by dark-field microscopy. The characteristic morphology of the leptospira is well preserved in formalized urine, but not in fresh urine. Fluorescent antibody (FA) staining can also be carried out on urinary sediment.
4. For isolation, cultivation, and identification: Demonstration in smears by FA and in sections by special stains. Leptospirae will remain viable in fresh kidneys kept at refrigerator temperature for at least 1 week.

    Not all of the procedures referred to above will be carried out in general service diagnostic laboratories.

Treatment

Treatment should be as early as possible. The following antibiotics have been effective: streptomycin, dihydrostreptomycin, and tetracyclines. An effective antibiotic combined with cortisone has been used to treat periodic ophthalmia.

Control

Because clinical leptospirosis is rare in horses, vaccination is not usually practiced.

EQUINE RESPIRATORY DISEASE

A number of viruses have the capacity to infect the equine respiratory tract; however, only a small number are responsi-

ble for significant clinical disease. They are equine rhinopneumonitis virus, equine influenza viruses, and equine arteritis virus.

Among the viruses that have been recovered from the
equine respiratory tract and whose disease significance is
questionable are reoviruses, equine herpesvirus-2, and parainfluenza viruses 1, 2, and 3. Adenoviral infections in im-
munocompetent foals are usually mild, but adenoviruses can
cause serious upper respiratory tract infections in Arabian
foals with combined immunodeficiency.

Streptococcus equi ssp. *equi* (formerly *S. equi*): The most
common bacterium causing upper respiratory disease in
horses.

Rhodococcus equi: Causes a suppurative pneumonia of foals
(see RHODOCOCCAL PNEUMONIA OF FOALS).

*Streptococcus zooepidemicus, Bordetella bronchiseptica,
Klebsiella pneumoniae, Actinobacillus equuli, Pasteurella multocida, P. caballi:* Some of the bacteria that
are sometimes associated with sporadic respiratory infections in horses, both as secondary invaders of viral infections, and also occasionally as primary pathogens.

Equine mycoplasmas: The significance in respiratory disease
is not yet known.

Aspergillus fumigatus: Regularly associated with gutteral
pouch mycosis.

Laboratory Diagnosis

If any of the four major viral diseases referred to above are
suspected, consult the separate discussions for information
on laboratory diagnosis.

If none of these four diseases appear to be involved,
nasal swabs and tracheobronchial aspirates should be submitted for viral and bacterial isolation.

Paired sera should be collected for serologic tests.

Treatment

Isolation of infected animals. Symptomatic and specific antimicrobial treatment if bacteria are involved.

Control

See the specific diseases for details.

EQUINE VIRAL RHINOPNEUMONITIS /
EQUINE ABORTION

Equine viral rhinopneumonitis is a usually mild upper respiratory infection caused by equine herpesvirus-1 (EHV-1). EHV-1 has the capacity to infect mares and produce abortion most frequently at 8–10 months. The respiratory infection is usually more severe in foals than in older horses.

Other syndromes attibuted to EHV-1 are a highly fatal viremia in foals less than 1 week of age and an encephalomyelopathy characterized by weakness, incoordination, and paralysis and death in young and adult horses.

Equine viral rhinopneumonitis occurs worldwide. There are asymptomatic carriers and the mode of infection is by the respiratory tract. The severity of the disease depends on the immune status of the animal.

Recent work suggests that the two syndromes, respiratory infection and abortion, are caused by two different viruses. EHV-1 is the proposed name for the herpesvirus causing abortion, whereas, EHV-4 is proposed for the respiratory strains. These are often referred to as EHV-1 subtype 1 and subtype 2, respectively.

Differential Diagnosis

Because horses usually recover uneventfully from the respiratory disease, the cause is not usually determined. In view of the threat this disease poses to pregnant mares, it is advisable to determine the precise cause of all respiratory diseases affecting horses. The need for definitive diagnosis becomes urgent when abortions occur.

Abortions due to equine viral arteritis (EVA) virus occur at any time during gestation, and the mare is clinically ill at the time of abortion. In addition, autolysis of the fetus is common with EVA virus infection. Other infectious agents do not usually cause multiple abortions. *Salmonella abortusequi* does not appear to be a cause of abortion in mares in North America.

Laboratory Diagnosis

Small, multifocal, yellow-white areas of necrosis throughout the fetal lung and liver are strongly suggestive.

SPECIMENS. Fresh fetus or fetal lung, liver, spleen, adrenal gland, and lymph nodes; nasal swabs in the respiratory form; and serum samples.

PROCEDURES/COMMENTS. Identification of EHV-1 in frozen sections of fetal tissues by fluorescent antibody staining is the most rapid and convenient means of diagnosis.

The viruses can be readily isolated, cultivated, and identified using cell cultures.

The finding of the typical inclusion bodies in fetal tissue is strongly supportive of a diagnosis. Fetal pulmonary edema and hepatic necrosis are characteristic.

Virus neutralization test for antibody in the mare is considered to be of diagnostic value.

Treatment
None.

Control
Isolation of aborting mares. New mares should be isolated from pregnant mares.

Immunity is usually of short duration. Live attenuated, as well as killed virus vaccines, are employed with conflicting reports as to their efficacy.

EQUINE VIRUS ARTERITIS / PINKEYE, EPIDEMIC CELLULITIS
Equine viral arteritis (EVA) is an infrequent, contagious disease caused by a togavirus (arterivirus) and in the acute form characterized by fever, an acute catarrhal inflammation of the upper respiratory tract, and abortion. The clinical signs, mainly attributable to infection of the small arteries, are variable. They include conjunctivitis, myalgia, edema of the limbs, colic, and diarrhea. A hive-like eruption of the skin of the abdomen and thorax may be seen.

The disease has been reported in some European countries and the United States where it appears to be widespread in standardbreds, but of low incidence in thoroughbreds. Most infections are mild or asymptomatic. The more severe disease occurs as outbreaks where horses are congregated, e.g., at shows, sales, racetracks, and breeding farms. Strains of the virus may vary in virulence.

The principal mode of infection is via the respiratory tract. However, infected stallions may shed virus from their semen for long periods and play a significant role in transmitting the disease.

Differential Diagnosis

Laboratory diagnosis is required to distinguish this disease from others with similar clinical signs such as equine viral rhinopneumonitis. The abortions in EVA may be multiple and usually take place between the 5th and 10th month of gestation and within days after exposure. The abortions in equine viral rhinopneumonitis infection usually occur after the 8th month.

Other causes of abortion (not usually multiple) are *Streptococcus zooepidemicus, E. coli, Rhodococcus equi,* and *Actinobacillus equuli. Salmonella abortusequi* does not appear to occur in North America.

Laboratory Diagnosis

SPECIMENS

1. Fresh fetus or portions of fetal lung, liver and spleen; nasal swabs from foals and horses. Portions of the above tissues fixed.
2. Serum.

PROCEDURES/COMMENTS

1. The virus can be grown and identified in cell cultures although not all laboratories are equipped to carry out these procedures. The absence of inclusion bodies in fetal tissues helps rule out equine viral rhinopneumonitis abortion. There are no characteristic gross or microscopic lesions.
2. Virus neutralization is the most commonly used test. Complement fixation and an enzyme-linked immunosorbent assay have also been employed. Infected horses show rapid serum conversion.

Treatment

None.

Control

An attenuated virus vaccine has been licensed for the use in the United States. Some states in the United States prohibit the introduction of horses from states with outbreaks.

General principles of infectious disease control, including segregation, should be applied.

EXUDATIVE EPIDERMITIS / GREASY PIG DISEASE

Exudative epidermitis is a severe, generalized, contagious dermatitis of young pigs (<10 weeks), which is caused by *Staphylococcus hyicus*. It is characterized by sudden onset; short-course (2–3 weeks), extreme dehydration; and often death.

Two principal forms are seen: a severe form with vesicle formation and a mild form that does not involve the whole body surface.

The disease probably occurs wherever there is intensive swine production. Whole litters may be affected. Poor management practices contribute to the disease.

Porcine parvovirus has been isolated from vesicular-like diseases of pigs that resemble exudative epidermitis, and it has been suggested that the latter is a dual viral-bacterial infection.

Differential Diagnosis

The marked exudative character of the disease is very suggestive.

Sarcoptic mange, parakeratosis (usually older pigs), swinepox, candidiasis (rare), and ringworm are among diseases that should be considered.

Laboratory Diagnosis

SPECIMENS. The surface of the skin is cleaned with soap and water or alcohol swabs to remove dirt and general debris. The lesions (vesicles in the severe form) are scraped to obtain material devoid of surface contamination. The scrapings can be submitted to the laboratory on a swab (in transport medium) or in a sterile vial.

Alternatively, a severely affected pig can be submitted.

PROCEDURES. Isolation and identification of *S. hyicus* and possible parvovirus.

Treatment

1. Broad-spectrum antibodies are used both for affected and contact pigs.

2. Antimicrobial susceptibility tests should be conducted on isolates of *S. hyicus.*

Control
1. Isolation of infected litters.
2. Prophylactic use of antimicrobial drugs if indicated.

FELINE CAMPYLOBACTERIOSIS
A considerable percentage of cats, like dogs, may be carriers of *Campylobacter jejuni.* However, there are differences of opinion as to whether or not this organism causes enteritis and diarrhea in cats. There is some evidence that it can cause diarrhea in kittens. The carrier cat sheds *C. jejuni* and thus can be a possible source of human infections. *C. coli* can also be recovered from cats, but its significance is not clear.

The laboratory diagnosis and treatment of feline campylobacteriosis is the same as for the canine disease (see CANINE CAMPYLOBACTERIOSIS).

FELINE IMMUNODEFICIENCY VIRUS INFECTION /
FELINE T LYMPHOTROPIC VIRUS INFECTION
Feline immunodeficiency virus (FIV) infection is caused by a lentivirus and characterized by a prolonged asymptomatic period of latent infection followed eventually by clinical disease. Among the clinical disorders seen are pneumonitis, rheumatoid-like arthritis, lymphoproliferative lesions, encephalopathies, and immune-complex disease leading to anemia, immunodeficiency, and chronic debilitation. Cats of all ages are susceptible.

The prevalence of FIV infection is not yet known but it would seem to be appreciable. Experiments with specific-pathogen-free kittens indicate that experimental infections are virus-positive for 2 years or longer.

Free-roaming male cats are at greatest risk of FIV infection. The principal mode of transmission would seem to be bites. The virus is present in saliva, blood, and cerebrospinal fluid.

In general the disease resembles AIDS, and cats with FIV infection are particularly prone to opportunistic infections. Even with supportive therapy, prognosis after clinical disease appears is about 2 years.

Differential Diagnosis

Given the great variation in clinical manifestations and signs, a reliable diagnosis of FIV infection can only be made by serologic means or virus isolation and identification. The latter is impracticable.

Cats with feline leukemia virus infection or feline sarcoma virus infection may also have FIV infection. All three diseases should be subject to laboratory diagnosis.

Laboratory Diagnosis

SPECIMENS. Serum or clotted blood sample.

PROCEDURE. An indirect fluorescent antibody test is used to detect FIV antibody. Kits for the enzyme-linked immunosorbent assay, used to detect antibody, are available commercially (see 12, Appendix A).

COMMENT. The presence of specific antibody signifies infection. Antigen detection assays have not been useful.

Treatment

Treatment of FIV infection with antiviral drugs is not yet practicable.

Symptomatic therapy with transfusions, fluids, and antimicrobial drugs is employed. In spite of such therapy, cats that develop clinical disease eventually succumb.

Control

As transmission of the disease is not fully understood, it is advisable to isolate infected cats.

No vaccine is available.

FELINE INFECTIOUS ANEMIA /

FELINE HAEMOBARTONELLOSIS

Feline infectious anemia is caused by the bacterium (rickettsia) *Haemobartonella felis* and is characterized by chronic or acute forms that lead to anemia. In the acute disease, clinical signs include temperatures ranging from 103 to 105°F, anorexia, jaundice, depression, weakness, and splenomegaly. In the chronic disease, the clinical signs are less severe with normal or subnormal temperatures.

The disease probably occurs worldwide. The modes of natural transmission are not known, although bloodsucking arthropods are probably involved. The disease occurs in a latent form in many cats and becomes clinical as a result of stresses or concurrent disease.

Differential Diagnosis

The disease should be considered when anemia and the clinical signs listed above are seen. Diseases in which anemia is encountered, such as feline leukemia, should be considered. In the southern United States, the protozoan disease feline cytauxzoonosis should be considered. A diagnosis of feline infectious anemia is dependent upon the demonstration of *H. felis* in blood smears.

Laboratory Diagnosis

SPECIMENS. A series of unclotted blood samples or blood smears taken over a period of several days.

PROCEDURES/COMMENTS. Demonstration of *H. felis* in blood smears stained by methods used for rickettsiae.
A number of smears are required because *H. felis* only appears in the blood periodically. A diagnosis is based upon the demonstration of the parasite, anemia, and the characteristic blood picture of a regenerative anemia.

Treatment

1. Blood transfusions depending upon the degree of anemia.
2. Tetracyclines for 2–3 weeks.
3. Various arsenical compounds are claimed to be effective.

Control

Control of external parasites. Blood-donor cats should be carefully screened to prevent the spread of feline infectious anemia.

FELINE INFECTIOUS PERITONITIS /
GRANULOMATOUS DISEASE COMPLEX

Feline infectious peritonitis (FIP) and pleuritis is a progressive, debilitating, febrile disease caused by a coronavirus and is manifested in two forms: The so-called "wet" form is characterized by a chronic fibrinous peritonitis, accumulation of peritoneal fluid, and gradual abdominal enlargement. The "dry," granulomatous, or nonexudative form usually involves the nervous system, eye, and abdominal and thoracic viscera. Depending on the form, clinical signs may include abdominal enlargement, depression, inappetence, fever, emaciation, anemia, and neurologic and ocular signs. In utero infections result in stillbirths and infected kittens.

Distribution is probably worldwide. The disease is contagious although the mode of transmission has not been established. The infection occurs in cats and larger felidae of all ages but is most frequent in animals 6 months to 5 years of age.

Feline enteric coronaviruses isolated from kittens with diarrhea and mild enteritis do not cause FIP.

Differential Diagnosis

The disease is suspected when there is a fever that doesn't respond to antibiotics, along with the presence of fluid exudates in the thoracic and peritoneal cavities. Cardiac failure and lymphosarcoma, i.e., diseases resulting in thoracic and abdominal cavity effusions, should be considered. Feline leukemia virus, feline immunodeficiency virus, and feline panleukopenia virus infections must also be considered. Laboratory confirmation is required.

Laboratory Diagnosis
SPECIMENS
1. Serum or a clotted blood sample.
2. Portions of lung, liver, kidney, and mesenteric lymph nodes with pleura and peritoneum.
3. Unclotted blood.

PROCEDURES/COMMENTS
1. The indirect immunofluorescence assay (IFA) test is conducted. A positive FIP-IFA test only means the animal has been exposed to the virus. However, there is some evidence that many serologically positive cats shed virus, probably from the respiratory and/or the intestinal tract. There would appear to be little difference in the susceptibility of a cat whether it has a titer of 1:5 or 1:600.

A positive FIP-IFA test (titers of 1:50 up to 1:6000), along with clinical signs of FIP, would strongly support a diagnosis of FIP.

The enzyme-linked immunosorbent assay (ELISA) for antibody may prove to be a simpler and more sensitive test.

Total protein as determined by electrophoresis is markedly elevated.

2. In the dead animal, the demonstration of FIP virus in typical lesions by specific fluorescent antibody staining is considered definitive. Enteric coronavirus cross-reacts with FIP virus.

3. In the live animal, changes in the blood such as moderate to severe anemia, neutrophilia, and a leukopenia are suggestive of FIP.

Commercial kits, ELISA, and IFA are available to test for antibodies to FIP (see 9,15, Appendix A).

Treatment
1. Generally ineffective.
2. Supportive care.

Control
1. If feasible, isolate serologically positive cats.
2. Efficacy is claimed for an intranasal, modified live virus vaccine.

FELINE LEPROSY
Feline leprosy is presumed to be an infectious disease caused by an as yet uncultivated mycobacterium and characterized by the formation of single and multiple granulomas or nodules (1–3 cm diameter) of the skin that develop over several months. They are painless, move freely, and some may be ulcerous and discharge a slight, serosanguineous exudate. The health of the cat is not usually affected and only rarely does the infection become generalized.

The causal mycobacterium has not yet been cultivated in artificial media. There is some evidence that it is identical to *Mycobacterium lepraemurium,* the cause of rat leprosy.

Occurrence is probably worldwide. The source of infection is infected cats and possibly rats through bites.

Differential Diagnosis

Nodules due to *M. fortuitum* and other opportunistic mycobacteria occur in the cat. Most cutaneous opportunistic mycobacterial infections are less nodular and tend to ulcerate.

Laboratory Diagnosis

SPECIMENS. Nodules are removed aseptically and submitted fresh and fixed.

PROCEDURES. Culture should be attempted although the causal agent of feline leprosy has not been grown on artificial media.

Smears and sections are stained by Gram and acid-fast procedures and examined for the characteristic organisms and microscopic pathologic changes.

COMMENTS. The presence of noncultivable, long, slender, acid-fast rods in the typical lesions and the absence of other bacteria or fungi strongly indicate a diagnosis of feline leprosy.

Treatment

Surgical removal of the nodules, which usually do not recur.

Streptomycin and isoniazid are toxic for the cat. Rifampin and clofazimine have been useful in some cases.

The human antileprosy drug dapsone has given variable results in the feline disease.

FELINE LEUKEMIA/SARCOMA COMPLEX

The feline leukemia/sarcoma complex is caused by a retrovirus (feline leukemia virus; FeLV) and has a variety of clinical and pathologic manifestations. Most clinical feline leukemia is seen in one of the following lymphosarcoma forms: alimentary, multicentric, thymic, and leukemic. There are also less-frequent myeloproliferative forms that are characterized by anemia, and several nonneoplastic diseases, all of which have been associated with FeLV. Infertility, greater susceptibility to infection due to thymic atrophy, and glomerulonephritis, probably due to antigen-antibody complexes affecting glomerular basement membrane, are examples of nonneoplastic diseases associated with FeLV.

A replication-defective mutant of FeLV, the feline sarcoma virus, is the cause of multicentric fibrosarcomas in young cats. These fibrosarcomas are rapid growing with multiple nodules involving the skin and subcutis. They are invasive and may metastasize to lungs and other tissues. Fibrosarcoma cells, like lymphoma cells of FeLV infection, express feline oncornavirus cell membrane–associated antigen (FOCMA).

The FeLV may be present in respiratory and oral secretions and is spread horizontally (e.g., licking) and vertically.

It is a commonly occurring worldwide disease with as many as 60% of urban cats infected, although only a small percentage will remain viremic (2–5%). Only a small number (about 2%) of infected cats develop the clinical disease.

Differential Diagnosis

The clinical signs vary with the different forms. General signs of lymphosarcoma (the most common) are lethargy, anorexia, and weight loss; other clinical findings are related to the anatomic location of the tumor.

Alimentary form: The cat may display vomiting and diarrhea.

Multicentric form: Generalized adenopathy, renal lymphosarcoma, splenomegaly, and hepatomegaly may be found.

Thymic form: Coughing, dysphagia, and dyspnea are common signs, and cyanosis may be present in advanced cases.

Leukemic form: The bone marrow is primarily involved and no tumor is evident. Pallor of the mucous membranes is frequent and lymphadenopathy, splenomegaly, and hepatomegaly may be present.

Myeloproliferative diseases: Are characterized by anemia.

Other neoplastic diseases and feline infectious peritonitis should be considered in the differential diagnosis.

Laboratory Diagnosis

When feline leukemia is suspected, a number of diagnostic procedures can be used, including histopathologic examination of biopsies, bone marrow examinations, and cytology of thoracic and abdominal fluids. Indirect immunofluorescent assay (IFA)–staining of blood smears and the enzyme-linked immunosorbent assay (ELISA) on serum are also applicable and the ones most commonly used.

The FeLV group specific antigen can be found in large amounts in the cytoplasm of infected leukocytes and in platelets. The soluble form is found in the plasma and serum of infected cats.

SPECIMENS
1. At least three blood smears.
2. Serum.

PROCEDURES/COMMENTS
1. For IFA (FeLeuk test) procedures on blood smears: This is a test for the p27 antigen in neutrophils and platelets. Positive immunofluorescence indicates infection; however, few positive cats develop clinical disease.
2. For ELISA (Leukassay test) on serum: This is also a test for the p27 antigen. Positive test indicates infection, although few positive cats develop clinical disease; approximately 80% of these die in 3 years.

   The ELISA test appears to be more sensitive than the IFA test. It has been recommended that, when on two occasions (12 weeks apart), cats are positive with the ELISA test but negative with IFA, they should be considered free of FeLV.

   For VNA (test for virus-neutralizing antibodies): Some commercial and university laboratories perform this test. Most cats with protective levels of VNA (≥ 10 by the focus inhibition assay) do not go on to develop FeLV-associated diseases.

   For FOCMA: This is an immunofluorescent procedure and titers $\geq$ 1:32 are thought to indicate protection.

   A number of commercial kits, employing ELISA or enzyme-immune assay, to detect antigen are available (see 4,7,9,12,16,20, Appendix A). A commercial kit, employing indirect immunofluorescence, to detect antibody is also available (see 15, Appendix A).

Treatment
1. Supportive therapy.
2. Chemotherapy may prolong life.
3. Surgical removal of the fibrosarcomas may be feasible.
4. Irradiation may also be helpful.

Control

The disease can be eradicated by serologic testing and the removal of positive cats, disinfection of potentially contaminated areas, and quarantine and testing of new additions. There should be an interval of at least 1 month before introducing negative cats to a formerly infected environment.

Some owners will elect to keep FeLV-positive cats that are asymptomatic. Such cats are a threat to negative cats and thus must be kept indoors, and they may later develop feline leukemia or feline leukemia–associated disease.

A killed virus vaccine derived from virus cultivated in a lymphoid cell line is available to elicit and increase protection against feline leukemia. Evaluation with ELISA and IFA tests are recommended prior to vaccination.

FELINE PANLEUKOPENIA / FELINE DISTEMPER, FELINE INFECTIOUS ENTERITIS

Feline panleukopenia is a highly contagious disease of cats caused by a parvovirus and characterized by sudden onset, fever, anorexia, depression, diarrhea, dehydration, marked leukopenia, and high mortality. Infection of kittens in utero or within a few days of birth leads to feline cerebellar ataxia.

This disease is worldwide in distribution and endemic in almost all cat populations. The virus causes disease in all members of the family Felidae and also infects raccoons, coatimundi, the ring-tailed cat, and mink. The virus is transmitted by contact with infected animals and fomites. Feline parvovirus is closely related to the canine parvovirus and the mink enteritis virus.

Differential Diagnosis

Feline infectious peritonitis, feline enteric coronavirus infection, feline leukemia, feline herpesvirus infection, feline calicivirus infection, and feline immunodeficiency virus infection should be considered.

Laboratory Diagnosis

SPECIMENS

1. Portions of small intestine, lung, kidney, lymph node, and spleen for histopathology. Also fetuses in abortions, and if cerebellar hypoplasia is suspected.

2. Unclotted blood for leukocyte count.
3. Portions of small intestine and spleen for fluorescent antibody (FA) staining.
4. Feces for electron microscopy.

PROCEDURES/COMMENTS
1. Type B intranuclear inclusions in intestinal epithelial cells are significant. The microscopic changes in the small bowel, which include crypt necrosis, villus loss, and collapse of the lamina propria, are diagnostic. The fetal brain is examined for evidence of cerebellar hypoplasia.
2. Leukopenia is suggestive.
3. Specific staining of small intestine and spleen with FA is reliable.
4. The presence of virus in feces can be determined by electron microscopy.
   Because the virus produces little or no cytopathic changes, virus isolation is not routinely carried out.

Treatment
1. Supportive to cope with dehydration and provide nutrients.
2. Broad-spectrum antibiotics may be used to cope with secondary bacterial infections.
3. Blood transfusions.

Control
1. Modified live virus vaccine is usually given at 9 and 14 weeks of age. Maternal antibodies may last as long as 3 months. Live vaccines are contraindicated in pregnant queens and in kittens under 4 weeks of age. Live vaccines offer faster protection, usually in 1–2 days.
2. Three injections of killed vaccines are required for initial immunization. Killed vaccines can be used in pregnant and young animals.
3. Exposed kittens can be given antiserum that protects for 2–4 weeks. Cats that recover from the infection are immune for life.
4. The virus is very resistant to environmental conditions and some common disinfectants. Sodium hypochlorite solution is very effective.

FELINE RESPIRATORY DISEASES / FELINE VIRUS RHINOTRACHEITIS, FELINE CALICIVIRUS INFECTION, FELINE PNEUMONITIS, FELINE MYCOPLASMA RESPIRATORY INFECTION

The principal infectious diseases of the feline respiratory system are discussed below. For practical reasons their differential diagnosis, laboratory diagnosis, treatment, and control are discussed together.

FELINE VIRUS RHINOTRACHEITIS (FVR)

Feline virus rhinotracheitis is a contagious disease caused by a herpesvirus and characterized by sudden onset, sneezing, fever, copious nasal discharge, and lacrimation. The disease is most severe in kittens. Abortion may be seen during the sixth week of gestation in pregnant queens. There may be ulcers on the tongue, necrosis of turbinates, ulcerative keratitis, and a severe panophthalmitis.

It is a frequently occurring, worldwide disease of cats. About one-half of respiratory disease in cats is caused by this virus, and many cats become latent carriers. In the latter, various stresses may trigger the excretion of the virus.

FELINE CALICIVIRUS INFECTION (FCI)

This is a highly contagious infection caused by a picornavirus and characterized by fever, rhinitis, conjunctivitis, palatine and/or glossal ulcerations, and nasal discharge. When bronchopneumonia develops, the mortality rate may exceed 30%. Abortion may occur in the queens.

It is worldwide in distribution and widespread in the cat population. The virus is transmitted by direct contact and ingestion. Infected cats become carriers and the virus is shed continuously from the pharynx and tonsils for months and sometimes for years.

FELINE PNEUMONITIS

This is a contagious disease caused by the bacterium *Chlamydia psittaci*, and characterized by upper respiratory infection with conjunctivitis and an ocular discharge that may become purulent.

It is worldwide in distribution and occurs frequently. Although it is diagnosed on occasion clinically, it appears to be infrequently confirmed in the laboratory.

FELINE MYCOPLASMA RESPIRATORY INFECTION
Mycoplasma felis causes an infrequent upper respiratory infection characterized by edema of the conjunctiva (chemosis) and rhinitis. *M. gateae* and *M. feliminutum* are recovered occasionally from the respiratory tract, but they are not considered important pathogens. The aforementioned species are widespread in the cat population and probably worldwide in distribution.

Differential Diagnosis
The four respiratory diseases referred to above share a number of clinical signs, thus making differential diagnosis difficult. Laboratory diagnosis is recommended for their differentiation. The least severe of the group is *M. felis* infection.

Laboratory Diagnosis
SPECIMENS
1. For all of the diseases: Nasal and ocular swabs in viral and bacterial transport media.
   In the dead animal: Portions of conjunctiva, nasal mucosa, trachea, and lungs.
2. Paired serum samples for FCI and FVR.
3. For feline pneumonitis: Smears from conjunctival scrapings for *Chlamydia psittaci.*

PROCEDURES/COMMENTS
1. Isolation and identification of the viruses that cause feline viral rhinotracheitis and feline calicivirus infection. These viruses grow well in cell cultures and produce characteristic cytopathic changes.

    The virus of FVR can be identified by the fluorescent antibody staining of smears from nasal and conjunctival scrapings and from frozen sections of lung.

    Mycoplasmas can be grown in special media but identification is time consuming and not carried out by most diagnostic laboratories.
2. Paired serum samples: Virus neutralization tests for FCI and FVR.
3. It is not usually feasible to isolate the agent of feline pneumonitis, but *C. psittaci* can be demonstrated in stained conjunctival smears.

Treatment

FVR and FCI: Symptomatic and supportive; local and systemic broad spectrum antibiotics for secondary bacterial infections.

Feline pneumonitis: Broad-spectrum antibiotics locally (nose and eyes) and systemically.

Feline mycoplasma respiratory infection: If the *M. felis* infection is severe, broad-spectrum antibiotics may be given locally and/or systemically.

Control

FVR and FCI: Live, attenuated virus vaccines; individual or combined. In FVR, maternal antibodies last from 2 to 11 weeks. Cats going to a show or being shipped should be vaccinated for FVR 2 weeks before the event. Pregnant queens should be vaccinated with only killed feline calicivirus vaccine. Maternal antibodies to FCI persist for up to 14 weeks.

Feline pneumonitis: Avianized inactivated *C. psittaci* vaccine is available. Isolation of sick cats.

FLAVOBACTERIUM

Members of this genus are found in soil and water. They are infrequent, opportunistic pathogens in humans, and it would seem reasonable to expect opportunistic infections in animals. *F. meningosepticum* causes meningitis, pneumonia, and septicemia, particularly in immunocompromised adult humans. Organisms are highly resistant to a variety of antibiotics.

FOOT ABSCESS OF SHEEP

This is a noncontagious disease, primarily of rams and ewes, that occurs when pastures are continually muddy and wet. The mode of infection is via wounds and cracks between the claws or around the coronet. The bacteria involved are primarily *Fusobacterium necrophorum* and *Actinomyces pyogenes*.

The disease is probably worldwide with many flocks involved. The incidence in herds may be as high as 25%. The hind feet are most commonly involved. Lambs are not usually affected.

There is pain, heat, and swelling in the region of the

wound with interdigital dermatitis and frequent spread of the suppurative process to the interphalangeal joint resulting in abscessation. Lameness is the cardinal clinical sign.

Differential Diagnosis

Contagious foot rot, contagious ecthyma, "scald" (epidermitis of the foot due to various irritants), postdipping lameness (infection of joints by various bacteria during dipping) should be considered.

Laboratory Diagnosis

The diagnosis is almost always made clinically.

SPECIMENS/PROCEDURES. Fresh pus is submitted for smears and cultures.

A highly presumptive diagnosis can be made on the basis of the clinical signs, abscessation, and the finding of organisms typical of *F. necrophorum* and other pyogenic organisms in smears. *F. necrophorum* is a strict anaerobe, and special efforts have to be made to isolate and identify it.

Treatment

Surgical drainage; antiseptic packs; amputation of the digit is sometimes indicated; antibiotics and sulfonamides.

Control

Avoidance, as much as possible, of conditions that lead to foot abscess such as contaminated dipping tanks and wet, muddy pastures. Control of interdigital dermatitis by the use of disinfectant footbaths. Bacterins containing *F. necrophorum* have been employed.

FOOT ROT OF CATTLE / INTERDIGITAL NECROBACILLOSIS

Foot rot of cattle is an acute or chronic, noncontagious disease primarily of adult cattle. It occurs most frequently in animals on wet, muddy pastures or pens. The cause is a synergistic infection of *Fusobacterium necrophorum* and *Bacteroides melaninogenicus.* Other pyogenic organisms such as *Actinomyces pyogenes, Bacteroides nodosus,* streptococci, and staphylococci may also be involved.

The mode of infection is usually via cracks and wounds of the skin between the claws or around the coronet. The suppurative, necrotic process may extend to involve the adjacent tissues and joints resulting in abscessation. Among the clinical signs are evidence of pain, swelling, fever, and marked lameness.

Differential Diagnosis

Ergotism, laminitis, fescue poisoning, bruising, and overgrown sole should be considered.

The season, the previous occurrence of the disease, and the lameness usually involving a number of animals, facilitate a reliable clinical diagnosis.

Laboratory Diagnosis

This is usually not sought (see FOOT ABSCESS OF SHEEP).

Treatment

Penicillin, broad-spectrum antibiotics, sulfonamides may be effective in some cases.

Surgical drainage; amputation of the digit may be necessary; antiseptic or astringent packs with bandaging; protective shoes; footbaths (10% zinc sulfate, formalin, and copper sulfate).

Control

Avoidance of injuries by providing pens and pastures that are level, well drained, and devoid of mud holes and stagnant water. Generous bedding should be provided for pens, and foot injuries should be attended to early.

FRANCISELLA

Species of this genus are small, gram-negative rods or coccobacilli. They are facultative intracellular parasites and the principal species are as follows:

Francisella tularensis: The principal cause of tularemia (q.v.).

F. novicida: Resembles *F. tularensis* genetically and was recovered from two humans with infections resembling tularemia. It has been proposed that this species be eliminated and considered a biogroup of *F. tularensis.*

F. philomiragia: A newly recognized species, less pathogenic than *F. tularensis,* does not require cystine for growth, and has been isolated mainly from immunocompromised humans and near-drowning victims. Isolations have also been made from water, muskrats, and other animals.

GARDNERELLA

Organisms of this genus are small, gram-negative coccobacilli or short rods. The only species recognized is *Gardnerella vaginalis,* which is considered a normal inhabitant of the genitourinary tract. It is occasionally implicated in genital (bacterial vaginosis) and urinary infections in humans.

Gardnerella vaginalis and *G. vaginalis*-like organisms have been recovered from the genital tract of mares by means of uterine swabs. Although some of the mares involved had reproductive inefficiencies, the pathogenic significance of these organisms for the horse is not yet known. They may also be normal inhabitants of the equine genitourinary tract.

GEOTRICHOSIS

Geotrichosis is an uncommon disease of cattle, dogs, fowl, and other species caused by the fungus *Geotrichum candidum* and characterized by small, granulomatous lesions that most often involve bronchi, lungs, kidney, wall of the digestive tract, and lymph nodes. Although the infection may be disseminated, usually only one or several organs or tissues are involved.

The disease is usually mild and the lesions, ordinarily unrelated to death, are found at necropsy or slaughter.

Geotrichum candidum, which occurs in nature, is sometimes implicated in otitis externa in the dog and mastitis in the cow.

Laboratory Diagnosis

SPECIMENS. Except for canine otitis and bovine mastitis, geotrichosis is rarely diagnosed in the living animal. Tissue sections and scrapings from lesions are the specimens examined in the necropsied animal.

PROCEDURES

Direct examination: Characteristic morphologic elements of the fungi can usually be seen in wet mounts of material from lesions.

Culture: Definitive diagnosis is dependent upon the isolation and identification of *G. candidum.*

Histopathology: Septate hyphae, yeast-like cells, and arthroconidia are seen in tissue sections.

Treatment

Because this infection is rarely diagnosed antemortem, treatment is not usually involved.

GLASSER'S DISEASE

Glasser's disease, which usually affects young pigs, is caused by *Haemophilus parasuis* and characterized by fever, depression, and the development of serofibrinous pericarditis, pleuritis and peritonitis, septic arthritis, and meningitis.

This infrequent disease probably occurs wherever pigs are raised in appreciable numbers. Whole litters are sometimes affected. Various stresses, such as weaning and shipping, may precipitate outbreaks. *H. parasuis* is carried as a commensal in the upper respiratory tract of some pigs and is often a secondary invader in swine influenza.

Differential Diagnosis

Several infectious agents may result in a polyserositis, but multiple cases are mainly caused by *Mycoplasma hyorhinis* or *H. parasuis*. Neurologic signs are seen in Glasser's disease but not usually in mycoplasmal polyserositis.

Other febrile diseases such as salmonellosis, hog cholera, African swine fever, *Streptococcus suis* infection, and erysipelas should be considered. Laboratory confirmation is required for definitive diagnosis.

Laboratory Diagnosis

SPECIMENS. Preferably a live, sick pig. Swabs for culture are taken from the various serous membranes, joints, and meninges.

PROCEDURES/COMMENTS. Because Glasser's disease and mycoplasmal polyserositis are so similar, attempts should be made to isolate mycoplasma as well as *H. parasuis*. Special media (or a staphylococcal streak) that provide the V factor must be used for the isolation of *H. parasuis*.

The lesions of Glasser's disease and *M. hyorhinis* polyserositis are grossly indistinguishable.

Treatment

Penicillin and streptomycin, and sulfonamides. Mycoplasmal polyserositis requires different treatment (see MYCO-PLASMA INFECTIONS OF SWINE).

Control

1. Isolation of infected animals.
2. Reduction of stresses; good husbandry.

GROUP EF4

These short, gram-negative rods are commensals in the mouth and nasopharynx of dogs and cats. They are commonly recovered from human wounds caused by dog or cat bites and do not appear to be pathogenic for animals.

GROUPS M5 AND M6

These bacteria designated M5 and M6 by the Centers for Disease Control resemble *Moraxella* spp. They are small, gram-negative coccobacilli that occur as commensals in the oropharynx of dogs. They have been isolated on a number of occasions from dog-bite wounds in humans but do not appear to be pathogenic for dogs.

GUTTURAL POUCH MYCOSIS

Guttural pouch mycosis is a disease of horses caused, after unknown primary incitants, by fungi of the *Aspergillus* genus (most commonly *Aspergillus nidulans*). It involves fungous invasion of the roof of the medial compartment of the guttural pouch.

The two most important clinical signs, in addition to the nasal discharge, are epistaxis due to fungal erosion of the wall of the internal carotid artery, and dysphagia due to neuritis of the laryngeal and pharyngeal nerves. Although most of the tissue damage is due to the fungi, the condition or circumstances that predispose to the fungal invasion are not known.

Differential Diagnosis

Cryptococcosis, tumors, and other infections of the upper respiratory tract should be considered.

Diagnosis is confirmed by observing with an endoscope the diphtheritic membrane involving the guttural pouch.

Laboratory Diagnosis
SPECIMENS
1. Parts of the lesion obtained with the biopsy attachment of the fiberoptic endoscope.
2. Swabs from discharging areas.

PROCEDURES/COMMENTS
1. For direct examination: Septate hyphae in wet mounts or stained sections suggest aspergillus infection.
2. For culture: Clinical material, swabs, and tissue are cultured for bacteria and fungi.

   Fungi other than *Aspergillus* may be isolated, but the latter are predominant in guttural pouch mycosis.

Treatment
Treatment is rather involved and a number of approaches are used.

Local: Infusions such as 10% povidoneiodine; other drugs including antifungal compounds have been used but not evaluated.

Systemic and oral: Among the drugs that have been used but not carefully evaluated are thiabendazole (oral), amphotericin-B (systemic), iodides (orally and intravenously). Drugs that may be effective are natamycin, clotrimazole, and 5-fluorocytosine.

Surgery.

HAEMOBARTONELLA
These rickettsial agents of the family Anaplasmataceae are parasites that reside in or on mammalian erythrocytes. They are spherical, coccoid, rod-like or ring-shaped bacteria. There are three principal species:

Haemobartonella felis: See FELINE INFECTIOUS ANEMIA.

H. canis and *H. bovis:* Cause only mild or inapparent diseases in their respective hosts.

HAEMOPHILUS SEPTICEMIA OF SHEEP
This disease, which has been reported from California, affects sheep of 6–7 months of age and is caused by *Haemophilus agni*. It is an acute, septicemic disease with high temperature, depression, and death, sometimes within 12 hours.

Lesions are seen only in the protracted cases. The mortality rate is nearly 100%.

Differential Diagnosis
Enterotoxemia and acute pasteurellosis should be considered.

Laboratory Diagnosis
SPECIMENS
1. A sick or recently dead lamb.
2. Fresh and fixed portions of brain (if CNS signs), liver, lung, spleen, and joint fluid if indicated.

PROCEDURES. Isolation and identification of *H. agni* from various organs and tissues.

COMMENTS. *Haemophilus agni* may be identical to *H. somnus* and to an organism called *Histophilus ovis. H. agni* is a fastidious organism requiring carbon dioxide for initial isolation.

Focal hepatic necrosis is characteristic of the disease.

Treatment
Penicillin and streptomycin; broad-spectrum antibiotics.

Control
No specific measures have been developed.

HAEMOPHILUS SOMNUS INFECTION OF CATTLE /
INFECTIOUS THROMBOEMBOLIC MENINGOENCEPHALITIS

Haemophilus somnus infection begins as a septicemia or bacteremia and is seen in four principal forms: (1) involvement of the central nervous system (CNS) (thromboembolic meningoencephalitis, TEM); (2) infection of the respiratory system with pneumonia, and heart muscle with myocarditis; (3) infection of joints; and (4) reproductive failure. The disease varies from acute TEM to subacute and chronic manifestations. More than one form may be seen in the same herd and even in the same animal. The neural form of the disease is almost always fatal.

It is probably worldwide but occurs most commonly where cattle are raised intensively, as in feedlots. Various stresses, such as transport, contribute to outbreaks. Other infections seen in cattle due to *H. somnus* are mastitis, conjunctivitis, otitis, and septicemia.

Differential Diagnosis

Diseases listed under BOVINE RESPIRATORY DISEASE (both viral and bacterial) should be considered; also listeriosis, polioencephalomalacia, and various bacterial encephalitides.

Such CNS signs as ataxia, blindness, and paralysis with coma followed by death, all in a course of several days, suggest TEM. Isolation and identification of the causal agent is necessary for a definitive diagnosis.

Laboratory Diagnosis

SPECIMENS. Fresh brain halved longitudinally; half for culture and the other half fixed for histopathology. Usually it is more convenient to submit the head of a sick or recently dead animal. Portions of lung and joint fluid if the respiratory or joint form is suspected. Semen samples and preputial washings of bulls are suitable for isolation if *H. somnus* is suspected.

Paired serum samples are submitted for serologic procedures.

PROCEDURES/COMMENTS. Isolation and identification of *H. somnus*. The organism is fastidious and requires 6–8% CO_2 for primary isolation. Blood agar is adequate for initial isolation; however, chocolate agar permits better growth of *H. somnus*.

The histopathologic changes in the brain in TEM are characteristic.

A strongly presumptive diagnosis of TEM can be made on the basis of finding the characteristic lesions in the brain, viz., multiple areas (0.5–1.5 cm in diameter) of focal necrosis; they are best seen when the brain is incised.

Agglutination, complement fixation, enzyme-linked immunosorbent assay, and agar gel immunodiffusion tests have been described for detection of antibody to *H. somnus*. They are mainly used for screening herds and are not conducted by all diagnostic laboratories.

Treatment

Penicillin, tetracyclines, cephalosporin, and sulfa drugs.

Control

Cattle showing clinical signs should be isolated.

Bacterins are available. The results of above-mentioned serologic tests for antibodies to *H. somnus* are used by some practitioners as a guide to whether or not the use of a bacterin is indicated and also to monitor increased exposure to the organism.

Avoid stresses and crowding as much as possible.

HISTOPLASMOSIS

Histoplasmosis is a noncontagious disease of domestic animals, humans, and other animals caused by the dimorphic fungus *Histoplasma capsulatum* and characterized by subclinical, chronic, and severe systemic infections.

It is a soil-borne infection of the reticuloendothelial system and is characterized by the formation of tubercle-like granulomas of the lymph nodes, internal organs, and intestinal tract. It is usually seen in either a predominantly pulmonary or intestinal form.

Worldwide in distribution, it is more frequent in certain geographic regions, e.g., in the United States, primarily in the northeast, central, and south-central states.

The organisms grow abundantly in shed bird feces, particularly that of starlings. It is not present in the intestine of live birds.

Differential Diagnosis

Blastomycosis, nocardiosis (mainly in the dog), canine actinomycosis, cryptococcosis, tuberculosis, and other diseases involving the lung and alimentary tract caused by various agents should be considered.

The disease is difficult to diagnose clinically. Radiographs of the thorax are helpful in the pulmonary form. The disease is most frequently diagnosed after necropsy by the histopathologic examination of tissue sections; however, laboratory tests make possible an antemortem diagnosis.

Laboratory Diagnosis
SPECIMENS

1. Urine sediment, excised lymph nodes, lymph node or liver biopsies, scrapings from ulcer base (skin or mucous membrane), bone marrow aspirate, or peripheral blood (buffy coat).

2. For pathology: Fresh and fixed portions of lung, liver, spleen, intestinal wall, skin, or any other tissue containing granulomas.
3. Paired serum samples, or several serial samples taken during the course of the disease.

PROCEDURES
1. Smears stained by the Giemsa, Wright, and fungal stains are suitable for demonstration of intraphagocytic yeast cells.
2. Culture and histopathologic examination.
3. For serology: Not all veterinary laboratories carry out serologic tests for histoplasmosis. The following tests are used in humans and can also be used in animals, although they have not been thoroughly evaluated in the latter:
   Complement fixation (CF): Increase in titer in serial or paired serum samples along with a positive immunodiffusion test indicates active infection.
   Immunodiffusion: Adjunct to CF test.
   Latex agglutination: Comparable in usefulness to the CF test.

   The tests just mentioned only become positive when the disease is well established, viz., at 2–4 weeks.

COMMENTS. Demonstration of the typical yeast cells in stained smears and sections is presumptive evidence of histoplasmosis.

   Isolation and identification of *H. capsulatum* is required for definitive diagnosis.

   The histoplasmin skin test is of little value in the diagnosis of the disease in animals.

Treatment

Amphotericin B is the drug of choice. Long-term use of the imidazoles (miconazole and ketoconazole) have shown promise but are still being evaluated. The prognosis in the disseminated disease is poor.

   Infected animals should be isolated although transmission to other animals and humans is not thought to occur.

Control

Prevention of exposure to *H. capsulatum* in the environment is ordinarily impracticable.

HYALOHYPHOMYCOSIS

This is an uncommon fungal disease of animals and humans caused by a large number of opportunistic fungi. These fungi have colorless walls (hyaline) and belong to a variety of genera including *Acremonium, Beauvaria, Fusarium, Penicillium, Paecilomyces, Scopulariopsis,* and others.

A wide variety of opportunistic infections have been reported in humans and to a lesser extent in animals. Among the many predisposing causes of these infections are trauma and neoplastic diseases. Infections may be localized or systemic.

The laboratory diagnosis involves the isolation and identification of the fungus. The latter may have to be done in a reference laboratory.

INCLUSION BODY RHINITIS OF SWINE /
CYTOMEGALOVIRUS INFECTION OF SWINE

Inclusion body rhinitis of swine (IBRS) is an acute infection primarily of young pigs and pregnant sows caused by a herpesvirus and characterized by the sudden onset of sneezing, dyspnea, hemotaxis, purulent nasal discharge, and the formation of inclusion bodies in the epithelial cells of the nasal mucosa. In severe cases, petechial hemorrhages in the kidney and myocardium are common. Severe anemia may occur in recovered pigs.

The virus is perpetuated in clinically inapparent infections. Infection is via the respiratory tract and congenitally. The incubation period is 7–10 days. Somewhat analogous cytomegalovirus infections are seen in other animal species.

The distribution is probably worldwide. It is a minor disease that occurs most commonly in pigs up to 12 weeks of age. Pigs usually recover completely.

Differential Diagnosis

The disease is mainly important because it can be confused with infectious atrophic rhinitis. The latter disease begins in nursing pigs, persists clinically, and results in turbinate atrophy. IBRS, in contrast, may affect both young and older pigs and complete recovery in several weeks is the rule.

Upper respiratory infections, infectious atrophic rhinitis, and swine influenza have some of the same clinical signs.

Laboratory Diagnosis
SPECIMENS
1. Live, sick pigs or their heads.
2. Exfoliated cells can be collected on nasal swabs for smears.
3. Nasal swabs and fresh nasal mucosa.

PROCEDURES
1. For histopathology and fluorescent antibody test: The disease is usually diagnosed by the demonstration of large intranuclear inclusions in sections or scrapings of the nasal mucosa or in exfoliated cells from the nasal mucosa.
2. For electron microscopy (EM): The virus can be seen by EM in negatively stained distilled water lysates of nasal mucosa.
3. For virus isolation: The virus can be cultivated and identified in primary porcine lung cultures.

Treatment
None.

Control
1. There is no vaccine.
2. Good husbandry.

INFECTIOUS BOVINE ABORTION
The microbial agents listed below have been documented as causes of abortion in cows and heifers. The diseases with which they are associated are discussed separately. See these discussions for details on laboratory diagnosis.

Bacteria: *Brucella abortus, Campylobacter fetus* ssp. *venerealis, C. fetus* ssp. *fetus, C. jejuni, Leptospira interrogans, Listeria monocytogenes, Actinomyces* (*Corynebacterium*) *pyogenes, Chlamydia psittaci, Ureaplasma diversum,* and others.

Fungi: *Mucor, Absidia, Rhizopus, Mortierella,* and *Aspergillus.*

Viruses: Infectious bovine rhinotracheitis virus and bovine virus diarrhea virus.

Protozoa: *Tritrichomonas foetus* and *Toxoplasma gondii.*

Laboratory Diagnosis

SPECIMENS/COMMENTS. The diagnostic procedures carried out are ordinarily based on the history, suspected disease, and results of the direct examinations of fetal and placental materials. These specimens are optimum for a comprehensive laboratory examination:

1. 10 ml of maternal blood for serologic tests. Preferably taken at the time of abortion and 2 weeks later. Collect from in-contact animals and those that have aborted.
2. 20 ml of maternal urine to which 1.5 ml of 10% formalin is added for leptospira.
3. Placenta with cotyledons; fresh for microbiology, and formalized for histopathology.
4. Uterine discharge on swabs if placenta is not available; colostrum for isolation of *B. abortus;* special transport medium for *Campylobacter.*
5. Fresh whole fetus (preferable) or fetal stomach contents.
6. Fetal lung and liver; fresh and fixed.

Commercial test kits are available to detect antibodies to *B. abortus* in cattle (see 12, Appendix A).

INFECTIOUS BOVINE KERATOCONJUNCTIVITIS /
PINKEYE, INFECTIOUS OPHTHALMIA, INFECTIOUS KERATITIS

Infectious bovine keratoconjunctivitis (IBK) is a contagious disease of cattle caused by *Moraxella bovis* and characterized by photophobia, lacrimation, conjunctivitis, and keratitis with such serious sequellae as corneal ulceration and opacity.

The disease is worldwide in distribution, most common in the summer and autumn, and aggravated by other microorganisms, insects, grass awns, and dust. Young and adult cattle are susceptible. The disease is perpetuated from year to year by asymptomatic carriers.

Differential Diagnosis

IBK can be confused clinically with the conjunctivitis caused by the viruses of infectious bovine rhinotracheitis (IBR) and malignant catarrhal fever. Mycoplasmal and ureaplasmal infections can predispose the animal to IBK. Laboratory confirmation should be carried out.

Laboratory Diagnosis

SPECIMENS/PROCEDURES. Conjunctival swabs should be taken for culture from several cases as early in the disease as possible. Because of the problem of overgrowth with contaminants, swabs in a transport medium should be taken to the laboratory as soon as possible. If feasible, the best cultural results are obtained by carefully inoculating blood agar plates in the field, directly after the swabs have been taken.

The recovery of *M. bovis* from cattle with the clinical signs and lesions of IBK constitutes a definitive diagnosis.

Treatment

Many treatments have been used. Powders and ointments containing various drugs administered locally. Penicillin and cortisone mixtures may be given subconjunctivally. Repeated applications are required.

Control

Animals should be kept in the shade and away from dust. Eye shades; ear tags with insecticides. Insect and fly control program; adequate level of vitamin A. Affected animals should be segregated. Vaccinate against IBK and IBR. If possible, mow pastures before grasses go to seed.

Autogenous bacterins have been used with variable success. A commercial bacterin is available. Vaccines containing pili of *M. bovis* appear to provide significant protection. Infection confers immunity for about 6 months.

INFECTIOUS BOVINE RHINOTRACHEITIS /
INFECTIOUS PUSTULAR VULVOVAGINITIS AND
BALANOPOSTHITIS, BOVINE COITAL EXANTHEMA, RED NOSE

Infectious bovine rhinotracheitis (IBR) is a contagious disease of cattle caused by bovine herpesvirus 1 and manifested in the following forms: (1) respiratory infection with nasal and ocular discharges; (2) encephalitis in 2- to 3-month-old calves; (3) an enteric form in young calves; (4) infectious pustular vulvovaginitis and balanoposthitis (IPV&B); and (5) abortion/stillbirths 2–3 months postinfection. It is an acute disease characterized by fever (104–107°F), dyspnea; edema, hemorrhages, and necrosis of the mucosa of upper respiratory tract. Deaths rarely exceed 5–10% of the affected animals. Stress may contribute to clinical disease.

It is probably worldwide in distribution and is endemic in many cattle-raising regions. It is most prevalent in the western United States.

Differential Diagnosis

Because of its different clinical manifestations it is advisable to seek laboratory confirmation of suspected IBR, regardless of the form. IBR virus may be accompanied by important secondary bacterial invaders giving rise to particularly severe respiratory infections.

Many infections should be considered, including those caused by the agents listed under BOVINE RESPIRATORY DISEASE. Pinkeye (*Moraxella bovis*) and calf diphtheria (*Fusobacterium necrophorum*) must be considered. Although IPV&B are clinically characteristic, definitive diagnosis requires identification of the IBR virus.

Laboratory Diagnosis
SPECIMENS
1. For virus isolation: Nasal, conjunctival, vaginal, and preputial swabs (the latter if there are genital signs). Tissues taken will depend on the form. Trachea, lung, and kidney; fluid from thoracic cavity of fetus, cotyledons, fetal liver, and kidney; brain and intestine.
2. For fluorescent antibody (FA): The tissues referred to above.
3. For serology: Paired serum samples.

PROCEDURES/COMMENTS
1. The IBR virus is readily isolated in cell cultures and identified.
2. FA staining can be used to identify virus in frozen sections of tissues.
3. Many normal cattle have antibody titers to IBR virus in the virus neutralization test. These titers and titers due to vaccination usually range from 1:4 to 1:32. A serologic diagnosis is made on the basis of a fourfold increase in titer between acute and convalescent sera.

Treatment

Antibiotics or sulfonamides for secondary bacteria.

Control

Live and inactivated vaccines alone or in combination with other viral or bacterial antigens. Clinical infection and live vaccines provide immunity for 2–4 years. Vaccinate at weaning time and at arrival at the feedlot. Vaccinate pregnant animals with care.

INFECTIOUS CANINE HEPATITIS

Infectious canine hepatitis (ICH) is a contagious disease, primarily of dogs, caused by canine adenovirus type 1 and characterized by anorexia; intense thirst; fever; tonsillitis; conjunctivitis; edema of the head, neck, and lower abdomen; vomiting; diarrhea; and abdominal pain. There is often a transient, occasionally permanent, corneal opacity in one or both eyes (blue eye). Central nervous system signs may include depression, disorientation, seizures, and terminal coma. Epistaxis and prolonged clotting time are often observed.

The disease is worldwide in distribution. The virus is ubiquitous and most dogs have been exposed to the ICH virus and have antibodies by 1 year of age. Infection with this virus can occur in foxes, coyotes, skunks, wolves, raccoons, bears, and guinea pigs. The disease in foxes is manifested primarily by an encephalitis.

Differential Diagnosis

Rapid onset and a prolonged bleeding time suggest ICH. The mortality rate may reach 90% in the acute disease. Less severe forms of the disease are also seen.

Distemper, parvovirus and herpesvirus infections, leptospirosis, toxoplasmosis, and warfarin poisoning should be considered.

Laboratory Diagnosis
SPECIMENS
1. Liver biopsy, urine, nasal swabs.
2. For pathology: Portions of the liver, spleen, and gall bladder; fresh and fixed.
3. Paired serum samples.

PROCEDURES/COMMENTS
1. Virus isolation and identification in cell cultures. Fluores-

cent antibody staining of liver biopsy material and cell cultures.
2. Examination of tissue sections for the characteristic inclusion bodies and other microscopic changes. The liver is usually mottled due to focal areas of necrosis.
3. Virus neutralization test. A fourfold increase in antibody titer is significant.

Treatment
1. Treatment is supportive: Blood transfusions, IV fluids, antibiotics.
2. Distemper-hepatitis-leptospira antiserum.

Control
Hygiene and isolation.

Vaccines containing ICH virus and usually one or more additional antigens are available. Maternal antibodies may be present for 14–16 weeks.

INFECTIOUS CANINE LARYNGOTRACHEITIS /
KENNEL COUGH, TRACHEOBRONCHITIS
Infectious canine laryngotracheitis is a highly contagious disease caused primarily by parainfluenza type 2 virus and characterized by a short course (7–10 days), fever, and a harsh, dry, hacking cough. Other signs include anorexia, nasal discharge, and in some cases pneumonia.

Canine reoviruses, canine herpesvirus, canine distemper virus and canine adenovirus 2 have been associated with some outbreaks. Parainfluenza type 2 infection with secondary invasion by *Bordetella bronchiseptica* can be particularly severe. *Mycoplasma cynos* and other bacteria may aggravate the primary virus infection.

The disease is widespread and is usually associated with hospitalization. *Bordetella bronchiseptica* is the most common bacterial secondary invader.

Differential Diagnosis
See CANINE RESPIRATORY DISEASE for a list of the microbial agents causing respiratory disease in the dog.

Laboratory Diagnosis
Ordinarily this disease is diagnosed clinically.

If the infection proceeds to pneumonia, a tracheal wash is submitted for viral and bacterial isolation and identification. Virus isolations can also be made from nasal and tracheal swabs. Antimicrobial susceptibility tests should be performed on significant bacterial isolates.

Although serologic tests are available for viral antibodies, they are not usually carried out.

Treatment
An antimicrobial drug for secondary bacteria, preferably based on antimicrobial susceptibility tests.

Control
Isolation of infected animals.

Vaccination against parainfluenza type 2 virus and *B. bronchiseptica* is recommended. Various vaccines are available, including intranasal ones.

INFECTIOUS EQUINE ABORTION
The principal microbial agents that cause abortion in the mare are listed in Table 2.10. Those associated with disease entities are discussed separately.

Table 2.10. Microbial agents that cause abortion in mares

Group	Agent
Viruses	Equine rhinopneumonitis virus
	Equine arteritis virus
Bacteria (usually sporadic abortions)	*Klebsiella pneumoniae*
	Streptococcus spp.
	Actinobacillus equuli
	Salmonella abortusequi (rare in United States)
	Leptospira interrogans
Fungi (rare)	*Aspergillus* spp.
	Mucor spp.
	Coccidioides immitis
	Others have been reported

Laboratory Diagnosis
SPECIMENS. The diagnostic procedures carried out are ordinarily based upon the history, suspected disease, and results of direct examinations of fetal and placental materials. These specimens are optimum for a comprehensive laboratory examination:

1. 10 ml of maternal blood for serologic tests, preferably taken at the time of abortion and 2 weeks later. Collect from in-contact animals and those that have aborted.
2. 20 ml of maternal urine to which 1.5 ml of 10% formalin is added for leptospira.
3. Placenta with cotyledons, fresh for microbiology and formalized for histopathology.
4. Uterine discharge on swabs if placenta is not available.
5. Fresh, whole fetus.
6. Fetal lung and liver, fresh and fixed.

INFECTIOUS NECROTIC HEPATITIS / BLACK DISEASE

Infectious necrotic hepatitis is an acute disease of sheep and rarely of cattle. It is caused by *Clostridium novyi* (type B), which produces a powerful necrotizing toxin in the necrotic liver tissue resulting from the migration of liver flukes.

It is worldwide in distribution and its occurrence is dependent upon the presence of the liver fluke *Fasciola hepatica*. The mode of infection is by ingestion of spores. Liver damage caused by tapeworms may also initiate the infectious necrotic hepatitis. Toxin is produced in the fluke-initiated necrotic lesion and absorbed into the blood, eventually causing death. Recovery from the disease is rare. Severe congestion of the blood vessels of the skin may result in blackening of the skin. Cutaneous edema may be present and it is usually sterile.

Differential Diagnosis

The disease is suggested by the history, including liver flukes; a short, fatal course usually involving adult sheep; necrotic areas in liver; and the black appearance of skin.

Consider acute fascioliasis, anthrax, blackleg, malignant edema, and clostridial enterotoxemia.

Laboratory Diagnosis

SPECIMENS

1. Portions of necrotic liver lesions, fresh and fixed.
2. Smears from the necrotic liver lesions.

PROCEDURES

1. Histopathologic examinations.
2. Fluorescent antibody (FA) staining of smears, and culture for isolation and identification.

3. Guinea pig inoculation can be used for the isolation of *C. novyi* from contaminated clinical materials.

COMMENTS. Identification of *C. novyi* by FA staining is rapid and reliable. Identification by cultural methods is slow and laborious.

The finding of the typical histopathologic changes in the liver lesions is highly suggestive.

Treatment
None.

Control
1. Elimination or reduction of liver flukes.
2. Treatment of sheep with a fasciolicide.
3. Annual vaccination with *C. novyi* type B bacterin or toxoid.

INFECTIOUS OVINE AND CAPRINE ABORTION
The microbial agents listed below have been incriminated as causes of abortions in sheep and goats. The diseases with which they are associated are discussed separately and should be consulted for details on laboratory diagnosis.

Campylobacter fetus ssp. *fetus*
Campylobacter jejuni
Chlamydia psittaci (agent of enzootic abortion of ewes)
Brucella ovis
Coxiella burnetii
Listeria monocytogenes, L. ivanovii
Salmonella abortusovis (not in North America)
Various *Salmonella* serovars
Bluetongue virus
Toxoplasma gondii

Some other bacteria may cause sporadic abortions.

Laboratory Diagnosis
SPECIMENS. The diagnostic procedures carried out are ordinarily based upon the history, suspected disease, and results of the direct examinations of fetal materials and placenta. These specimens are optimum for a comprehensive laboratory examination:

1. 5–10 ml of maternal blood for serologic tests, preferably taken at the time of abortion and 2 weeks later. Collect from in-contact animals as well as those that have aborted.
2. 20 ml of maternal urine to which 1.5 ml of 10% formalin is added for leptospira.
3. Placenta with cotyledons, fresh for microbiology and formalized for histopathology.
4. Uterine discharge on swabs if placenta is not available; special transport medium for *Campylobacter* (see 2, Appendix A).
5. Fresh, whole fetus or fetal stomach contents.
6. Fetal lung and liver, fresh and fixed.

INFECTIOUS PORCINE ABORTION

The microbial agents listed below have been incriminated as causes of abortion in sows. The diseases with which they are associated are discussed separately. See these discussions for details on laboratory diagnosis.

> *Brucella suis*
> *Leptospira interrogans,* principally serovar *pomona*
> *Erysipelothrix rhusiopathiae*
> Other bacteria cause sporadic abortions
> Hog cholera virus
> Pseudorabies virus
> Porcine parvovirus*
> Enteroviruses* (SMEDI viruses)
> *Associated with stillbirths and mummification but not abortion.

Laboratory Diagnosis

SPECIMENS. The diagnostic procedures carried out are ordinarily based upon the history, suspected disease, and results of the direct examinations of fetal and placental materials. These specimens are optimum for a comprehensive laboratory examination:

1. 10 ml of maternal blood for serologic tests, preferably taken at the time of abortion and 2 weeks later; collect from in-contact animals as well as those that have aborted.
2. 20 ml of maternal urine to which 1.5 ml of 10% formalin is added for leptospira.

3. Placenta with cotyledons, fresh for microbiology and formalized for histopathology.
4. Uterine discharge on swabs if placenta is not available.
5. Fresh, whole fetuses.
6. Fetal lung and liver, fresh and fixed.

KITTEN MORTALITY COMPLEX

The term kitten mortality complex (KMC) is used to describe a group of specific disease syndromes in kittens and adult queens. The exact cause of KMC has not been determined; however, it has been speculated that the feline infectious peritonitis virus may play a significant etiologic role.

The KMC was first described recently in the United States. Two major syndromes have been recognized: reproductive problems in queens and kitten deaths due to acute congestive heart failure. The reproductive problems include repeat breeding, fetal resorption, abortion, stillbirths, and congenital birth defects. In addition, respiratory disease, endometritis, and circulatory disorders have been observed in adult cats with KMC.

LACTOBACILLUS

These long, slender, pleomorphic, gram-positive rods, which are part of the normal flora of the mouth, vagina, and intestinal tract of animals, are rarely pathogenic. The presence of large numbers of lactobacilli in vaginal secretions indicates a healthy vagina.

Cultures of *L. acidophilus,* sometimes in milk (sweet acidophilus milk), have been administered to animals and humans to treat intestinal disorders. The idea is to replace the "undesirable" intestinal bacteria.

LEGIONELLA

Legionella pneumophila, the causal agent of Legionnaire's disease in humans, is the most important species in this genus. These fastidious, gram-negative, small rods are widely distributed in many water-associated environments.

Although infections in animals would appear to be rare, antibodies to *L. pneumophila* have been detected in cattle, sheep, horses, antelopes, and buffaloes.

The organism was first propagated in laboratory animals and embryonated chicken eggs. Specially formulated selective media are now available for its cultivation. A direct fluorescent antibody procedure can be used for rapid identification of the organism.

LISTERIA

Species of this genus are small, motile, gram-positive, non-sporeforming, facultatively anaerobic rods.

The species now recognized are as follows:

Listeria monocytogenes: See LISTERIOSIS. This is the principal pathogenic species.

L. ivanovii: This is the only species other than *L. monocytogenes* that is naturally pathogenic for animals and humans. It can cause abortion in sheep but the extent of infections is not known. There is a carrier state in animals and humans.

L. innocua: It has been isolated from plants, soil, and animal and human feces.

L. welshimeri: It has been recovered from vegetation, soil, and animal feces.

L. seeligeri: It has been isolated from animal feces, vegetation, and soil.

L. murrayi: Its habitat is probably soil and vegetation.

L. grayi: Soil and vegetation are thought to be its habitat.

LISTERIOSIS / CIRCLING DISEASE, LISTERELLOSIS

Listeriosis is a noncontagious disease of sheep, goats, cattle, swine, horses, chickens, turkeys, rodents (both wild and laboratory), and humans. It is mainly caused by *Listeria monocytogenes* and is often sporadic but multiple cases also occur. In general, it is characterized by a neural form seen most often in ruminants with fully developed stomachs and a visceral or septicemic form occurring most often in monogastric animals. *L. monocytogenes* is an important cause of abortion in sheep and cattle. The disease is seen particularly in winter and early spring; all ages are susceptible. Keratoconjunctivitis and ophthalmitis have been described in cattle and sheep. Several cases of bovine mastitis caused by this organism have been reported. *Listeria ivanovii* has been reported to cause abortion in sheep.

The disease is worldwide in distribution. The organism is carried as a commensal by many animals and is shed in the feces of wild rodents. The neural form of the disease, the form most often seen in practice, may frequently be brought on by various stresses or the feeding of spoiled silage. Organisms multiply when the pH of silage rises above 5.5.

Differential Diagnosis

The presence of neurologic signs, including circling, along with a history of feeding silage, will suggest listeriosis. Because there are other diseases with neurologic signs, laboratory confirmation should be sought.

Visceral listeriosis is not usually diagnosed antemortem.

Abortions are usually single in cattle but may be multiple in ewes.

Rabies, thromboembolic meningoencephalitis, enterotoxemia, brain abscesses, sporadic bovine encephalitis, polioencephalomalacia, and various other encephalitides should be considered.

Laboratory Diagnosis

SPECIMENS

1. Neural form: Brain stem; visceral form: portions of liver; abortion: fetus and placenta.
2. Visceral or septicemic form: Brain stem fixed; formalized portions of the liver.
3. Paired serum samples.

PROCEDURES/COMMENTS

1. Isolation and identification. Repeated culturing (cold enrichment) may be necessary.
2. Histopathologic examination. Microabscesses in the brain stem strongly suggest listeriosis.
3. A tube agglutination test is performed in some diagnostic laboratories to confirm abortion due to *L. monocytogenes*. The test is usually interpreted as follows:
   suspicious: 1:160
   positive: ≥1:320

A definitive diagnosis is made on the basis of the isolation and identification of *L. monocytogenes*.

Treatment

1. Treatment is usually of little value after neurologic signs are seen.
2. The drugs of choice are the tetracyclines at a maximum dosage level.

Control
1. Avoid spoiled silage.
2. Vaccines are not used in North America.

LYME DISEASE

Lyme disease is a noncontagious, multiorgan infection, primarily of humans, caused by the tick-borne spirochete *Borrelia burgdorferi* and characterized by a skin eruption (erythema chronica migrans) followed weeks or months later by a migratory arthritis. Cardiac and neurologic abnormalities may also develop; the disease may persist for months.

The tick vector in the United States is *Ixodes dammini*. The disease has been reported from Australia, Europe, Japan, and the former U.S.S.R.

There have been a number of reports of Lyme disease in dogs in a number of states where the human disease occurs and *I. dammini* is found. That the canine disease is widespread in the United States is suggested by serologic surveys. Canine infections are generally milder than the human disease, with usually a history of fever, inappetence, lethargy, and sudden onset of lameness associated with pain in two or more joints. The episodes of lameness, which vary from one to several, occur at intervals of roughly 1 month to 1 year. Some infected dogs have developed renal disorders.

Arthritis, encephalitis, and uveitis have been recognized in horses. In cattle, abortion, arthritis, myocarditis, nephritis, and pneumonitis have been reported.

Laboratory Diagnosis
SPECIMENS. Serum.

PROCEDURES/COMMENTS. The organism has been difficult to demonstrate by microscopy and difficult to culture. At present the indirect fluorescent antibody test, fluorescence immunoassay (FIA), and an enzyme-linked immunosorbent assay (ELISA) for antibodies to *B. burgdorferi* are the most useful diagnostic procedures. High antibody titers have been observed in dogs considered to have Lyme disease. Such high titers along with a history of arthritis and intermittent lameness in endemic areas would strongly suggest Lyme disease. However, it must be kept in mind that dogs with subclinical infections may also have appreciable antibody titers.

An ELISA for antibody detection is commercially available (see 16, Appendix A).

Treatment

Tetracyclines, penicillin, cephalosporins, and erythromycin are used in acute cases. May require prolonged antibiotic therapy.

Control

Tick control is very important. Commercial bacterins appear to protect dogs; two doses are given intramuscularly with an interval of 2–3 weeks. Annual revaccination is recommended.

MADUROMYCOSIS / EUMYCOTIC MYCETOMA

Maduromycotic mycetomas (subcutaneous mycotic abscesses) consist of granulomatous processes, which may be fibrotic and cystic, and are produced by several species of fungi. Microcolonies that are frequently pigmented can sometimes be seen grossly in lesions and exudates.

There are several reports of these infrequent infections in horses, cattle, dogs, and cats. The lesions occur most commonly on the extremities but may be found involving the nasal mucosa (e.g., bovine nasal granuloma), the peritoneum, and the skin in various locations.

Incision of the lesions reveals discrete brown or black fungous microcolonies embedded in a large mass of granulation tissue. The following species of fungi have been recovered:

Pseudallescheria boydii
Curvularia geniculata
Cochliobolus spicifer
Helminthosporium spp.
Madurella mycetomatis

The first species mentioned is a hyaline, nonpigmented fungus while the other four are dematiaceous (black or brown pigment) fungi.

Some additional species and genera have been recovered from human maduromycosis.

Differential Diagnosis

The lesions of this disease resemble somewhat those of phaeohyphomycosis. A highly presumptive diagnosis of maduromycosis can be made if the characteristic grains or microcolonies are seen in lesions and exudates. Precise diagnosis is dependent upon the demonstration, isolation, and identification of the causative fungus.

Laboratory Diagnosis

SPECIMENS. For direct examination, culture, and histopathology, use material from the lesions. Biopsy and portions of lesions, fixed.

PROCEDURES. The characteristic grains or microcolonies can be seen grossly. The microcolonies are selected and examined in wet mounts for the characteristic fungal elements. The fungi grow readily on Sabouraud agar in 2–3 weeks at room temperature.

The finding of grains and the fungal elements in tissue sections confirms the etiologic role of the fungus.

TREATMENT

Surgical intervention if indicated. The success of treatment depends on the nature and extent of the lesions. Fibrotic and cystic lesions resist drug penetration. Drugs that may be useful are iodides, amphotericin B, 5-fluorocytosine, ketoconazole, and thiabendazole.

MALIGNANT CATARRHAL FEVER / SNOTSIEKTE, BOVINE EPITHELIOSIS, MALIGNANT HEAD CATARRH

Malignant catarrhal fever (MCF) or African MCF is usually an acute, highly fatal disease of cattle and water buffaloes caused by a herpesvirus and characterized by the development of a catarrhal and mucopurulent inflammation of mucous membranes usually manifested in five different syndromes or forms: peracute, head and eye, intestinal, benign, and chronic.

Although presumed to be viral the causal agent of the European and American MCF has not been isolated and characterized. Sheep are thought to be carriers of this postulated virus. The virus of African MCF has been isolated and characterized (see MALIGNANT CATARRHAL FEVER [AFRICAN] in Section 3).

The head and eye form is the most common. Among the signs, depending on the form, are profuse mucopurulent discharge, erosions of the oral and nasal mucosa, severe keratoconjunctivitis, high fever (105–108°F), severe diarrhea, convulsions, excitability, and tremors. Fatality rate is 100%.

Occurrence is worldwide; the incidence in a herd is usually low. Sporadic cases are seen most often, but outbreaks can occur. Sheep are subclinically infected and may serve as a reservoir of infection. Blue and black wildebeests are natural hosts of the African disease; cattle are secondary hosts. The disease occurs commonly in spring and fall in Europe and North America.

Differential Diagnosis

The disease is most often tentatively diagnosed as MCF based upon its sporadic occurrence and the recognition of the syndromes described above. MCF resembles, in some respects, bovine virus diarrhea, rinderpest, bluetongue, infectious bovine rhinotracheitis, foot-and-mouth disease, and vesicular stomatitis.

Laboratory Diagnosis
SPECIMENS
1. Fresh leukocytes (buffy coat), fresh spleen, lymph nodes, tonsils, thyroids, and adrenals.
2. Brain; portions of liver, kidney, spleen, lymph nodes, adrenals, and lesions of the alimentary tract, fixed in formalin.

A diagnosis is usually made on the basis of clinical signs and the finding of characteristic histopathologic changes (essentially a vasculitis).

PROCEDURES/COMMENTS
1. The virus has been isolated from the wildebeest in Africa but not from North American or European cattle. Rabbits inoculated with infected tissue suspension develop central nervous system signs and die within a month.
2. The finding of characteristic histopathologic changes, including vasculitis and lymphocytic infiltration and proliferation in most organs, along with typical clinical signs, is usually the basis for a diagnosis.

Treatment
None.

Control

If MCF is a continuing problem, cattle should not be exposed to possible carrier sheep. No vaccine is available. Solid immunity occurs if an animal survives natural infection.

MALIGNANT EDEMA

Malignant edema is an acute, often fatal, toxemic disease seen most often in cattle, sheep, goats, swine, and horses. It is caused by *Clostridium septicum* and characterized by a gangrenous process beginning in a wound and usually involving skeletal muscle.

It is worldwide in distribution, and most common in cattle and sheep; infrequent in swine and horses. The organism is shed in the feces of many animals, thus, spores are widely present in the soil.

Differential Diagnosis

The gangrenous process begins at the site of the wound and spreads in tissues, most commonly in muscles. Cases are sporadic unless a number of animals have been wounded, e.g., lambs from docking. Unlike blackleg, the age range is wide. The following are characteristic of the lesions in muscle: red rather than black, gelatinous, little gas, and pits on pressure.

Blackleg, anthrax, and gas gangrene due to other causes are among the diseases that should be considered.

Laboratory Diagnosis
SPECIMENS
1. In the dead animal, a portion of the muscle and smears prepared from the lesion.
2. In the live animal, material may be taken from the lesion with a syringe for smears and culture.

PROCEDURES. Fluorescent antibody (FA) staining of smears is quick and reliable. Because of its accuracy and rapidity, FA staining has largely replaced culture. The latter is expensive and time consuming.

COMMENTS. It is very important that the specimen (muscle) be fresh, for other clostridia may invade the lesions within a few hours after death, particularly in warm weather.

It should also be kept in mind that *C. septicum* is a rapid postmortem invader.

Identification of *C. septicum* by FA staining or by culture from fresh lesions constitutes a definitive diagnosis of malignant edema.

Treatment
1. Penicillin, tetracyclines.
2. Supportive therapy.

Control
Bacterins containing *C. septicum* and *C. chauvoei* and sometimes other clostridia are used widely in cattle and sheep.

MORAXELLA
Moraxella species are small, gram-negative, nonmotile rods.

Moraxella bovis: See INFECTIOUS BOVINE KERATO-CONJUNCTIVITIS.

M. lacunata: Has been isolated from aborted equine fetuses, septicemia in a goat, and from canine and feline clinical specimens.

M. phenylpyruvica: Has been recovered from the genitourinary tract of cattle, sheep, and swine; from the brain of sheep and cattle; and from the intestinal tract of goats.

MYCOBACTERIUM
The mycobacterial diseases caused by *Mycobacterium bovis* and *M. paratuberculosis* are discussed separately.

Some additional species of these small, acid-fast rods are capable of causing infections in domestic animals; however, they are mainly of importance because they can sensitize animals to tuberculin. Most of the species occur in nature. Some of the species and the infections they cause in animals are listed below:

Mycobacterium kansasii: Has been isolated from the lymph nodes of swine, cattle, and other animals.

M. scrofulaceum and *M. xenopi:* Have been recovered from the lymph nodes of animals.

M. avium (M. avium, intracellular complex): In addition to the strains causing avian tuberculosis, several serotypes infect and cause tuberculosis in swine and other animals.

M. fortuitum: Can cause skin infections of cats characterized by ulceration or nodule formation; lymph node infection and mastitis in cattle; joint and respiratory infection in pigs, and pneumonia in dogs.

M. smegmatis: Has been recovered from cows with mastitis.

Other rapid-growing mycobacteria have been isolated from ulcerative dermatitis in cats and occasionally dogs.

MYCOPLASMA INFECTIONS OF DOGS AND CATS

The mycoplasmas that have been recovered from dogs and cats along with the diseases attributed to them are listed below:

Dogs. *Mycoplasma cynos:* Pneumonia. This mycoplasma is considered a cause of a rapidly spreading respiratory infection. By itself it may have little significance, but in combination with other bacteria and viruses a severe pneumonia may result (see CANINE RESPIRATORY DISEASE).

M. spumans: Has been associated with canine polyarthritis.

M. canis: Has been associated with urogenital disease.

M. maculosum, M. edwardii, M. molare, M. opalescens: Other species that have been recovered from the dog and whose significance is uncertain.

Cats. *M. felis:* Conjunctivitis and pneumonia. This species causes a unilateral or bilateral conjunctivitis that begins with papillary hypertrophy of the conjunctival surface and results in a deep-red, velvet appearance. If untreated, a mucoid exudate develops within a week and there may be pseudomembrane formation.

M. felis: Has also been implicated in polyarthritis in the cat.

M. gatiae and *M. feliminatum:* Also recovered from cats, but their significance is uncertain.

Differential Diagnosis

Dogs. Pneumonia caused by bacteria other than *Mycoplasma,* and fungal and viral pneumonia (see CANINE RESPIRATORY DISEASE).

Cats. Conjunctivitis and pneumonia caused by various viruses and bacteria (see FELINE RESPIRATORY DISEASES).

MYCOPLASMA INFECTIONS OF SHEEP AND GOATS

Several *Mycoplasma* spp. cause important diseases of sheep and goats.

These infections are referred to briefly below.

Contagious caprine pleuropneumonia: This acute serofibrinous pleurisy and pneumonia, which may involve almost entire lobes, is characterized by red and gray hepatization with characteristic hemorrhagic infarction. A severe arthritis may be a sequella of the bacteremia, which has been attributed to *Mycoplasma mycoides* ssp. *capri, M. ovipneumoniae,* and *M. mycoides* ssp. *mycoides* (large colony). This disease occurs in Europe, Asia, Africa, and there is recent evidence that it occurs in the United States. The small-colony form of *M. mycoides* ssp. *mycoides* is the causative agent of contagious bovine pleuropneumonia.

Contagious agalactiae: An acute, subacute, or chronic disease of sheep and goats that is caused by *M. agalactiae.* Other mycoplasmas, viz., *M. mycoides* ssp. *mycoides* (large colony) and *M. capricolum* are claimed to cause similar syndromes. It is characterized by a bacteremia (after ingestion) with localization and inflammatory activity in the udder, uterus, joints (arthritis), and eyes (conjunctivitis). There is an interstitial mastitis that without treatment may lead to extensive fibrosis. It occurs in Mediterranean countries as well as in some regions of Europe, Africa, and Asia.

Polyarthritis in sheep and goats: Probably the most common and geographically widespread mycoplasmosis in these species. It is most often caused by *M. capricolum.*

Keratoconjunctivitis in sheep and goats: A widespread disease caused by *M. conjunctivae* and *M. oculi. M. mycoides* ssp. *mycoides* (large colony) has been reported to cause epizootics that are characterized by septicemia, polyarthritis, and pneumonia with high morbidity and mortality in kids. The organism is usually acquired from the milk of shedding females.

Other disease manifestations: In sheep and goats, various mycoplasmas have been associated with enzootic pneumonia (*M. ovipneumoniae* in sheep), vulvovaginitis, infertility, and central nervous system disorders.

Laboratory Diagnosis

Laboratories should be contacted in advance, for not all have the capability of isolating and identifying mycoplasmas. Specimens may have to be sent to reference laboratories.

SPECIMENS. In collecting material, keep in mind that these organisms are fragile and specimens must be refrigerated and delivered to the laboratory within 48 hours.
1. For culture: This will depend on the disease, e.g., portions of lungs, milk, joint fluid, eye swabs, etc.
2. For histopathology: Portions of affected tissues, fixed.
3. For serology: If feasible, acute and convalescent sera.

PROCEDURES. These will involve culture and identification, and serologic procedures, such as agglutination, enzyme-linked immunosorbent assay, and complement fixation tests.

Treatment

Erythromycin, tylosin, spectinomycin, and tetracyclines have been found effective in some of these infections.

Control

Sanitary measures and the isolation of infected animals to prevent spread. Efforts should be directed at minimizing stress.

A variety of live, attenuated, and inactivated vaccines have been used with variable success.

MYCOPLASMA INFECTIONS OF SWINE

Mycoplasma spp. cause the important diseases of swine listed below. The most widespread of these diseases, enzootic pneumonia, is discussed separately. All of the porcine mycoplasmas can exist as commensals in the upper respiratory tract.

Mycoplasmal polyserositis of young pigs (1–5 weeks): Is caused by *M. hyorhinis* and is characterized by arthritis and serofibrinous serositis involving the pleura, pericardium, and peritoneum. The disease is precipitated by various stresses, such as shipment, and often involves all or most of a litter.

Septic arthritis of feeder pigs: Is caused by *M. hyosynoviae* and results in lameness, which seriously interferes with weight gains and finishing. Generally only a small percentage of pigs are affected.

Enzootic pneumonia of swine: The primary cause is *M. hyopneumoniae* (*M. suipneumoniae*). It is dealt with under ENZOOTIC PNEUMONIA OF SWINE.

Differential Diagnosis

Mycoplasmal polyserositis: Distinguish from chlamydial arthritis, Glasser's disease, *Streptococcus suis* infections, and various infections of piglets.

Septic arthritis: Is caused by *M. hyosynoviae.* Consider erysipelas; arthritis due to other bacteria such as streptococci, staphylococci, and *Actinomyces pyogenes;* and chlamydial polyarthritis.

Laboratory Diagnosis

Definitive diagnosis is dependent on the isolation and identification of the specific mycoplasma.

SPECIMENS

1. For culture: Mycoplasmal polyserositis — a sick or recently dead pig; portions of affected lungs, pericardium and fluid from the pericardial sac, and thoracic and abdominal cavities; joint fluid. *M. hyosynoviae* arthritis — joint fluid.

    Specimens for culture must be refrigerated and reach the laboratory within 48 hours.

2. For serology: Paired serum samples.

PROCEDURES/COMMENTS

1. For culture: Mycoplasmas are fragile, fastidious organisms that require special media and procedures for isolation and identification. Identification to species is accomplished by the serum growth inhibition test, complement fixation test, enzyme-linked immunsorbent assay, fluorescent antibody procedures, etc. These tests are not available in most diagnostic laboratories.

2. *M. hypopneumoniae* is particularly difficult to isolate and cultivate. The complement fixation test has been used to identify exposed and infected pigs.

Treatment

Tylosin, tetracyclines, and erythromycin are among the most effective drugs. Corticosteroids, along with an antibiotic, have been effective in treating *M. hyosynoviae* infections.

Control

Good management with the avoidance of stresses will mitigate the occurrence of mycoplasmal polyserositis and arthritis. The treatment and control of enzootic pneumonia of swine is dealt with separately.

MYCOPLASMA, UREAPLASMA, AND *ACHOLEPLASMA* INFECTIONS OF CATTLE

Many species of mycoplasmas, ureaplasmas, and acholeplasmas have been recovered from cattle. The diseases known to be caused by these agents are tabulated (see Table 2.11) under MYCOPLASMAS, UREAPLASMAS, AND ACHOLEPLASMAS. See also BOVINE RESPIRATORY DISEASE and CONTAGIOUS BOVINE PLEUROPNEUMONIA in Section 3.

Laboratory Diagnosis

SPECIMENS. These will depend upon the disease. Materials from lesions and affected tissues should be refrigerated and delivered to the laboratory within 48 hours. If ureaplasmas are suspected, samples should reach the laboratory within 24 hours. If they can't be delivered to the laboratory within these times, they should be maintained in the frozen state until delivered to the laboratory.

Paired serum samples may be useful.

PROCEDURES/COMMENTS. The procedures are essentially the same as those described for the recovery of swine mycoplasmas (see MYCOPLASMA INFECTIONS OF SWINE). Special media are required and some species of mycoplasmas have special nutritional requirements.

An indirect hemagglutination test and an enzyme-linked immunosorbent assay are available in some laboratories to detect antibodies against certain mycoplasmal infections.

Ureaplasmas have different nutritional requirements than mycoplasmas and thus a special medium is required.

Mycoplasmas frequently occur on mucous membranes as commensals, thus their isolation alone does not necessarily indicate significance.

Although some diagnostic laboratories have the capability of culturing mycoplasmas they are not usually able to speciate them. This is done in reference laboratories.

Treatment

This will depend upon the infection. The drugs most frequently used are spectinomycin, erythromycin, tetracyclines, and tylosin.

Control

This will depend upon the disease. Frequently all that can be done is to apply appropriate sanitary measures and isolate infected animals to prevent spread. Cattle are vaccinated with an attenuated strain of *M. mycoides* ssp. *mycoides* to prevent contagious bovine pleuropneumonia.

MYCOPLASMAS OF HORSES

Several species of mycoplasmas have been recovered from horses but as yet no disease has not been attributed to them (see MYCOPLASMAS, UREAPLASMAS, AND ACHOLE-PLASMAS).

MYCOPLASMAS, UREAPLASMAS, AND ACHOLEPLASMAS

Many of the mycoplasmas are discussed separately under the various diseases they cause. However, a number of species either cause less frequent infections or have not yet been proved to have pathogenic significance. All of the currently named mycoplasmas, ureaplasmas, acholeplasmas, and their disease status are listed in Table 2.11 to help clinicians assess the probable significance of isolates.

Table 2.11.   Disease status of all currently named mycoplasmas, ureaplasmas, and acholeplasmas

Animal	Disease	Organisms
Cattle	Pneumonia	*Mycoplasma mycoides* ssp. *mycoides*
		M. bovis
		M. dispar
		Ureaplasmas
	Arthritis	*M. bovis*
		M. bovigenitalium

Table 2.11. (*continued*)

Animal	Disease	Organisms
	Mastitis	M. bovis
		M. californicum
		M. canadense
	Abortion	M. bovis
	Vaginitis	M. bovigenitalium
		Ureaplasmas
	Seminal vesiculitis	M. bovis
		M. bovigenitalium
	Uncertain	M. bovirhinis
		M. alkalescens
		M. arginini
		Acholeplasma modicum
		A. laidlawii
		M. bovoculi
		M. verecundum
		M. alvi
Swine	Pneumonia	M. hyopneumoniae
	Arthritis	M. hyorhinis
		M. hyosynoviae
	Uncertain	M. flocculare
		M. sualvi
		M. hyopharyngis
		A. axanthum
		A. granularum
Sheep and goats	Pneumonia	M. ovipneumoniae
		M. mycoides ssp. *capri*
	Arthritis	M. mycoides ssp. *mycoides*
	Mastitis	M. agalactiae
		M. putrefaciens
	Conjunctivitis	M. conjunctivae
	Arthritis	M. capricolum
	Uncertain	M. arginini
		M. oculi
Horse	Uncertain	M. equigenitalium
		M. equirhinis
		M. subdolum
		M. felis
		M. arginini
		M. salivarium
		A. equifetale
		A. hippikon
		A. laidlawii
Dogs	Pneumonia	M. cynos
	Uncertain	M. spumans
		M. maculosum
		M. edwardii
		M. molare
		M. canis
		M. opalescens
Cats	Conjunctivitis	M. felis
	Pneumonia	M. gateae
		M. felis
		M. feliminutum

Source: Adapted from Stalheim, O.H.V. 1990. Mycoplasmas of animals. In *Diagnostic Procedures in Veterinary Bacteriology and Mycology,* 5th ed. Ed. G. R. Carter and J. R. Cole, Jr. New York: Academic Press.

NASAL ASPERGILLOSIS / CANINE NASAL ASPERGILLOSIS

Nasal aspergillosis is a chronic fungal disease, principally of dogs (rarely in cats and horses), and usually caused by the colonization of *Aspergillus fumigatus* in the nasal cavity and paranasal sinuses.

The disease is characterized clinically by a persistent unilateral or bilateral nasal discharge, sometimes bloody or purulent (secondary bacteria), sneezing, open-mouth breathing, and such less commonly seen signs as facial and palatal swelling, loss of appetite, and depression. Ordinarily the disease does not become systemic, although if untreated it results in an intractable process with extensive local tissue damage.

Dogs of the mesocephalic and dolichocephalic types are more often affected than the brachycephalic breeds.

Penicillium spp. can cause a disease of the nasal passages of dogs that is similar to nasal aspergillosis but much less frequent.

Differential Diagnosis

Nasal tumors, cryptococcosis, ehrlichiosis (epistaxis), allergic and infectious rhinitis should be considered.

Laboratory Diagnosis

Radiography, blood count, and tests for immune deficiencies may be helpful. Isolation and identification of *A. fumigatus* with repeated recovery of the fungus is definitive.

SPECIMENS

1. For direct examination and culture: Swabs of the nasal cavity and curretted material from the lesion.
2. For histopathology: Curretted material and biopsies, fixed.
3. For serology: 3–5 ml of serum.

PROCEDURES/COMMENTS

1. For direct examination: Wet mounts are examined for fungal elements.

   For culture: Swabs and curretted material are cultured for bacteria and fungi.

   Aspergillus and *Penicillium* spp. can be cultured from a considerable percentage of canine nares. The amount of culture (number of colonies), relative purity, and presence on repeated culturing should be considered.

2. For histopathology: Sections are examined for fungal elements and characteristic tissue changes.

3. For serology: The agar gel immunodiffusion test is performed using an extract of *Aspergillus* as antigen. The test is not quantitative and is reported as positive or negative. Some uninfected dogs will give a positive test, but a positive test is supportive of a diagnosis when other diagnostic procedures such as culture, histopathology, and radiography indicate the disease. An immunodiffusion test can also be performed for *Penicillium*.

An enzyme-linked immunosorbent assay is also available in some diagnostic laboratories.

Treatment

Each case requires individual attention. Treatment may involve surgical currettage, local and systemic antifungal medication, and in some instances immune stimulation. Among the drugs used locally are Lugol's iodine, thiabendazole, amphotericin B, and natamycin; drugs used systemically are thiabendazole, 5-fluorocytosine, amphotericin B, and ketoconazole.

NECROBACILLOSIS

The term necrobacillosis is commonly used to describe those lesions or diseases with which *Fusobacterium necrophorum* is associated. This anaerobic, nonsporulating, gram-negative bacterium is present as a commensal in the intestinal tract and on mucous membranes of many animals. Infections are endogenous, frequently secondary, and characterized by necrosis. The organism invades and multiplies in the anaerobic environment provided by damaged tissue.

Fusobacterium necrophorum may be isolated from numerous infections initiated by a variety of wounds and injuries in domestic animals. Some of the well-known diseases with which *F. necrophorum* is associated are CALF DIPTHERIA (q.v.), NECROTIC RHINITIS (q.v.), FOOT ROT OF CATTLE (q.v.), FOOT ABSCESS OF SHEEP (q.v.), and BOVINE LIVER ABSCESSES (q.v.).

Diagnosis is usually based on clinical signs, appearance,

and the often foul odor of lesions. Infections are frequently mixed and *F. necrophorum,* a fastidious anaerobe, is often difficult to isolate.

NECROTIC RHINITIS / BULLNOSE

This uncommon disease results from injuries to the mouth and snout caused by nose ringing, eruption of teeth, or the clipping of teeth. Bacteria, particularly *Fusobacterium necrophorum,* invade the necrotic tissue resulting in an inflammatory process that may extend to tissues of the upper jaw, snout, and face. Infections are usually mixed.

The disease is most often seen where sanitary and general management practices are poor.

The appearance and clinical signs of this disease are so characteristic, that a laboratory diagnosis is not usually sought.

NEISSERIA

These are aerobic, gram-negative cocci that occur singly or in clumps. They are commensals on the mucous membranes of the nasopharynx and conjunctiva of animals. The *Neisseria* spp. that are frequently associated with animals are listed below:

N. canis: Is isolated from the nasopharynx of dogs and cats.

N. flavescens and *N. sicca:* Are isolated from the oropharynx of normal dogs.

N. lactamica: Is recovered from the conjunctival sac of healthy dogs.

N. ovis: Is associated with keratoconjunctivitis in goats.

NOCARDIA

These are gram-positive, nonmotile, nonsporeforming, saprophytic bacteria found widely in the soil. They are variably acid-fast rods with occasional branching and aerial hyphae. Important *Nocardia* spp. are listed below:

N. asteroides: See NOCARDIOSIS.

N. caviae (syn.: *N. otitidiscaviarum*): Occasionally causes bovine mastitis.

N. brasiliensis: Causes nocardiosis in humans and occasionally mastitis in bovines.

NOCARDIOSIS

Nocardiosis is a chronic, noncontagious, sporadic disease of dogs, cattle, cats, swine, goats, sheep, horses, humans, and occasionally other animals. It is caused by a soil-borne organism *Nocardia asteroides* and characterized by thoracopulmonary (dogs particularly), mastitic (cow), and mycetoma (skin, subcutis) forms.

The organism is found widely in the soil and the disease is worldwide in distribution. *N. asteroides* enters by wounds (mycetoma), inhalation (thoracopulmonary), and the teat canal (mastitis). In the latter form, the organisms are usually introduced when asepsis is not practiced in treatment. A suppurative infection, called bovine farcy, involving the lymphatics of the extremities and head region has been attributed to *N. asteroides*. It appears to be confined to tropical regions.

Differential Diagnosis

Similar mycetomas are seen in actinomycosis (dog), cryptococcosis (skin lesions), and blastomycosis (skin lesions). The thoracopulmonary form in the dog can be confused with canine actinomycosis and other pulmonary infections. Nocardial mastitis (also caused occasionally by *N. caviae* and *N. brasiliensis*) is characterized by a chronic granulomatous process.

Laboratory confirmation is required.

Laboratory Diagnosis
SPECIMENS

1. Fresh pus and exudate taken aseptically from lesions; excision may be necessary.
2. In the thoracopulmonary form, thoracocentesis and a tracheal wash are used to collect material.
3. Milk is submitted if nocardial mastitis is suspected.

PROCEDURES/COMMENTS. A strongly presumptive diagnosis of nocardiosis can be made on the basis of demonstration of a gram-positive filamentous, partially acid-fast organism in smears. A definitive diagnosis depends on the isolation and identification of *N. asteroides*.

Treatment

Surgical debridement and drainage of lesions are useful. Advanced nocardiosis does not usually respond well to treatment. The early disease may respond to prolonged treatment with trimethoprim-sulfonamide, tetracyclines, sulfadiazine, or novobiocin. *Penicillin is not effective.* Early nocardial mastitis has responded to nitrofurazone and novobiocin; however, if the disease is advanced, the cows are usually sacrificed.

Control

Prompt treatment of wounds in order to avoid sepsis.

NONENTERIC INFECTIONS OF NEONATAL CALVES AND LAMBS

Diseases referred to by such names as navel ill, omphalitis, joint ill, and septic polyarthritis are less common in calves and lambs than in young foals. The mode of infection, clinical signs, and disease manifestations are much the same as in foals.

As with the analogous infections in foals, diagnosis depends upon the isolation and identification of the causative organisms. Treatment, control, and prevention are basically similar.

NONENTERIC INFECTIONS OF NEONATAL FOALS

The major diseases of this category are known by such names as navel ill, omphalitis, septic polyarthritis, and sleepy foal disease, and may be prenatal, perinatal, or postnatal in occurrence. The mode of infection is usually by the umbilicus, ingestion, or inhalation. Availability of colostrum has a major influence on these infections.

SLEEPY FOAL DISEASE

This is frequently an acute disease of very young foals. It is caused by *Actinobacillus equuli* and is characterized by diarrhea shortly after birth and such later manifestations as meningitis, suppurative nephritis, pneumonia, and arthritis resulting from a bacteremia.

The following bacteria are also frequently involved in infections of foals:

Pyogenic streptococci; particularly *Streptococcus equi* ssp. *zooepidemicus*
Escherichia coli
Staphylococcus aureus
S. intermedius
Klebsiella spp.
Actinomyces pyogenes
Salmonella serovars

The organisms listed above, in addition to being associated with diarrhea (*E. coli, Klebsiella, Salmonella*), can cause general infections in young foals characterized by fever, bacteremia, septicemia with omphalitis, arthritis, pneumonia, pleuritis, and peritonitis.

Differential Diagnosis

Because of the variety of potential causative agents and clinical signs, a definitive diagnosis can only be made by the isolation and identification of the pathogen.

Laboratory Diagnosis

SPECIMENS/PROCEDURES. For culture and histopathology: Selection of materials will depend upon the disease. In the live animal, feces, unclotted blood for culture (5–10 ml), joint fluid, and transtracheal aspirates if pneumonia is suspected. If a necropsy is performed, portions of affected tissues and vital organs, both fresh and fixed, should be submitted.

The organisms that cause these various infections can be isolated and identified without difficulty. The gross and microscopic pathologic changes may offer supportive evidence in a diagnosis.

Treatment

This is usually administered empirically before the results of the antibiotic susceptibility tests are received. Broad-spectrum antibiotics such as chloromycetin and tetracyclines have been effective. Good supportive care.

Control

Prophylactic administration of broad-spectrum antibiotics in some situations. Good sanitary practices at parturition.

NONENTERIC INFECTIONS OF PIGLETS

These infections have been given a variety of names including navel ill, joint ill, omphalitis, infective or pyemic arthritis, and polyarthritis.

A variety of causes can contribute to microbial infections in young pigs. These include insufficient colostrum and milk, and poor management practices. However, some infections occur from year to year in herds in spite of good husbandry practices. Piglets are most often infected postnatally, usually via the umbilicus or by ingestion. Animals die of a septicemia or as a result of damage due to the localization of organisms in various organs and tissues after a bacteremia.

The following are the most common agents causing these infections:

E. coli

Streptococcus spp.; several serologic groups have been implicated (see STREPTOCOCCI)

Staphylococcus aureus

S. intermedius

Actinomyces pyogenes

Salmonella serovars

Actinobacillus suis

Differential Diagnosis

The clinical signs are generally similar for each of the various causative agents.

Laboratory Diagnosis

Sick or recently dead pigs are usually submitted. Vital organs and joints are usually cultured. A specific diagnosis is dependent upon the isolation and identification of the organism or organisms involved.

Treatment/Control

This is essentially the same as for NONENTERIC INFECTIONS OF NEONATAL FOALS.

OVINE BRUCELLOSIS / EPIDIDYMITIS OF RAMS

Brucellosis of sheep, frequently called epididymitis of rams, is caused by *Brucella ovis* and is characterized in the ram by epididymitis, orchitis, and infertility and uncommonly in ewes by placentitis and abortion. The disease is usually seen in sheep 1 year of age or older.

Occurrence is probably worldwide; transmission is by coitus and direct contact. Infected rams may shed *B. ovis* in the semen for months and thus perpetuate the disease.

Differential Diagnosis

The disease should be suspected if there are clinical signs of epididymitis and orchitis. Bacteria other than *B. ovis* cause epididymitis in young or puberal rams (see OVINE EPIDID-YMITIS: GENERAL).

Campylobacter abortion (see OVINE GENITAL CAM-PYLOBACTERIOSIS), enzootic abortion of ewes, and toxoplasmosis should be considered.

Laboratory Diagnosis
SPECIMENS

1. Aseptically collected semen; fetal cotyledons and fetus; testicle and epididymis.
2. Serum. It is advisable to collect a number of samples from rams and ewes.
3. Air-dried smears of semen/cotyledons.

PROCEDURES/COMMENTS

1. Isolation and identification of *B. ovis*. Several semen samples should be cultured as the organism may be shed intermittently.
2. Complement fixation (CF) test: A titer of 1:10 or greater is considered positive. The CF test is considered more reliable than culture for detecting *B. ovis* infection. An enzyme-linked immunosorbent assay is used by some laboratories.
3. The modified acid-fast or Koster's stain is used to stain smears for *B. ovis*.

Treatment

Not usually practiced.

Control

Segregation of noninfected stock, particularly young rams. Test and removal or isolation of reactors. Because ewes are not involved in transmission, they are not removed or routinely vaccinated. Vaccination of rams with a killed *B. ovis* adjuvant bacterin is sometimes practiced.

OVINE EPIDIDYMITIS: GENERAL
The name "epididymitis of rams" (see OVINE BRUCELLOSIS) usually denotes a specific disease of sheep 1 year of age or older caused by *Brucella ovis* and characterized in the ram by epididymitis and infrequently in the ewe by placentitis and abortion.

Epididymitis occurs commonly in puberal rams and is frequently associated with bacteria other than *B. ovis*. The most frequently occurring are *Actinobacillus seminis, Histophilus ovis,* and *Actinobacillus actinomycetemcomitans.* Other less commonly associated bacteria are *Actinomyces pyogenes, Corynebacterium pseudotuberculosis, Pasteurella haemolytica, P. multocida, Streptococcus* and *Staphylococcus* spp.

Laboratory Diagnosis
SPECIMENS. Testicle and epididymis; semen.

PROCEDURES/COMMENTS. Isolation and identification of the bacteria involved from lesions. Recovery from semen only is not definitive, for some of the organisms mentioned above can occur as commensals in the genital tract.

Treatment
Antimicrobial treatment may be of value early but not if there is appreciable suppuration.

Control
Rams that don't respond to treatment are removed.

OVINE GENITAL CAMPYLOBACTERIOSIS / VIBRIONIC
ABORTION OF SHEEP, OVINE GENITAL VIBRIOSIS
Ovine genital campylobacteriosis (OGC) is a contagious, nonvenereal disease of sheep caused by *Campylobacter fetus* ssp. *fetus* and is characterized by multiple abortions in flocks during the last 8 weeks of pregnancy.

Distribution is worldwide but OGC is more prevalent in certain regions such as the Rocky Mountain area of the

United States. *C. fetus* ssp. *fetus* occurs as a commensal in the intestine of some cattle, sheep, and humans. The mode of transmission is by ingestion.

Differential Diagnosis

Because there are a number of causes of abortion in ewes (see INFECTIOUS OVINE AND CAPRINE ABORTION) including listeriosis, chlamydiosis, salmonellosis, and toxoplasmosis, laboratory confirmation is required.

The time of abortion and the characteristic fetal lesions may be suggestive of OGC.

Laboratory Diagnosis
SPECIMENS
1. Fresh whole fetus (preferably) or fetal stomach contents.
2. A number of serum samples from normal ewes and ewes that have aborted.

PROCEDURES/COMMENTS
1. For culture: A definitive diagnosis is made on the basis of the isolation and identification of *C. fetus* ssp. *fetus*. Positive fluorescent antibody–stained smears provide reliable identification of *C. fetus*. This stain does not distinguish between subspecies.

   Organisms with morphology and motility resembling *Campylobacter* can be demonstrated in the fetal stomach contents by negative staining and by phase microscopy.

   For pathology: The fetal liver may show small, gray necrotic foci. The fetus and fetal membranes may be edematous and body cavities may contain red-tinged fluid. These findings are supportive of a diagnosis of OGC.

   For serology: Some laboratories carry out an agglutination test.

   Negative: Most animals with low titers (1:20, 1:40).

   Positive: High titers from several animals including ones that have aborted.

Treatment

Ewes that have aborted should be segregated. During an outbreak, bacterin, penicillin, and streptomycin are given to pregnant ewes.

Control

Bacterins. Tetracyclines are sometimes fed during the last 8 weeks of pregnancy.

PAPILLOMATOSIS

Papillomatosis, or warts, is a disease principally of cattle, horses, dogs, and goats. It is caused by host-specific papillomaviruses and is characterized by the formation of benign tumors involving the skin and oral mucous membrane. The warts vary in size from occasionally large cauliflower-like growths in cattle to the small elevated tumors or warts in dogs.

The virus is resistant and remains viable for long periods of time in contaminated kennels, stanchions, fences, etc. Transmission is by direct and indirect contact. The disease is self-limiting and sometimes will clear up spontaneously.

Some characteristics of the warts seen in domestic animals are given briefly below:

BOVINE PAPILLOMATOSIS

Young cattle (usually less than 2 years old) are most severely affected with warts that appear mainly on the head, neck, and shoulders. The udder and teats are less frequently affected. The warts may be large, pendulant, or cauliflower-like in shape. Occasionally they occur on the penis and the vaginal mucous membrane, leading to breeding difficulty. At least six distinct papovavirus types have been identified as causing bovine papillomas. There is evidence that the kind of lesion seen depends on the particular virus type involved.

EQUINE PAPILLOMATOSIS

Warts are usually seen in horses up to 3 years of age, involving mainly the nose and lips. The papillomas vary in size and usually disappear within 2 or 3 months. Congenital papillomas occur on the head, neck, back, and croup of newborn foals that are infected in utero.

CANINE PAPILLOMATOSIS

Canine warts are usually found on the mucous membrane of the lips, mouth, tongue, and pharynx of young dogs. Although highly contagious, the warts usually disappear spontaneously in several months.

Skin warts, which may be caused by another papillomavirus, are mostly seen in older dogs. Cutaneous papillomas do not regress spontaneously. Dogs more than 2 years of age are usually immune to oral papillomatosis.

GOAT PAPILLOMATOSIS
Warts involving the skin, udder, and teats have been reported in goats.

Differential Diagnosis
A clinical diagnosis is made on the basis of the characteristic lesion.

Laboratory Diagnosis
A laboratory diagnosis is not usually necessary.

Treatment
Chemical treatment and surgery are sometimes used.

Commercial and autogenous vaccines, prepared with wart tissue, have been used for treatment with variable results.

Control
Autogenous wart vaccines are used for prophylaxis in cattle as well as in horses and dogs. Commercial wart vaccines are available for cattle and dogs. Their value is difficult to assess as warts often disappear spontaneously.

PAPULAR DERMATITIS OF HORSES
Papular dermatitis of horses is a benign disease thought to be caused by a virus and characterized by the production of firm papules of the skin (up to 2 cm in diameter) that do not progress to vesicles and pustules, but do result, finally, in a dry crust with alopecia. There is not appreciable systemic involvement.

The virus is probably spread by biting arthropods and the course ranges from 10 days to 6 weeks with uncomplicated recovery.

Papular dermatitis of horses has been reported only from Australia and the United States.

Because the disease is benign, it may frequently go undiagnosed. Attempts should be made to isolate and demonstrate virus from material collected from papules and vesicles.

PARAINFLUENZA-3 INFECTION OF CATTLE

Parainfluenza-3 (PI-3) virus, a paramyxovirus, is considered to be one of several primary causes of the bovine respiratory disease (BRD) complex (shipping fever, pneumonic pasteurellosis). See BOVINE RESPIRATORY DISEASE for a list of the other agents that can be involved.

Without secondary invaders, PI-3 virus causes a usually mild respiratory disease of cattle, horses, sheep, and possibly swine. Stresses such as those encountered in shipping, along with secondary bacterial invaders, lead frequently to severe BRD, which is most commonly a pneumonic pasteurellosis.

The virus is probably worldwide in distribution and occurs widely in cattle populations. Consequently, many animals have antibodies as a result of exposure. The virus is spread primarily by direct contact.

Differential Diagnosis

The diagnosis of PI-3 infection is only significant if it contributes to a diagnosis of more serious BRD. Diagnosis of the latter can only be complete if lungs or tracheal washes are also examined for such microorganisms as *Pasteurella haemolytica, P. multocida, Actinomyces pyogenes, Haemophilus somnus, Mycoplasma* spp., bovine herpesvirus 1, bovine virus diarrhea virus, bovine respiratory syncytial virus, etc.

Laboratory Diagnosis

Laboratory diagnosis should be directed to BRD rather than PI-3 infection alone.

SPECIMENS
1. Nasal swabs, tracheal washes, and portion of lungs.
2. Paired serum samples.

PROCEDURES/COMMENTS
1. Virus isolation is rarely carried out. The virus is not always present when BRD has reached the stage of a clinical bronchopneumonia. Fluorescent antibody test on frozen

lung sections is very reliable. Cultures should be attempted for potential bacteria.

2. Antibody titers (hemagglutination inhibition) in normal cattle in temperate zones will vary from 1:4 to 1:256. A fourfold increase in titer between acute and convalescent sera indicates infection.

Treatment

There is no treatment for PI-3 infection.

Control

Killed and live attenuated vaccines in various combinations with other agents are available. Presence of maternal antibodies in calves may affect active immunization.

PARATUBERCULOSIS / JOHNE'S DISEASE

Paratuberculosis is a contagious disease of cattle, sheep, and goats caused by the acid-fast organism *Mycobacterium paratuberculosis* and characterized by a long incubation period (up to 2 years), thickening of the intestinal wall, and recurring fetid diarrhea leading to emaciation and death. The genital tract of the male and female may be infected.

The disease in sheep and goats is widespread in some countries and is similar to the bovine disease except that diarrhea is less pronounced and the thickening of the intestinal wall is not as marked. It is progressive and proceeds to extreme emaciation and ultimately death.

The disease is worldwide in distribution and occurs widely in dairy and beef cattle with considerable variation in incidence from herd to herd. Because there is no national eradication program in the United States for this disease, it is difficult to determine its precise incidence. The organism is a facultative, intracellular parasite and the immune response is predominantly cell mediated.

Animals are infected by ingestion of food and water contaminated by feces. Calves may be infected in utero. The incidence of subclinical cases with intermittent shedding of *M. paratuberculosis* in feces is as high as 15%.

Differential Diagnosis

Emaciation with recurring fetid diarrhea is highly suggestive of paratuberculosis. Diarrhea is not a constant sign of the disease in sheep and goats. Salmonellosis, coccidiosis, parasitism, and molybdenum poisoning should be considered.

Laboratory confirmation is required.

Laboratory Diagnosis

Culture and identification of the causal organism is the most reliable means of diagnosis.

SPECIMENS/PROCEDURES

1. For culture: The preferred tissues for the isolation and cultivation of *M. paratuberculosis* are taken from the ileocecal junction and adjacent lymph nodes. Other portions of the intestinal tract can be submitted but the chances of isolation are less than from the aforementioned tissues. Feces should be rinsed from tissues before shipment. Clean tap water is satisfactory. Refrigerate if delay is anticipated. Do not use chemical preservatives.

   In the living animal, the fecal specimen is taken from the rectum using a dry, single-service glove. Approximately 0.5 ounce is placed in a suitable container (small jar or 1-ounce ointment tin is convenient). Seal with masking tape and ship to the laboratory in an insulated container. *Do not freeze samples.*

2. For staining: At necropsy, thin smears are made from the mucosa in the region of the ileocecal valve. In the live animal, smears are made from the feces (fluid) and from the mucosa pinched from the rectal wall. Smears are usually submitted to a diagnostic laboratory for acid-fast staining. An involved but effective procedure is to obtain tissue from mesenteric nodes in the region of the ileocecal valve by laparotomy. Smears and sections are stained and examined for mycobacteria.

3. For serology: Serum for the complement fixation test if such procedure is carried out by the laboratory. This test and the johnin test are mainly useful in detecting infected herds.

   An agar gel immunodiffusion test is used to detect antibodies in cattle, sheep, and goats. It is rapid, inexpensive, and most useful in confirming a clinical case of Johne's disease. The test is not useful for screening herds for the presence of Johne's disease, for many false negatives occur. A USDA-licensed test kit (see 13, Appendix

A), which uses the agar gel immunodiffusion procedure, is available.

COMMENTS. Cultivation and identification of *M. paratuberculosis* is the most reliable means of diagnosis. The organisms take 6–8 weeks to grow on culture media.

It is often difficult to demonstrate the organisms in smears. Rectal smears are only positive in advanced cases, usually less than 25% of infected animals.

The complement fixation test, because of false positive reactors, is not as reliable as culture.

The intravenous johnin test will detect about 80% of cases found positive by culture.

Enzyme-linked immunosorbent assay and tests measuring cell-mediated responses have shown promise in detecting early infections. Other serologic procedures are inefficient in this regard.

A species-specific DNA probe is available for rapid identification of *M. paratuberculosis* in bovine feces (see 12, Appendix A). The test may not be available in many diagnostic laboratories because of cost.

Treatment
None.

Control
Although difficult, control and eradication programs are employed in some countries.

Vaccination is practiced in some countries but not in North America. It sensitizes animals to johnin.

PASTEURELLA
Species of this genus are small, gram-negative rods or coccobacilli. Most occur as commensals and they vary greatly in their potential to cause disease. A number of new species have been added in recent years.

Pasteurella multocida: See Microbial Diseases Foreign to North America, HAEMORRHAGIC SEPTICEMIA; ENZOOTIC PNEUMONIA OF SHEEP AND SWINE; BOVINE RESPIRATORY DISEASE; ATROPHIC RHINITIS OF SWINE; etc. This is a serologically and biochemically heterogeneous species that occurs as a commensal in many animal species. It has the capacity to cause primary and secondary infections in all domestic animals, but particularly in cattle, swine, sheep, and goats. In addition to the diseases referred to above, it is causally involved in mastitis in cows and ewes, abortion, meningitis, encephalitis, and many other sporadic infections in all the domestic animals.

Three subspecies are now recognized: *P. multocida* ssp. *multocida* includes most of the strains causing significant disease in domestic animals; *P. multocida* ssp. *septica* has been recovered from dogs, cats, birds, and human beings; and *P. multocida* ssp. *gallicida* has been recovered from avian species. Because of the small differences among these subspecies, many laboratories may continue to identify strains by the species name only.

P. haemolytica: See BOVINE RESPIRATORY DISEASE, ENZOOTIC PNEUMONIA OF SHEEP, etc. This is also a serologically and biochemically heterogeneous species that often occurs as a commensal in cattle, sheep, and goats. It has a primary or secondary role in pneumonia of cattle, sheep, and goats; it is the primary cause of mastitis of ewes and septicemia of lambs. *Pasteurella haemolytica*–like organisms have been isolated from swine with enteritis; their pathogenic significance is not yet known.

P. pneumotropica: A commensal in the nasopharynx of rodents, dogs, and cats. Its potential for causing disease in cats and dogs is low.

P. aerogenes: Is part of the normal flora of the porcine intestine and rarely causes disease. It will eventually be reclassified.

P. dagmatis: A commensal of the oro- and nasopharynx of cats and dogs. Local and systemic infections have been described in humans as a result of animal bites. These strains are identical to a biotype of *P. pneumotropica*. It is not a significant cause of disease in cats and dogs.

P. canis: Many strains previously described as *Pasteurella*-like conform to this new species. It occurs in the canine oral cavity and has been responsible for bite infections in humans. It is not a significant cause of infections in dogs.

P. stomatis: A commensal in the respiratory tract of cats and

dogs. It does not appear to be important in infections in
the latter species.

P. caballi: This new species is a commensal in the upper respiratory tract of horses and is considered to have a causal
role in upper respiratory infections and pneumonia in
that species. It has also been recovered from a variety of
sporadic infections including wound infections, fistulous
withers, and a mesenteric abscess.

P. granulomatis: Isolated from lechiguana, a severe, progressive, fibrogranulomatous disease of cattle reported from
Southern Brazil.

P. anatis, P. gallinarum, P. avium, P. langaa: Species that
have been recovered only from avian species.

PHAEOHYPHOMYCOSIS / CHROMOMYCOSIS

Phaeohyphomycosis denotes an infrequent fungal infection
of humans, dogs, and horses and is caused by a number of
species of fungi. The infections, which begin in wounds or
abrasions, result in nodular and frequently ulcerating lesions
of the feet and legs with regionally granulomatous lymphadenitis.

These species of fungi have been incriminated: *Dactyla-
ria gallopava, Exophiala* spp., *Scolecobasidium humicola, S.
tshawytschae, Drechslera* spp., and *Fonsecaea pedrosoi.*

Differential Diagnosis

Phaeohyphomycosis should be suspected when chronic, granulomatous lesions resulting from wounds are seen involving
the feet, legs, and regional lymph nodes. Definitive diagnosis
depends upon the demonstration, isolation, and identification of the causative fungus.

Laboratory Diagnosis

SPECIMENS. Material from granulomatous and/or ulcerous
lesions, biopsies, or portions of lesions; fresh and fixed.

PROCEDURES. The characteristic brown-pigmented fungal
elements can be seen in wet mounts and sections of
lesions in phaeohyphomycosis. The fungi, which are slow
growing (up to 1 month), can be cultivated without difficulty
on Sabouraud agar at room temperature. Identification may
require the aid of a reference laboratory.

The finding of the fungal elements in tissue sections confirm the etiologic role of the fungus.

Control

1. Surgical excision in some cases.
2. Amphotericin B, locally and systemically.
3. Thiabendazole has been used successfully in humans; 5-fluorocytosine has also been effective in human cases.

PLAGUE

Plague is an acute, often fulminating disease of humans and rodents (including rats, squirrels, marmots, gerbils, and others) and is caused by the gram-negative organism *Yersinia pestis;* it is transmitted by fleas. Humans are considered accidental hosts. The disease transmitted from rodents to humans is called bubonic plague, and plague transmitted from human to human is termed pneumonic plague (spread by aerosol). Sylvatic plague is the name used for the plague that is endemic in woodland rodents in the American Southwest and some other countries. It is contracted from the bites of infected fleas and gives rise to bubonic plague in humans.

Domestic animals, with the exception of the cat, are relatively resistant to *Y. pestis.* However, natural infections have been reported in dogs, camels, elephants, buffaloes, and deer. A small number of acute cases of plague have been reported in cats in the southwestern United States. Characteristics of the disease have been high fever, abscessation of lymph nodes, and a mortality of approximately 50%. In several cases, there was transmission to humans.

Humans can become infected by (1) exposure to infected fleas on rodents brought home by cats; (2) exposure to infected fleas picked up and carried by dogs and cats; (3) direct contact with infected dogs, cats, and possibly other animals; and (4) fleas from infected cats, rats, other rodents, etc.

Differential Diagnosis

The possibility of feline plague should be kept in mind in areas of the sylvatic disease. Cats showing lymphadenopathy with abscesses should be particularly suspect.

Special precautions, including flea treatment and the use of gloves and masks, should be taken if plague is suspected.

Laboratory Diagnosis

If plague is suspected, exudate from abscesses should be sent to a special laboratory equipped to deal with the diagnosis of this dangerous pathogen. The location of such laboratories can be obtained in the United States through the Public Health Service. The animal should be treated for fleas and kept under strict isolation pending the results of the laboratory examination. A mask and gloves should be used when handling the animal.

The organism can be identified by specific fluorescent antibody staining in exudates. It can also be isolated, cultivated, and identified without difficulty.

If the specimen is highly contaminated, guinea pig inoculation is helpful for recovery of plague bacilli.

Treatment

Tetracyclines are effective if administered early enough. As mentioned above, special precautions must be taken if plague is suspected.

Control

Control of disease transmission largely depends on control of sylvatic reservoirs. The use of insecticides should precede the elimination of rodents, for otherwise the dislodged fleas seek human hosts. Vaccination and chemoprophylaxis are useful for preventing human exposures.

PORCINE EPERYTHROZOONOSIS

Porcine eperythrozoonosis is caused by the rickettsia (bacterium) *Eperythrozoon suis* that is transmitted from pig to pig by bloodsucking insects. The infection, which is usually subclinical, can on occasion produce a disease characterized by icterus, hemolytic anemia, inappetence, fever, and weakness in neonatal and stressed feeder pigs. Delayed estrus, early embryonic death, and abortions in late gestation have also been attributed to this agent.

It is probably worldwide in distribution. The incidence of the clinical disease is low; the extent of subclinical infections appears to be considerable. The severity of the disease appears to be dose related.

Differential Diagnosis

Nutritional anemias and anemias in association with various infections are among the diseases that should be considered.

A clinical diagnosis should be confirmed by laboratory tests.

Laboratory Diagnosis

SPECIMENS/PROCEDURES

1. For antibody (indirect hemagglutination and complement fixation tests): 10 cc clotted blood samples should be submitted from suspected cases.
2. For parasite demonstration: Obtain blood smears from a number of animals.
3. For packed-cell volume: Microhematocrit tubes of blood are taken from a number of suspected pigs.

COMMENTS

1. Indirect hemagglutination:
      Negative: titer less than 1:40
      Suspicious titer: 1:40 to 1:80
      Positive > 1:80
2. Giemsa-stained blood smears are definitive when positive. They also serve to distinguish normochromic anemia (eperythrozoonosis) from hypochromic anemia (iron deficiency). The disadvantage of blood smears is that the parasitemic stage may be missed.
3. Besides being able to determine the packed-cell volume, the microhematocrit tubes allow observation of icteric serum.

Treatment

1. Tetracyclines.
2. Hematinics.

Control

1. Reduction, if feasible, of bloodsucking insects.
2. Disinfection of surgical instruments and hypodermic needles from pig to pig.

PORCINE EPIDEMIC DIARRHEA

Porcine epidemic diarrhea (PED) is caused by a porcine coronavirus that is antigenically distinct from transmissible gastroenteritis (TGE) virus, and hemagglutinating encephalomy- elitis virus of pigs. PED is characterized by acute diarrhea, vomiting, and dehydration. The virus affects all age groups. Morbidity is very high in suckling pigs and mortality may reach 50% or higher.

Clinically, PED is indistinguishable from TGE. A defini- tive diagnosis can be made by fluorescent antibody staining of frozen sections of affected intestinal tissue.

PORCINE LEPTOSPIROSIS

Leptospirosis of swine occurs worldwide and is caused by several serovars of *Leptospira interrogans,* although serovar *pomona,* commonly called *L. pomona,* is the most common. It is characterized by disease that varies from a very mild form to an acute infection with fever, jaundice, hemorrhage, neurologic signs, and death. Many sows may abort late in pregnancy or pigs may be born weak or dead. A very acute leptospirosis is sometimes seen in young pigs due to *L. ictero- hemorrhagiae.* Serious infections can occur in humans, par- ticularly in farmers, veterinarians, and slaughterhouse work- ers.

There is a high incidence of subclinical infections in which the organisms can be shed for months in the urine from infected kidneys. The reservoir for *L. pomona* includes cattle, swine, skunk, and opossum. The other species, more correctly called serovars, that can also cause swine lepto- spirosis, viz., *L. grippotyphosa, L. canicola, L. bratislava,* also have a reservoir in wildlife.

A relatively new serovar *L. bratislava* has been one of the predominant serovars in swine in England and Ireland. Serologic studies conducted in recent years indicate that *L. bratislava* is also widespread in swine in the United States.

Transmission is by direct or indirect contact, with urine being the usual source of leptospira. The organisms can read- ily cross the skin and mucous membranes.

Differential Diagnosis

Brucellosis, pseudorabies, and porcine parvovirus and en- terovirus infections are among the diseases that should be considered.

Laboratory Diagnosis
SPECIMENS
1. For demonstration of leptospira: Fresh fetus; kidney and liver from adults and neonates; 20 ml of urine plus 1.5 ml of 10% formalin.
2. For isolation and culture: Fresh fetus; kidney and liver from adults and neonates; fresh urine diluted 1:10 in 1% bovine serum albumin.
3. For histopathology: Fixed tissues (see 2).
4. For serology: Serum samples taken at the time of abortion and 2 weeks later; also from some unaffected animals in the herd.

PROCEDURES/COMMENTS
1. Leptospira can sometimes be demonstrated by dark-field microscopy in fetal tissues, and kidney and liver of adults and neonates but most readily in urine. If formalin is not added to the urine, the leptospira become unrecognizable in several hours.
2. Isolation and culture in appropriate media is not commonly carried out.
3. Leptospira can be demonstrated in kidney and liver sections with silver impregnation stains.
4. A fourfold increase in titers of paired sera strongly suggests leptospirosis. Lower titers in apparently unaffected animals in the same herd would also suggest leptospirosis.

Treatment
Tetracyclines administered in the feed have been effective.

Control
1. Sows are sometimes treated prophylactically with tetracyclines for 2 weeks prior to farrowing.
2. Bacterins, usually polyvalent, are available.

PORCINE PARVOVIRUS INFECTION
Porcine parvovirus infection is considered one cause of fetal mummification and the birth of dead and/or weak pigs, particularly in gilts and young sows. The virus crosses the placenta and infects the fetus. The age of the fetus at the time of infection determines the degree of fetal damage. The virus causes infertility and congenital defects. If infection occurs

between 30 and 70 days after conception, mummified fetuses result. If infection takes place after 70 days gestation, weakened and/or stillborn piglets often result. There is a possibility of developing immune tolerance and a life-long carrier state as a result of very early infection of the fetus. Pregnant sows may not show any signs of the disease except reproductive failure.

The disease is probably worldwide in occurrence, and the incidence is high in swine herds in North America. The virus is shed in the feces, and the mode of infection is by ingestion of water and food contaminated with feces and other infectious discharges.

Differential Diagnosis

Brucellosis, leptospirosis, enterovirus infection, and pseudorabies infection should be considered. Because a number of different agents can cause mummification, stillbirths, and the birth of weak pigs, a laboratory diagnosis should be sought.

Laboratory Diagnosis
SPECIMENS
1. For fluorescent antibody (FA) staining: Fetal lung, kidney, liver, and spleen; whole fetus as fresh as possible; dead or stillborn pigs, and mummified fetuses.
2. For serology: Fetal serum or fluid extracted from fetal tissues.
3. For virus isolation: Same tissues as for FA staining listed in 1 above.

PROCEDURES/COMMENTS
1. Because the tissues of fetuses and stillborn pigs are often decomposed, the FA staining procedure is usually more effective than virus isolation.
2. Fetal serum and fetal tissue extracts can be tested for hemagglutinating activity and specific antibody. Because the virus is widespread, titers are found widely in sows and are not considered of value in diagnosis.

Hemagglutination inhibition (HAI) test is an important test to distinguish it from other viruses. Also, the HAI test is used to distinguish piglets that were infected in utero (HAI titer > 1:256 at 3 months) from those that

have maternal antibody (HAI titer < 1:256).
3. The virus is difficult to isolate and cultivate.

Treatment
None.

Control
Pigs from infected herds should not be introduced to herds that are free of the disease. If gilts are introduced to an infected herd they should be allowed to acquire immunity (virus exposure) before breeding. This can be promoted by maintaining a gilt pool with a wide age range.

Some indication of the animals at risk can be determined by serologic testing of gilts and young boars.

Live and inactivated vaccines are available.

PORCINE PYELONEPHRITIS
Porcine pyelonephritis is caused by a gram-positive, anaerobic, rod-shaped bacterium *Eubacterium suis*. The disease is characterized by cystitis and pyelonephritis in all ages of pigs and appears to be an ascending type in sows. This organism was formerly known as *Corynebacterium suis*.

The disease has been recognized most frequently in breeding sows in Europe; it also occurs in North America, Canada, Mexico, Australia, and no doubt other countries. Boars may carry *E. suis* as normal flora in the preputial diverticulum and serve as the source of infection.

Laboratory Diagnosis
This disease is most often recognized at necropsy.

SPECIMEN
1. Urine and/or vaginal discharge for culture. Proper collection and submission of specimens for anaerobic culture are necessary for isolation of *E. suis* (see Section 1).
2. Smears of urinary sediment and pus may be submitted for direct examination.

PROCEDURE/COMMENTS
1. Urine and/or vaginal discharge are cultured aerobically and anaerobically for isolation and identification of *E. suis*. Recovery of *E. suis* is difficult if specimens are sub-

mitted in an aerobic environment.
2. Presence of a large number of gram-positive, slender rods in the urinary sediment or pus smear is a good indication of *E. suis* infection.

Control

Penicillin therapy in early stages of infection is effective. Treatment is rarely successful in advanced cases.

POTOMAC HORSE FEVER / EQUINE MONOCYTIC
EHRLICHIOSIS, EQUINE EHRLICHIAL COLITIS

Potomac horse fever (PHF) is an apparently noncontagious disease of horses caused by the rickettsia *Ehrlichia risticii* and characterized by fever, anorexia, leukopenia, listlessness, and usually, diarrhea. The mortality rate is estimated to be approximately 30%. Laminitis may be a complication. Ulcerative gastroenteritis is the most visible lesion at necropsy.

The disease was first reported in Maryland but is now known to occur throughout the eastern United States and in other regions of the country. It has also been reported from France and India.

It is seasonal, occurring from May to October, and is thought to be transmitted by biting arthropods. The reservoir host is not known.

Differential Diagnosis

The diseases that most resemble PHF clinically are salmonellosis, equine clostridiosis, and colitis-X. Because diarrhea is not always present, other infectious febrile diseases may resemble PHF. The disease can only be diagnosed with certainty by laboratory means.

Laboratory Diagnosis
SPECIMENS
1. Acute and convalescent sera are preferred.
2. Unclotted blood or blood smear for direct examination.

PROCEDURES
1. The indirect fluorescent antibody (IFA) test and the enzyme-linked immunosorbent assay for the detection and titration of antibodies are available in a number of laboratories.

2. Demonstration of the morulae of *Ehrlichia* in stained blood smears (in monocytes and neutrophils) is indicative of PHF. Because of the irregular presence of the rickettsiae in smears, this procedure is not usually carried out.

COMMENTS. There is no serologic cross reaction between the ehrlichia of this disease and *E. equi.* Serologic procedures (IFA) are used almost exclusively for the diagnosis of PHF.

While the IFA test does not discriminate between present and past exposure, horses that react positively and have characteristic clinical signs should be considered to have PHF.

The organism can be isolated, cultured, and identified in macrophage cultures although this is a specialized diagnostic procedure.

Treatment

Tetracyclines are effective in many cases if administered early enough. Early fluid supportive therapy is beneficial.

Control

Although the mode of transmission is not known, it is thought to be via biting arthropods. Ticks and blackflies are prevalent during the peak period of the disease, i.e., from May to late June in east central United States. Efforts should be directed at reducing exposure to biting insects and eliminating ticks. A bacterin is available.

POXVIRUSES

Poxviruses are large DNA viruses grouped in the family Poxviridae. These viruses cause mainly skin lesions that are characterized by the formation of papules, followed by vesicles, pustules, and finally scabs.

The following diseases caused by poxviruses are discussed separately: COWPOX (orthopoxvirus), PSEUDO-COWPOX (parapoxvirus), SWINEPOX (suipoxvirus), BOVINE PAPULAR STOMATITIS (parapoxvirus), SHEEP-AND GOATPOX (capripoxvirus), LUMPY SKIN DISEASE (capripoxvirus), and CONTAGIOUS ECTHYMA (parapoxvirus). Other poxviruses are the following:

Vaccinia virus (orthopoxvirus): Cattle and humans are the hosts of this virus. Cattle usually acquire the virus from humans vaccinated with the vaccinia virus. Vesicles, followed by crusting, are seen on the teats and udders of infected cows. Vesicles may rupture during milking and become infected with secondary bacteria. Since smallpox vaccination with this virus has been discontinued, the disease in cattle and humans appears to no longer exist.

Catpox virus (orthopoxvirus): Causes infrequent, acute, or chronic skin infections in domestic and exotic cats and other felids. The infection, which has been reported in Europe mainly, may result in a single skin lesion with rash or multiple skin lesions. Occasionally, the virus may cause serious respiratory disease in cats. There are reports of transmission to humans. Definitive diagnosis is by virus isolation and identification, or by direct fluorescent antibody staining of clinical material.

PROGRESSIVE PNEUMONIA OF SHEEP AND GOATS
/ MAEDI-VISNA

Progressive pneumonia is a contagious, nonfebrile disease of adult sheep and goats, most commonly in animals more than 2 years of age, and involves the central nervous system and/or respiratory tract. It is caused by a retrovirus (lentivirus) and is characterized by a chronic, insidious course with such signs as dyspnea, circling, trembling, deviation of the head, emaciation, progressive paresis, and finally death.

The name Maedi has been given to the pneumonic form; visna refers to the neural form.

It has been reported from all continents except Australia and is sporadic in occurrence. The virus is present in respiratory secretions and feces and the mode of infection is by droplets (inhalation) and ingestion. The virus will survive at least 4 months at refrigerator temperature.

Differential Diagnosis

The incubation period and the course may each be as long as 2 years. Signs depend on whether the animal has the pneumonic form, the neural form, or both.

Pulmonary adenomatosis, enzootic pneumonia, rabies, listeriosis, louping ill, scrapie, caseous lymphadenitis with pulmonary involvement, verminous pneumonia, and brain abscessation should be considered.

Laboratory Diagnosis

SPECIMENS

1. Serum samples from advanced cases and in-contact animals.
2. In the Maedi form: Portions of lung, fresh and fixed.
3. In the Visna form: Portions of the cerebrum and cerebellum, fresh and fixed.

PROCEDURES. The following procedures are only performed in specialized laboratories and not in all diagnostic laboratories:

1. Serum neutralization test is helpful in advanced cases. Complement fixation test is preferred over virus neutralization test for serodiagnosis, since complement-fixing antibody appears early in the disease.
2. Virus isolation and identification in cell cultures using fresh lung and brain.

   Histopathologic examination of affected lung and brain. Significant changes include interstitial pneumonia with lymphoid nodules, and in the brain a periventriculitis with demyelination.

Treatment

None.

Control

The disease is controlled by eradication procedures involving removal and slaughter or temporary segregation of infected animals and finally restocking with serologically negative animals.

PROTOTHECA

These are microscopic, colorless achlorophyllic algae of the family Chlorellaceae. They are ubiquitous in nature and are occasionally recovered from clinical specimens in which they are not usually significant. Some are infrequent opportunists that would appear to produce disease only if host resistance is impaired. *Prototheca* have been reported to cause bovine mastitis, localized infection in cats, and disseminated protothecosis in dogs.

Laboratory diagnosis

Laboratory diagnosis involves isolation, cultivation and identification, and/or demonstration of algal cells in unstained wet mounts and stained smears.

Treatment

Amphotericin B and ketoconazole have shown promise in human infections.

PSEUDOCOWPOX / PARAVACCINIA, MILKER'S NODULES

Pseudocowpox is a widespread, frequently occurring, mild disease caused by a parapoxvirus. It is characterized by the formation of small papules on the udder and teats that progress to vesicles, sometimes pustules, and finally scabs within 1 or 2 weeks.

Granulomas develop under the scabs and may persist for several months giving the affected teats a roughened aspect. The disease will usually spread through the herd. It is worldwide in occurrence.

The infection can also spread to milkers, with development of painless purplish nodules on the fingers and hands. Although itchy, the nodules disappear in a few weeks without causing any serious discomfort.

Differential Diagnosis

The disease is frequently not considered significant enough to warrant veterinary attention and is often allowed to run its course. Warts, cowpox (apparently rare in North America), and bovine ulcerative mammillitis should be considered.

If a diagnosis is made, it is most often based on clinical signs rather than on laboratory findings.

Laboratory Diagnosis
SPECIMENS/PROCEDURES

For culture and electron microscopic (EM) examination: Fluid from vesicles.

The virus can be cultivated and identified in cell cultures. A presumptive diagnosis can be made by identifying parapoxviruses in vesicular fluid and scrapings from lesions by electron microscopy.

Treatment
Local, with ointments and astringents.

Control
Good sanitary milking practices. Special measures to prevent spread within a herd are not usually effective.

PSEUDORABIES / AUJESZKY'S DISEASE, MAD ITCH, INFECTIOUS BULBAR PARALYSIS

Pseudorabies is primarily a disease of swine, rodents, and infrequently many other animal species, caused by a herpesvirus (porcine herpesvirus-1). It is characterized in older swine by a usually inapparent infection and in younger pigs by an acute, fatal encephalitis.

When other species, including farm animals, dogs, cats, and rabbits, are infected, usually as single cases, there is an intense pruritis at the entry site of the virus with self-mutilation followed by an acute fatal encephalitis.

It is endemic in the swine of many countries. Adult swine are the principal reservoir of the virus. It occurs frequently in the United States but not in Canada and Australia. The incidence varies with regions.

Differential Diagnosis
Incoordination of the hind limbs, paddling movements, and convulsions in young pigs are characteristic. Intense pruritis and encephalitic signs in other animals, usually single cases, are suggestive of pseudorabies. Other diseases in which neurologic signs are seen should be considered in the various animals: e.g., in pigs Teschen and Teschen-like diseases, and vomiting and wasting disease. The possibility of rabies and bacterial meningitis caused by *Streptococcus suis* and other bacteria should always be considered. Laboratory confirmation is recommended.

Laboratory Diagnosis
SPECIMENS
1. From all species, submit one half of the brain (fresh) after longitudinal bisection, skin, and subcutaneous tissue (except pigs) at the site of the pruritis, and portions of the cord. The other half of the brain and portions of the cord should be fixed for histopathology. Portions of lung, ton-

sil, spleen, and kidney should be submitted from pigs in addition to the brain and cord.

2. Serum samples from swine to determine whether or not pigs have been exposed.

PROCEDURES/COMMENTS

1. Demonstration of the virus in frozen sections by the fluorescent antibody (FA) procedure indicates infection. This may be followed by virus isolation and identification, but FA demonstration is sufficient.

2. A positive virus neutralization test, even at the lowest titer, indicates exposure to the virus but not necessarily infection. An enzyme-linked immunosorbent assay is also available for the detection of antibodies to pseudorabies virus. A positive reaction in the screening test indicates infection.

Several commercial test kits are available to detect antibodies in the serum or plasma (see 3,6,9,12,16,19, Appendix A).

A skin test (delayed hypersensitivity) has been used successfully to detect infection in adult pigs.

A diagnosis of pseudorabies can be made on the basis of finding the characteristic inclusion bodies of the disease in histopathologic sections.

Treatment

None.

Control

Herds may be kept free of pseudorabies by adding only serologically negative pigs.

Live attenuated and inactivated virus vaccines are available to reduce losses in herds in which the disease is a continuing problem. Vaccination does not necessarily prevent infection or shedding of the virus.

PULMONARY ADENOMATOSIS / JAAGSIEKTE, OVINE PULMONARY ADENOMATOSIS

Pulmonary adenomatosis is a chronic, contagious disease of sheep and goats caused by a virus (probably a retrovirus) and characterized by a progressive pneumonia and a long incubation period (months to years). The most characteristic pathologic feature is the presence of alveolar adenomata.

The disease occurs infrequently in North and South America, Europe, Asia, and Africa. A high morbidity has been reported in Iceland.

Differential Diagnosis

Chronic progressive pneumonia, verminous pneumonia, enzootic pneumonia, and other chronic pneumonias and pulmonary tumors should be considered.

Laboratory Diagnosis

SPECIMENS. Portions of affected lungs, fresh and fixed.

PROCEDURES. The virus is not readily cultivable, but viral and other microbial isolations should be carried out for differential purposes. The characteristic microscopic tissue changes, adenomatous proliferation of alveolar epithelial cells, and the absence of inclusion bodies help differentiate it from chronic progressive pneumonia.

COMMENTS. A diagnosis is usually based upon the history and clinical findings, along with the results of microbial and pathologic examinations.

Treatment

None.

Control

The disease has been controlled in Iceland by isolation and slaughter methods. Tissue vaccines have shown some promise.

PYTHIOSIS / MYCOTIC SWAMP CANCER, FLORIDA HORSE LEECHES, OOMYCOSIS

Pythiosis is a chronic skin disease of horses, cattle, and dogs caused by the fungus *Pythium insidiosum* (formerly called *Hyphomyces destruens*) and characterized by the formation of fibrogranulomatous skin lesions, ulcers, and necrosis. Fistulous tracts may be seen in advanced cases. The fungus gains entrance via wounds involving the hoof, hock, fetlock, head, neck, and lips. Several cases of intestinal pythiosis have been described in the horse.

The disease, which was originally called phycomycosis, is seen mainly in tropical and subtropical areas including Australia, New Guinea, India, Japan, Indonesia, and South America. A number of cases have been reported in southern United States.

Laboratory Diagnosis

SPECIMENS/PROCEDURES/COMMENTS. Affected tissue or biopsies, fresh and fixed, or smears from clinical material for direct examination. Pythiosis is suspected if hyphae are demonstrable in stained sections and smears from characteristic lesions.

Cultivation and identification is rather involved and may require the assistance of a mycologist. Characteristic zoospores, seen in cultures, aid in identification.

An immunodiffusion test is available in some reference laboratories.

Treatment

Surgery and amphotericin B.

Q FEVER

Q fever is a mild, acute, febrile disease of humans and animals caused by the rickettsia *Coxiella burnetii* and characterized in humans by an influenza-like disease with pneumonitis and such various manifestations as chronic endocarditis, pericarditis, hepatitis, and systemic infection. The mortality is less than 1% in treated cases with the exception of elderly patients and those with hepatitis or endocarditis.

Q fever is found worldwide and the reservoir of *C. burnetii* is ticks, cattle, sheep, goats, and some wild animals including bandicoots, kangaroos, caribou, and bison. The disease in wild animals is transmitted via body fluids and ticks. The disease in domestic animals, particularly cattle, sheep and goats, is transmitted via milk, discharges, placenta, and feces. Dust and aerosols derived from the latter infectious materials serve to infect humans as well as animals. The survival of *C. burnetii* in the environment is probably due to endospore-like forms. The disease in wild and domestic animals is ordinarily mild although abortion has been reported in cattle, sheep, and goats.

The disease in animals is significant mainly because it serves as a source of infection for humans.

Laboratory Diagnosis

Coxiella burnetii infection is rarely diagnosed clinically in animals. It is infrequently detected in the laboratory as a cause of abortion. The laboratory diagnosis of the disease in humans is carried out in Public Health Laboratories.

SPECIMENS. The specimen most frequently indicated is placenta in the case of *C. burnetii* abortion.

PROCEDURES. *Coxiella burnetii* can be demonstrated in the cells of affected tissues by direct immunofluorescence. Special stains (Gimenez, etc.) are also employed to demonstrate the organism in cells although they do not differentiate *C. burnetii* from *Chlamydia psittaci.* Isolation and identification of the organism is not carried out in many laboratories.

Complement fixation and microagglutination tests are useful when paired sera are submitted although very few laboratories carry out these tests.

RABIES / HYDROPHOBIA

Rabies is a fatal (rare exceptions) encephalitis of all warm-blooded mammals caused by a rhabdovirus (lyssavirus) and manifested mainly in either a furious or dumb (paralytic) form. The infection usually originates in a bite wound and ascends a nerve trunk to the cord and brain. The incubation period is variable and, on occasions, has been longer than 6 months.

The disease is worldwide except for Australia, New Zealand, the British Isles, Hawaii, the Scandinavian countries, Cyprus, and Japan. It is frequently endemic in wild animals including the skunk, fox, raccoon, wolf, bobcat, and coyote. There are also periodic epidemics among wild animals. Asymptomatic salivary gland infections occur in vampire bats resulting in prolonged viremia. Insectivorous bats may also be infected.

Four serotypes of lyssavirus are recognized. Serotype 1 is responsible for classical rabies. The virus is shed in the saliva from infected salivary glands. The disease almost always results from the bites of infected or rabid animals. Several cases in humans have resulted from aerosol exposure.

Although susceptible to common disinfectants and ultraviolet light, the virus retains its viability in tissues for several weeks at room or refrigerator temperatures.

Clinical Signs

The signs listed below are for the dog; however, the signs in other domestic and wild animals are similar. The incubation period is usually 2–8 weeks but can be several months. The course is 3–10 days.

Prodromal form: Animals show apprehension, anxiety, and changes in temperament and behavior. Severe pruritis may develop at the site of exposure. This stage lasts from 1 to 3 days.

Furious form: Aimless wandering; bumps into objects; excitement; irritability; bites or attempts to bite animals, people, and inanimate objects; depraved appetite; bark altered; muscle paralysis, salivation, convulsions, ataxia, paralysis, and death.

Paralytic form: This form is most common. Lethargic and hides; doesn't usually bite; muscular tremors; perceived difficulty in swallowing; terminal paralysis.

Inapparent form: This form has been observed in dogs, cats, skunks, and bats. These animals may seroconvert, survive, and serve as a source of the virus for extended periods. Bats may be asymptomatic or have protracted clinical signs with transmission of the virus for months. There have been two known recoveries in humans.

Differential Diagnosis

Canine distemper, pseudorabies, canine hepatitis, listeriosis, cryptococcosis, toxoplasmosis, and other infections of the central nervous system should be considered. Poisons such as lead, strychnine, and various pesticides.

Laboratory Diagnosis

Rabies can only be definitively diagnosed by laboratory means. After human exposure to a dog or cat suspected of having rabies, the dog or cat may be killed and submitted to the laboratory immediately, or be confined for 10 days. If suspicious signs develop, the animal should be killed and submitted to the laboratory for tests.

Check first with your local Public Health Laboratory or whichever laboratory does rabies diagnosis.

SPECIMENS

1. The entire carcass or head.
2. Live animal.

PROCEDURES/COMMENTS

1. The fluorescent antibody (FA) procedure is widely used and is the preferred method. It is used on animals that have died or been killed and is recommended for the immediate examination of wild animals that cannot be readily held for observation. Smears of the hippocampus major are usually employed, but they can also be made from the salivary gland. Mice are inoculated with selected negative specimens. Correlation of 99.9% between FA and mouse inoculation results is reported.

2. Demonstration of Negri bodies in the neurons of the hippocampus major using Giemsa and Sellers' stains. They are more apt to be found in animals that die of rabies. If Negri bodies are not seen, mice are inoculated intracerebrally with a suspension of brain.

3. In the living animal, a biopsy taken from the skin of the face (including tactile hair) and stained with FA reagents is recommended for a rapid diagnosis. This is not a standard test and should not be used in unvaccinated animals where there has been human exposure.

Treatment

None.

Control

A variety of live attenuated and inactivated vaccines are available.

Avian flury strain: A modified live virus (MLV) vaccine. The high egg passage can be used in dogs, cats, and cattle. The low egg passage can only be used in dogs.

Cell culture MLV vaccines: Cause fewer allergic reactions than the avian strain. They are given intramuscularly to take advantage of the large amount of nervous tissue in the muscle. There have been postvaccinal reactions in cats.

Inactivated nerve tissue vaccines: Have been made from goats and mice. The goat origin vaccine may cause postvaccinal paralysis. The mouse brain vaccine, because of its lack of myelin, does not cause postvaccinal paralysis and is highly antigenic.

Maternal antibodies from vaccinated females will protect most neonates until 3 months of age. There are several types of vaccines but the first injection should be given at 3 months and the second injection at 1 year of age. Animals should be revaccinated every 2–3 years.

Decisions frequently have to be made by veterinarians regarding human exposure. It is important to remember that the virus can be in the saliva of infected animals from 1 to 13 days before clinical signs occur. The location and severity of the bite are quite important. Persons bitten in the face by a stray animal should begin treatment immediately if the animal cannot be found. When the animal is available and has not been vaccinated, it should be sacrificed and the brain examined by the FA test.

Inactivated human or animal cell culture vaccines, rabies immune globulin, and antirabies serum (equine) are widely used for prophylaxis in humans.

REOVIRUS INFECTIONS

Reovirus infections of domestic animals are usually inapparent or mild.

Bovine reovirus infection is widespread in North America and characterized by mild respiratory infections in calves. Complications may occur due to secondary bacterial infections.

Equine reovirus infection is characterized by a cough and nasal and ocular discharges with no fever.

Canine reovirus infection is characterized by a mild or inapparent upper respiratory infection.

The feline reovirus causes gingivitis, conjunctivitis, and lacrimal photophobia in domestic cats.

Reoviruses are transmitted primarily by direct contact or by aerosol.

Laboratory Diagnosis

Isolation and identification of the virus in cell cultures. Virus neutralization and hemagglutination inhibition tests on paired serum samples are useful for diagnosis of feline and bovine reoviral infections. In view of the usually mild character of these infections, they no doubt frequently go unrecognized.

RHINOSPORIDIOSIS

Rhinosporidiosis is a chronic disease of horses, mules, cattle, dogs, and humans caused by the fungus *Rhinosporidium seeberi* and characterized by the formation of polyps on the nasal and ocular mucosa. They may be sufficiently large and numerous to interfere with respiration.

The fungus, which has not been cultivated on artificial media, is thought to occur in water as a free-living organism. It is presumed to gain entry to the nasal mucosa via wounds.

Although the disease is worldwide in distribution and occurs occasionally in the United States, most cases are seen in tropical and subtropical countries.

Differential Diagnosis

Finding the typical polyps will suggest a diagnosis of rhinosporidiosis; however, other fungi occasionally cause nasal granulomas. Definitive diagnosis depends upon the demonstration of the characteristic large sporangia in sections of the polyps or in nasal discharge.

Laboratory Diagnosis

SPECIMENS. For direct examination and culture: Nasal discharge and surgically removed polyps, fresh and fixed.

PROCEDURES/COMMENTS
1. Nasal discharge and material from polyps are examined in wet mounts for the presence of the characteristic fungal elements.
2. Stained sections of polyps are examined for the sporangia and spores.
3. Nasal discharge and ground polyps are cultured on bacterial and fungal media.

A definitive diagnosis depends on the demonstration of the characteristic fungal elements in polyps. The organism does not grow on artificial media.

Treatment

Surgical removal of polyps is usually curative. When there is recurrence, drugs such as dapsone (long term) and ketoconazole have been effective.

RHINOVIRUS INFECTIONS

Rhinoviruses cause inapparent to usually mild infections in cattle and horses. They are probably most important in providing entree to secondary bacteria.

Rhinovirus infection of cattle is characterized by serous nasal discharge, fever, coughing, anorexia, hyperpnea, dyspnea, or pneumonia. It is not an economically important disease of cattle; however, secondary bacterial infection may result in significant economic losses (see BOVINE RESPIRATORY DISEASE).

In horses, rhinoviruses cause an upper respiratory tract infection that may become severe as a result of invasion by secondary bacteria (see EQUINE RESPIRATORY DISEASE). The complicated disease is characterized by fever, cough, nasal discharge, lymphadenitis, and abscess of the maxillary lymph glands.

Laboratory Diagnosis

Virus neutralization test with paired sera; virus isolation and identification employing cell cultures.

RHODOCOCCAL PNEUMONIA OF FOALS /
CORYNEBACTERIAL PNEUMONIA OF FOALS

Rhodococcal pneumonia, caused by *Rhodococcus equi* (formerly *Corynebacterium equi*), affects foals usually 1–3 months of age and is characterized by fever, coughing, anorexia, and a bronchopneumonia with multiple, usually large, abscesses in the lungs and bronchial lymph nodes. The course is up to 2 weeks and the mortality is high in young foals.

In foals older than 3 months, a subacute form of the disease with a longer course is seen. Septicemia has been reported in 1-month-old foals. The organism can occasionally be recovered from the equine cervix. Extrapulmonary infections occur occasionally in older horses.

Rhodococcus equi is a small, pleomorphic, gram-positive rod that occurs in soil, manure, and litter. The organism is carried as a commensal in the alimentary tract of some male and female horses. Infection is by ingestion or inhalation. Pulmonary migration of helminth larvae may predispose to infection. Occurrence of this pneumonia is probably worldwide.

Differential Diagnosis

The younger foals are affected most severely; pneumonia, dyspnea, fever, anorexia, and finally emaciation. There are loud, moist rales on auscultation; the course is usually 1–2 weeks.

Respiratory infections caused by other agents, e.g., streptococci and various viruses including those of equine rhinopneumonitis and viral arteritis (see EQUINE RESPIRATORY DISEASE).

Laboratory Diagnosis

SPECIMENS. Cervical swabs from the mare; transtracheal aspirate; portions of lung and lymph nodes containing abscesses, or swabs from excised abscesses; nasal swabs, although there is not usually a nasal discharge.

PROCEDURES. Definitive diagnosis depends on isolation and identification of *R. equi*.

Treatment

Penicillin is the preferred drug, but if abscesses are established, treatment is usually unsuccessful. Large doses of penicillin, erythromycin, gentamycin, or one of the rifamycins given for several weeks have been effective.

Control

1. Vaccines are not available. Autogenous vaccines have not been effective.
2. Long-acting penicillin is used on foals shortly after birth when an outbreak is in progress. Colostrum is important.
3. Mares should not be allowed to foal on contaminated premises or quarters and foals should not be kept in such an environment.
4. Anthelmintics for helminths.

RHODOCOCCUS

Members of this genus are gram-positive, variably acid-fast, and occur as coccoid and rod forms. Only two species are known to be pathogenic for animals.

Rhodococcus equi (formerly *Corynebacterium equi*): see RHODOCOCCAL PNEUMONIA OF FOALS. It is isolated frequently from lesions simulating tuberculosis in the cervical and pharyngeal lymph nodes of swine. It is an infrequent cause of metritis and abortion in mares, and diarrhea in neonatal and older foals.

R. sputi: Has been recovered from mesenteric lymphadenitis in swine.

ROCKY MOUNTAIN SPOTTED FEVER

Rocky Mountain spotted fever is a febrile disease, principally of humans, caused by *Rickettsia rickettsii*. The human infections vary from mild to quite severe and fatal. Young sheep and dogs are susceptible but the disease is usually mild or subclinical, although there have been recent reports of some severe infections in young dogs. These resembled canine ehrlichiosis clinically.

The reservoir of the agent is principally wild rodents, hares, rabbits, and the ticks (at least six species in the United States) that feed on them. Most infections in humans and animals result from tick bites, although bites cannot always be found. Tick feces and fluids contain the organism, which can penetrate the skin and conjunctivae. Dogs may bring infected ticks into contact with humans.

The organism multiplies in endothelial cells resulting in thrombosis and hemorrhages. When small peripheral blood vessels are involved, there is a widespread skin rash.

Most cases in the United States occur in eastern United States; it is infrequent in the Rocky Mountain regions. The disease also occurs in Canada, Mexico, and Central and South America.

Differential Diagnosis

Other febrile diseases and particularly canine ehrlichiosis should be considered. A thrombocytopenia has been a consistent finding in the canine disease.

Laboratory Diagnosis

This is carried out in some diagnostic laboratories where the disease occurs.

SPECIMENS. Because the agent is highly infectious for humans, blood and tissues should be handled with great care. Paired serum samples are required, for many dogs will have titers in endemic regions; skin biopsies.

PROCEDURES. The serologic procedures recommended for canine sera are the microimmunofluorescent, enzyme-linked immunosorbent assay, and latex agglutination tests. A fourfold increase in IgG titer is considered significant.

Demonstration of rickettsia in fluorescent antibody-stained preparations of skin biopsies is significant.

Treatment
Tetracyclines and chloramphenicol are effective.

Control
Prevention in dogs requires tick control. No vaccine is available.

ROTAVIRUS AND CORONAVIRUS INFECTIONS OF CALVES

These viruses are important causes of enteric infection and diarrhea in young calves.

Rotavirus usually affects calves up to 7 days of age, whereas coronavirus infects calves from 1 day to 3 weeks of age. Both viruses are responsible for disease characterized by a profuse, watery diarrhea of sudden onset, which shortly results in extreme dehydration.

These infections occur most commonly in dairy calves and are probably worldwide in occurrence. Both viruses can be recovered from the intestine of many normal calves. The viruses are shed in the feces and the mode of infection is by ingestion. Insufficient colostral antibody is thought to contribute to the development of these infections.

Enteropathogenic *E. coli* may act in concert with either of these viruses in causing diarrhea, particularly after the intestinal mucosa has been rendered vulnerable by necrosis and the loss of epithelial cells.

Differential Diagnosis
Enteric diseases of young calves should be considered (see ENTERIC INFECTIONS OF YOUNG CALVES). Definitive diagnosis requires laboratory procedures.

Laboratory Diagnosis
SPECIMENS. Segments of intestine including spiral colon, ileum, and jejunum, fresh and fixed. Feces are of value if collected shortly after the onset of clinical signs.

PROCEDURES/COMMENTS. The most convenient and effective procedure is the fluorescent antibody (FA) staining of fecal smears (primarily for rotavirus) and frozen sections of intestine. The viruses are identified by specific FA staining.

An enzyme-linked immunosorbent assay on feces is also used for rapid diagnosis of rotavirus by several laboratories. A latex agglutination test is also commercially available (see 1, Appendix A).

The demonstration of rotaviruses and coronaviruses in fecal suspensions by electron microscopy is also useful.

The finding of characteristic histopathologic changes, including villus atrophy, blunting, and fusions, is supportive.

Treatment

Antibiotics for *E. coli* (after susceptibility test).

Control

Adequate colostrum. Isolation. Good management and sanitation. Rotaviruses and coronaviruses are relatively resistant in the environment.

Parenteral immunization of cows and heifers prior to parturition with a live rotavirus and coronavirus vaccine is widely practiced. An inactivated *E. coli* bacterin is sometimes included.

ROTAVIRUS INFECTIONS OF FOALS

Rotavirus has been incriminated as a cause of enteritis and diarrhea in foals. It is most serious during the first 2 weeks of life and is characterized by depression, a greenish watery diarrhea, dehydration, and reluctance to nurse. It is usually mild and of short duration unless complicated by concurrent bacterial infection. A chronic form occurs in 10–40% of infected foals up to 8 months of age causing intermittent diarrhea.

Differential Diagnosis

For other diseases that should be considered in the differential diagnosis, see ENTERIC INFECTIONS OF YOUNG FOALS. *E. coli, Salmonella* and *Actinobacillus equuli* infections are of particular significance.

Laboratory Diagnosis

The virus can most readily be demonstrated in feces within 24–48 hours of the onset of diarrhea.

The characteristic virus can be seen by the examination of feces with the electron microscope.

An enzyme-linked immunosorbent assay has also been used to detect virus in the feces. An equally sensitive latex agglutination test is also available (see 1, Appendix A).

The virus is difficult to isolate and cultivate.

Treatment

Fluids for the dehydration; antibiotics for complicating bacteria; and general supportive measures.

Control

Foals are usually protected by an adequate amount of colostrum. Affected foals should be kept in isolation.

ROTAVIRUS INFECTIONS OF LAMBS

There are reports of rotaviruses causing a diarrheal syndrome in neonatal lambs. The disease is similar to that caused by rotaviruses in calves, pigs, and foals. Because the rotaviruses are related antigenically, the fluorescent antibody reagent used for the calf disease can also be used in lambs. The same kind of specimens are submitted as for calves. As in other rotavirus infections it is important to obtain specimens within 1 or 2 days of the onset of disease.

The laboratory diagnosis is essentially the same as for ROTAVIRUS INFECTION OF CALVES (q.v.).

ROTAVIRUS INFECTIONS OF PIGLETS

Rotavirus infects piglets in the age range of 1–8 weeks, most often 3–8 weeks, producing a diarrhea resembling that of transmissible gastroenteritis of moderate severity. Enterotoxigenic strains of *E. coli* may also be involved in the etiology.

Although worldwide in distribution, not enough information is available to be precise as to actual distribution and occurrence. Rotaviruses are common in the intestines of many normal animals. Infections probably result from several factors including stress, poor sanitation, and inadequate colostral immunity.

Differential Diagnosis

Some of the diseases and agents that should be considered are listed under ENTERIC INFECTIONS OF PIGLETS. Because several agents can cause clinically indistinguishable diarrheal disease, a laboratory diagnosis should be sought.

Laboratory Diagnosis

SPECIMENS

1. For fluorescent antibody (FA) staining: Mucosal smears are made from the duodenum, jejunum, and ileum of a piglet that has had diarrhea for less than 24 hours. Frozen sections of duodenum, jejunum, ileum, and spiral colon are equally useful.
2. For electron microscopic examination: Feces from a piglet with diarrhea of no longer than 24 hours duration.

PROCEDURES/COMMENTS

1. The FA procedure is rapid and reliable. If it is thought that an enterotoxic *E. coli* is involved, appropriate cultures and tests should be made (see COLIBACILLOSIS OF PIGS).
2. The characteristic morphology of the virus in feces can be seen with the electron microscope. The virus is difficult to cultivate.

Treatment

1. Antibiotic treatment for secondary bacteria such as *E. coli*.
2. Fluid therapy.

Control

1. Attention to management including comfort and sanitation.
2. Sufficient colostrum.

SALMONELLOSIS

Salmonellosis is a contagious disease of domestic and wild animals caused by over 2000 serovars (serotypes are occasionally referred to as species) of *Salmonella* (see ENTEROBAC-TERIACEAE) and manifested by one of the following three syndromes: septicemia, acute enteritis, or chronic enteritis.

There are frequently a number of asymptomatic carriers in a herd that shed salmonellae intermittently.

The disease is worldwide in distribution and particularly widespread in livestock subject to intensive production methods. Various stresses can trigger cases and outbreaks. Young animals frequently develop the septicemic form, whereas acute and chronic enteritis is seen most commonly in adult animals. The asymptomatic carrier serves as a reservoir of the disease; some species show a host predilection (Table 2.12).

Table 2.12. **Some important salmonellae and their frequent hosts**

Organism	Host
Salmonella choleraesuis	Swine
S. newport	Cattle
S. dublin	
S. typhimurium	Cattle, swine, horses
S. enteritidis	Laboratory animals
S. abortusequi	Horses

Many different serovars have the capacity to infect farm animals. Dogs and cats are relatively less subject to salmonella infections; however, working greyhounds are frequently affected. Salmonellosis is frequently a problem in equine clinics.

Differential Diagnosis

Because salmonellosis resembles clinically a number of other diseases, a laboratory diagnosis is required. Coccidiosis, hog cholera, colibacillosis, bovine virus diarrhea, mycotoxicosis, arsenic poisoning, enterotoxemia, parasitism, and swine dysentery are important diseases that should be considered. Potomac horse fever and colitis-X must be considered in equines.

Laboratory Diagnosis

SPECIMENS/PROCEDURES. Feces taken from the rectum are satisfactory for culture. Feces collected on a swab are sufficient in an animal showing clinical signs; however, to detect carriers, up to 10 g of feces should be cultured. Three negative fecal cultures on successive days will usually indicate the animal is not infected. From necropsied animals (sick or dead) portions of intestine, liver, spleen, lung, and lymph nodes are cultured.

Formalized portions of the above-mentioned tissues are appropriate for histopathology.

COMMENTS. It is not usually difficult to recover salmonellae from animals that have died as a result of salmonellosis. Salmonellae recovered from lymph nodes and vital organs are especially significant. The finding of the characteristic lesions of salmonellosis is supportive.

Carrier animals shed salmonellae intermittently and, as mentioned above, three negative cultures on successive days will usually indicate there is no infection.

Treatment

Antimicrobial drugs are used after susceptibility tests are conducted, although their value is questionable. Strains that are resistant to more than one drug are common. Fluid and electrolyte administration. It may not be possible to eliminate the carrier state.

Control

Efforts should be directed toward minimizing exposure, particularly to infected and carrier animals.

Killed and live attenuated (European) vaccines, and autogenous bacterins have been used with variable success.

SALMON POISONING COMPLEX

Salmon poisoning complex (SPC) is an acute infectious disease of dogs (also some wild animals) contracted from eating fluke-encysted salmon (occasionally other fish), caused by *Neorickettsia helminthoeca* (and sometimes the Elokomin fluke fever agent). These rickettsial agents are present in the liver fluke *Nanophyetus salmincola,* the cysts of which occur in salmon. The rickettsia from the ingested liver flukes released into the gut of dogs and other animals infect the lymphatic structures of the intestine resulting in a hemorrhagic enteritis often leading to death. It is an acute, febrile disease with mortality reaching as high as 90%. The intermediate hosts of the rickettsia are snails and fish.

The disease occurs in the western coastal United States and Canada, from northern California to Alaska. Dogs of all breeds and ages are susceptible. Dog-to-dog transmission has not been proved.

Differential Diagnosis

The geographic region and a severe disease after eating fish suggest SPC. Signs may include diarrhea, vomiting, passage of blood, and dehydration.

Leptospirosis, infectious canine hepatitis, distemper, hookworm infection, parvovirus infection, and salmonellosis are some of the diseases to be considered.

Laboratory Diagnosis
SPECIMENS
1. Feces are submitted for examination for fluke eggs.
2. A moribund or dead dog should be submitted for necropsy examination and smears.

PROCEDURES/COMMENTS. The finding of the ova of *N. salmincola* in the feces supports a diagnosis of SPC. A definitive diagnosis can be made on the basis of demonstrating the rickettsia in smears from lymph nodes of the alimentary tract, tonsils, thymus, or spleen.

Supportive of a diagnosis are the gross and microscopic pathologic changes of SPC, including hemorrhagic enteritis, marked lymphadenopathy, hyperplasia, and focal necrosis with organisms demonstrable by rickettsial stains.

Treatment

Sulfonamides, tetracyclines, or chloramphenicol. Praziquantel given in a single dose has been effective in dogs and coyotes. Supportive treatment.

Control

Avoid uncooked fish as dog feed.

SCRAPIE

Scrapie is a chronic, degenerative disease of the central nervous system of sheep and goats now thought to be caused by a prion (see below) and characterized by a long incubation period (6 months to 5 years), incessant itching, depression, muscular tremors, ataxia, incoordination, excitability, and death.

The disease occurs in Europe, Asia, Africa, and South and North America (infrequent). It is almost always transmitted from parent to offspring. Lateral transmission is probably rare.

There is evidence that scrapie is caused by prions, i.e., small particles of protein that are smaller than the smallest viruses. The scrapie agent is particularly resistant to chemicals and radiation that kill viruses.

Differential Diagnosis

Advanced scrapie is clinically characteristic and there is often a history of previous cases in the flock. Animal health officials should be notified if scrapie is suspected.

Maedi-visna, pseudorabies, louping ill, and external parasitism are among the diseases that should be considered.

Laboratory Diagnosis
SPECIMENS/PROCEDURES
1. For animal inoculation: Portions of brain and cord, fresh.
2. For histopathology: Portions of brain and cord, fixed.

COMMENTS. Diagnosis is usually based upon the characteristic clinical signs and histopathologic changes in the brain and cord. The diagnostic microscopic lesion involves the vacuolation of neurons.

For confirmation, mice and sheep are sometimes inoculated with fresh brain and cord.

Treatment
None.

Control
This usually involves quarantine and slaughter of all infected sheep and goats or all bloodline-related animals in a flock.

SHAKER FOAL SYNDROME
This syndrome is caused by intoxication attributable to toxins produced by *Clostridium botulinum* type B (see BOTULISM). This disease of foals occurs sporadically in the United States. Severe muscular weakness, prostration, and the inability to rise are the principal clinical signs. Animals die of respiratory failure. See BOTULISM for Laboratory Diagnosis and Treatment.

SPORADIC BOVINE ENCEPHALOMYELITIS /
BUSS DISEASE

Sporadic bovine encephalomyelitis (SBE) is an infrequent disease, mainly of young cattle, caused by a strain of *Chlamydia psittaci* and characterized by a neurologic form in which there is a meningoencephalitis and a chronic form in which fibrinous pericarditis, pleuritis, and peritonitis may be seen. When neurologic signs are seen, the disease usually terminates fatally. The course varies from days to weeks and the morbidity and mortality rates may reach 50%.

Little is known of the epidemiology of SBE. It has been reported in South Africa, Japan, some European countries, and the United States.

Differential Diagnosis

Listeriosis, pseudorabies, rabies, encephalomalacia, malignant catarrhal fever, and encephalitis due to various bacteria are among the diseases that should be considered.

Laboratory Diagnosis
SPECIMENS

1. For smears, culture, and histopathology: Brain, half fresh and half formalized; portions of affected pericardium, pleura and lung, and peritoneum.
2. For complement fixation: Paired serum samples; or samples from affected and nonaffected cattle in the same herd.

PROCEDURES/COMMENTS. Smears made from brain, pericardium, pleura, lung, and peritoneum are stained and examined for chlamydia. The finding of chlamydia from characteristic lesions is highly presumptive. The characteristic histopathologic changes, which include a purulent inflammation of the meninges and parenchyma of the brain, also support a diagnosis of SBE.

A definitive diagnosis depends upon the isolation and identification of *C. psittaci*. This may be beyond the scope of many diagnostic laboratories.

A fourfold increase in titer of paired serum samples in the complement fixation test strongly indicates a diagnosis of SBE. A moderate to high titer in a sick or recovered animal with low or negative titers in nonaffected animals supports a diagnosis of SBE.

Treatment

Tetracyclines or tylosin at high dose levels given early in the disease.

Control

None.

SPOROTRICHOSIS

Sporotrichosis is usually a chronic disease of horses, mules, dogs, cats, pigs, rats, foxes, and camels caused by the soil-borne fungus *Sporothrix schenckii* and characterized by suppurative nodules involving mainly the skin, subcutis, superficial lymphatics, and lymph nodes. Dissemination to internal organs occurs occasionally, particularly in the dog.

The disease is worldwide in distribution, and the organism lives in nature, being present in soil and decaying wood and vegetation.

The portal of entry is most commonly by cutaneous wounds of the limbs. In horses, the infection often begins in the lower part of the leg and spreads upward via the lymphatics resulting in a chain of small, often suppurating, nodules.

Differential Diagnosis

The disease in the horse and mule resembles in appearance ulcerative lymphangitis (*Corynebacterium pseudotuberculosis*) and epizootic lymphangitis (*Histoplasma farciminosum*). Nocardiosis, canine actinomycosis, cutaneous glanders, and mycetomas caused by various fungi are other diseases that should be considered.

Laboratory confirmation should be sought.

Laboratory Diagnosis

Humans can readily be infected if infectious material enters the skin via cuts or abrasions.

SPECIMENS/PROCEDURES/COMMENTS

1. For direct examination: The cigar-shaped bodies that occur in lesions are very difficult to demonstrate in stained smears and wet mounts. Fluorescent antibody staining has increased the success of direct examination. The cigar-shaped bodies (yeast form) are reported to be easier to demonstrate in feline lesions.

2. For culture: This dimorphic fungus can readily be cultivated and identified; *S. schenckii* takes from 1 to 3 weeks
to grow.
3. For serology: Serologic tests have been little used in the
animal disease. In humans the agglutination and immunodiffusion tests are recommended for diagnosis.

Treatment

1. Potassium and sodium iodide are used orally and intravenously; they are almost always effective.
2. Amphotericin B, griseofulvin, flucytosine, and natamycin
have been used effectively.
3. Ketaconazole and itraconazole have shown promise.

STAPHYLOCOCCI

Staphylococci are among the most important pyogenic organisms causing disease in animals. Bovine mastitis caused by
Staphylococcus aureus is discussed separately as is exudative
epidermitis caused by *S. hyicus*.

The staphylococci have been reclassified in recent years
into a number of distinct species. The most important of
these are listed below with their principal hosts and associated diseases.

Staphylococcus aureus: Among the infections that have been
attributed to this species are botryomycosis (infrequent
chronic granulomatous lesions of the udder of the mare,
cow, and sow and the spermatic cord of horses); mastitis
in the cow, ewe, and sow; pyoderma and cellulitis in
horses; pyemia in lambs; arthritis; subcutaneous abscesses; septicemia; wound infections; urinary tract infections; and nosocomial infections.

Staphylococcus intermedius: This organism causes a variety
of infections in dogs, including pyoderma, otitis externa,
mastitis, eye infections, urinary tract infections, folicu-
litis, and furunculosis. It also causes mastitis in cows.

Staphylococcus hyicus: It causes exudative epidermitis (q.v.)
or "greasy pig disease" in pigs. It has also been implicated in septic arthritis of pigs, dermatitis of donkeys
and horses, and dermatitis and mastitis of cattle.

Staphylococcus epidermidis: It is ordinarily a commensal on
the skin that can on infrequent occasions cause low-
grade infections.

STRANGLES

Strangles is an acute contagious disease of young equidae caused by *Streptococcus equi* ssp. *equi* (formerly *S. equi*). It begins as a rhinitis and pharyngitis and is characterized later by abscesses in lymph nodes, particularly the intermandibular and parapharyngeal, draining the upper respiratory and buccal mucosa. In rare instances, the disease may be generalized and terminate in death. Among infrequent sequellae are variably disseminated abscesses, guttural pouch involvement, and purpura hemorrhagica (type III hypersensitivity).

It is worldwide in distribution. A small number of horses are asymptomatic carriers. The disease occurs when young or highly susceptible animals are exposed to carriers. This most often happens when horses from different locations are brought together, e.g., at horse shows and race tracks.

Bastard strangles is an infrequent chronic form with disseminated abscesses.

Differential Diagnosis

A diagnosis is usually made on the basis of the characteristic clinical signs; however, laboratory confirmation is recommended.

Laboratory Diagnosis

Fresh pus for culture is taken on a swab from an excised mature abscess.

PROCEDURES/COMMENTS. The isolation and identification of *S. equi* ssp. *equi* provides a definitive diagnosis. Older discharging abscesses may yield *S. equisimilis,* which is a secondary invader.

Treatment

Penicillins and sulfonamides are very effective. Abscessation can be prevented by early treatment.

Control

Isolation of horses to be added to a herd. Bacterins are useful but should be used with care as severe local reactions sometimes occur. It is claimed that a vaccine consisting largely of the M protein of *S. equi* ssp. *equi* results in less severe reactions.

STREPTOCOCCAL LYMPHADENITIS OF SWINE /
JOWL ABSCESSES, CERVICAL LYMPHADENITIS OF SWINE, CERVICAL ABSCESSES OF SWINE

This benign, contagious disease is caused by *Streptococcus porcinus* (groups E,P,U,V) and affects, most frequently, feeder swine and is characterized by the development of one or more heavily encapsulated abscesses involving the cervical lymph nodes.

The disease is worldwide and endemic in many swine herds where, in the absence of immunization, it may manifest itself clinically in successive generations of feeder pigs.

Many pigs carry the organism in their tonsils and the mode of infection is by ingestion.

Differential Diagnosis

The disease can be readily diagnosed clinically on the basis of the abscessed cervical lymph nodes.

Laboratory Diagnosis

Laboratory diagnosis is not frequently carried out.

SPECIMENS/PROCEDURES. For culture: Preferably fresh pus is taken from an excised lymph node.

A definitive diagnosis is made on the basis of the isolation and identification of *S. porcinus*.

Treatment

The streptococci are susceptible to many antimicrobial drugs including penicillin and tetracyclines; however, treatment is of little value after abscesses develop.

Control

The disease is often introduced by carrier pigs, including those with visible abscesses. Early-weaned pigs should be kept free of possible carrier older pigs and affected older pigs. Serologic tests (agglutination) have been used to detect carriers.

Modified live vaccines administered orally or intranasally by spray are used in 10-week-old pigs.

STREPTOCOCCI

In addition to specific diseases such as strangles (q.v.) and streptococcal lymphadenitis of swine (q.v.), a number of species or varieties of streptococci cause infections in domestic animals. They are listed below with the infections with which they have been most commonly associated.

Streptococcus pyogenes (group A): Principal cause of streptococcal disease in humans. May rarely cause bovine mastitis with possible dissemination to humans. It occasionally causes lymphangitis in foals.

S. agalactiae (group B): This streptococcus and *Staphylococcus aureus* are the most important and frequent causes of bovine mastitis (see BOVINE MASTITIS). *S. agalactiae* is a pathogen that can be eliminated from herds. Infection is mainly spread by the milker's hands or by contaminated teat cups. *S. agalactiae* also causes mastitis in sheep and goats, and has been associated with several canine neonatal deaths, and kidney and uterine infections in cats.

S. dysgalactiae (group C): It causes mastitis in cows and polyarthritis in lambs.

S. dysgalactiae ssp. *equisimilis* (formerly *S. equisimilis*) (group C): Occasionally associated with strangles, wound infections, genital infections, and mastitis in the horse; cause of various infections in swine, cattle, dog, and fowl.

S. equi ssp. *equi* (formerly *S. equi*) (group C): Strangles (q.v.) and other infections of the horse; genital and udder infections in the mare.

S. equi ssp. *zooepidemicus* (formerly *S. zooepidemicus*) (group C): Primary cause of genital infections in the mare and navel infections in foals. This streptococcus is associated with cervicitis, metritis, and mastitis in cattle; arthritis, abortion, and septicemia in swine; fibrinous pleuritis, pericarditis, and pneumonia in lambs; and mastitis in goats.

Enterococcus faecalis, E. faecium, E. durans (formerly *S. faecalis, S. faecium,* and *S. durans*) (group D): These cocci are common inhabitants of the intestinal tract of animals and humans. *E. faecalis* may cause urinary infections in various animals and endocarditis in chickens.

S. suis (groups D,R,S): Frequently causes meningitis, septicemia, pneumonia, and arthritis in pigs of all ages. Other conditions in pigs such as local abscesses, endocarditis, encephalitis, polyserositis, and peritonitis are less frequently seen. It is also associated with abortion in sows. *S. suis* may cause meningitis, arthritis, septicemia, diarrhea, and deafness in humans. Of the 23 serotypes (based on capsular antigens) *S. suis* type 2 appears to be the predominant serotype in North America.

S. uberis (groups C,D,E,P,V): Causes bovine mastitis; found in the vagina and tonsils of cattle.

S. porcinus (groups E,P,U,V): Causes abscesses of mandibular, pharyngeal, and other lymph nodes in pigs (see STREPTOCOCCAL LYMPHADENITIS OF SWINE).

S. pneumoniae (Syn.: *Diplococcus pneumoniae,* no group): An important cause of pneumonia in guinea pigs, it has been implicated in respiratory infections in calves, monkeys, rabbits, and rats. There are several reports of bovine mastitis caused by pneumococci; septicemia and septic arthritis have been reported in the domestic cat.

S. canis (group G): Causes genital, skin, and wound infections in dogs.

Additional groups of streptococci:

Group G: Mastitis in cows; lymphadenitis in cats.

Group H: Causes rare infections in cattle.

Group L: Causes infections in dogs, pigs, and cattle.

Group M: Various infections in dogs.

Groups O and P: Uncommon infection in farm animals.

Viridans group of streptococci: Streptococci of this serologically heterogeneous group are almost always alpha-hemolytic and nonpathogenic. Rare urinary tract infections have been reported in animals.

Anaerobic streptococci: Are found as commensals in the alimentary and upper respiratory tracts. They may occur alone or in mixed infections, and it seems likely that they will be found, as in humans, in infections associated with operative procedures or wounds involving the gastrointestinal or genitourinary tract.

Nutritionally variant streptococci: Have special nutritional requirements and are isolated from a variety of clinical specimens taken from horses, cattle, and sheep. Their significance in disease processes is not always clear.

SWINE BLUE EYE DISEASE

Swine blue eye disease (SBED) is a rare disease that is caused by a paramyxovirus and is characterized by central nervous system (CNS) disorders, reproductive failures, corneal opacity, and high mortality. Ataxia, weakness, rigid hind legs, muscle tremors, and abnormal posture are some of the signs seen. Infertility in boars has been attributed to severe orchitis and epididymitis caused by the virus. The disease is most common from March to July.

Outbreaks of disease have only been reported in several states of Mexico. Periodic recurrences have been observed on farms with continuous systems of swine production. The disease appears to be self-limiting. Subclinically infected pigs are the main source of the disease. Dogs, cats, rabbits, and mice can be infected experimentally with the virus.

Differential Diagnosis

SBED must be differentiated from other diseases resulting in encephalitis and reproductive failure. These include pseudorabies; Teschen and Teschen-like diseases; porcine parvovirus infection; and stillbirths, mummification, embryonic death, and infertility, referred to as SMEDI and caused by porcine enteroviruses (see ENTEROVIRUS INFECTIONS IN SWINE).

Laboratory Diagnosis

Clinical signs in piglets, such as CNS disorders, corneal opacity, reproductive failure in sows, or orchitis and epididymitis in boars, may suggest SBED.

SPECIMENS

1. Nasal and occular discharges collected during the first 3–5 days of infection; fresh brain and tonsil.
2. Brain, reproductive organs, and eye formalized for histopathology.
3. Serum samples.

PROCEDURES

1. Virus can be isolated in PK-15 cell monolayers. Cytopathic effects are characterized by syncytium formation. A direct fluorescent antibody procedure is used to identify the virus in cell cultures.

2. The presence of nonsuppurative encephalitis, anterior uveitis, keratitis, orchitis, and epididymitis may also contribute to a presumptive diagnosis.
3. Hemagglutination inhibition, virus neutralization, and enzyme-linked immunosorbent assays have been developed to detect specific SBED antibody.

Treatment
None.

Control
Good management practices including herd quarantine, cleaning and disinfecting sties, and serologic testing and eliminating the affected pigs.

Initial trials with a killed virus vaccine have been promising.

SWINE BRUCELLOSIS
Swine brucellosis is a contagious disease almost always caused by *Brucella suis* and characterized by abortion, birth of stillborn and weak pigs, and infection of the testicles and accessory sex glands of the male leading to varying degrees of infertility in both sexes.

Probably worldwide in distribution; incidence in the United States is probably low.

Differential Diagnosis
Leptospirosis, porcine parvovirus infection (mainly mummified fetuses), and pseudorabies. A number of agents can cause sporadic abortions in swine.

Laboratory Diagnosis
Swine brucellosis is usually diagnosed by the brucellosis card test.

SPECIMENS
1. Serum samples from a number of animals in a herd.
2. Fetus; fetal stomach contents; testicles.

PROCEDURES
1. Brucellosis card test (preferred) or other agglutination tests.

2. Isolation and identification of *B. suis.*

COMMENTS. *B. suis* can be demonstrated in smears from infected fetal cotyledons by Koster's or the modified acid-fast stain.

An individual serum sample is not sufficient for the card test or other agglutination procedures, for some infected pigs do not develop appreciable titers; therefore, serum samples should be taken from a number of animals.

Treatment
None.

Control
Test, segregation, and slaughter. Elimination of the disease may be difficult. It may be advisable to start with a brucellosis-free herd and only add animals from herds that are also disease free. The United States has a plan for the validation of brucellosis-free herds.

SWINE DYSENTERY / BLACK SCOURS, BLOODY SCOURS, VIBRIONIC DYSENTERY

Swine dysentery is a contagious disease caused by *Serpulina hyodysenteriae* (formerly *Treponema hyodysenteriae*) in association with gram-negative anaerobic bacteria (e.g., *Fusobacterium necrophorum, Bacteroides fragilis*) and *Campylobacter coli.* Disease is manifested by a bloody diarrhea that may terminate in death or in a chronic form characterized by a diphtheritic inflammatory process involving the mucosa of the cecum, large intestine, and rectum.

The disease is worldwide in distribution and most common in pigs that are raised intensively. The infection is perpetuated by asymptomatic carriers, and the mode of transmission is by the ingestion of fecal material from infected pigs. Frequency of exposure and dosage of organisms are important in the establishment of the disease.

Differential Diagnosis
Salmonellosis, hog cholera (swine fever), stomach ulcers, chronic scours, and acute trichuriasis should be considered. Laboratory confirmation is recommended.

Laboratory Diagnosis
SPECIMENS
1. For stained smears, dark-field examination, and culture: A live, sick pig for necropsy. Smears are made from the colonic mucosa. Fresh material from the colonic mucosa is examined by dark-field microscopy. Material may also be taken from the colonic mucosa or colon content for culture if the laboratory performs this procedure.

    If a live, sick pig cannot be submitted, a tied off, fresh portion of the colon can be submitted refrigerated. Smears from the colonic mucosa may also be submitted.
2. For gross and microscopic examination: A live, sick pig or formalized portions of affected colon and cecum.

PROCEDURES/COMMENTS
1. Isolation and identification of *S. hyodysenteriae* is preferable, although with experience the organism can be identified in the smears and in wet mounts by dark-field examination. *S. hyodysenteriae* must be distinguished from the nonpathogenic porcine spirochete *S. innocens*. Fresh material is required for culture. Microbial susceptibility tests are not ordinarily carried out.
2. A provisional diagnosis can be made on the basis of history, clinical signs, and characteristic gross pathological changes.

Treatment
Drugs are administered via the feed. The principal drugs are carbadox, virginiamycin, tylosin, furazolidone, sodium arsanilate, and lincomycin.

Control
1. Good management and sanitary practices to reduce exposure. In herds free of disease, new stock should be screened for swine dysentery before introduction to the herd.
2. A commercial bacterin consisting of killed *S. hyodysenteriae* is available.

SWINE ERYSIPELAS
Swine erysipelas is a contagious disease principally of swine, less frequently of sheep and poultry, caused by *Erysipelothrix*

rhusiopathiae (*E. insidiosa*) and characterized by an acute septicemic form and by chronic skin, arthritic, and cardiac (endocarditis) forms. Any combination of the various forms may be seen in the same herd.

The disease is worldwide in distribution. Besides pigs, there are outbreaks in poultry and a nonsuppurative polyarthritis in lambs and calves. The infection in humans is usually localized and is called erysipeloid. The organism occurs on the skin of fish.

E. rhusiopathiae: A small gram-positive rod, it is relatively resistant and can survive and multiply in the soil of some regions, probably because of its alkaline condition. There are asymptomatic carriers and the mode of infection is by ingestion.

E. tonsillarum: A nonpathogenic commensal of the tonsils of normal swine.

Differential Diagnosis

This depends on the various manifestations:

Acute form: High temperature, depression, anorexia. Death often occurs shortly after signs are seen.

Skin form: Less severe, fever may be present, may be some loss of condition. Raised diamond- or square-shaped red to purple areas that later become gangrenous resulting in large scabs.

Arthritic form: May occur in absence of other forms, but sometimes with one of the other chronic manifestations. Lameness; stifle and hock joints often involved; progresses to a marked periarticular fibrosis.

Cardiac form (valvular endocarditis): May be a sequel to the acute form or the skin form. It is progressive and accompanied by dyspnea, passive congestion with resulting skin discoloration of extremities, debilitation, stunted growth, abnormal heart sounds, and sudden death.

Hog cholera (swine fever), salmonellosis, acute enzootic pneumonia, Glasser's disease, African swine fever, and arthritis caused by various organisms are among the diseases that should be considered.

Laboratory Diagnosis
SPECIMENS

1. Acute: Heart blood, portions of kidney, spleen, and liver.

2. Arthritic and cardiac: Swabs from affected joints, and affected tissues.
3. Blood smears in the acute septicemic disease. If feasible it is advisable to submit one or two sick pigs for necropsy examination.

PROCEDURES/COMMENTS
1. A definitive diagnosis is based upon the isolation and identification of *E. rhusiopathiae* by cultural methods. The organism is not usually recoverable from the skin lesions.
2. The finding of the typical small, gram-positive rods in fresh blood smears is supportive of a diagnosis.

   The finding of characteristic gross and microscopic pathologic changes in the chronic forms of the disease supports a diagnosis.

Treatment
1. Penicillin given early is the drug of choice.
2. Tylosin and tetracyclines are also effective.

Control
1. Live and killed vaccines are of value and are widely used.
2. Hyperimmune serum can be used for treatment and passive protection.

SWINE INFERTILITY AND RESPIRATORY SYNDROME / PORCINE REPRODUCTIVE AND RESPIRATORY SYNDROME, BLUE EAR DISEASE

Swine infertility and respiratory syndrome (SIRS) is a recently described viral disease of swine that is characterized in sows by abortion and stillborn fetuses, and in piglets by respiratory infection. The first signs of infection are fever, anorexia, with edema and cyanosis of the teats, ears, and tail. Up to 20% of affected sows farrow prematurely and up to 20% abort in the late stages of gestation. Farrowing at term results in fetuses that may be live, mummified, or stillborn. Initial rise in stillborn rate may reach up to 50% of piglets, followed by a peak in mummified fetuses. Survivors are weak and may die within a week.

SIRS has been reported from the Netherlands, Germany,

United States, United Kingdom, and Spain. Large numbers of
herds have been involved. Spread is thought to be mainly by
direct and indirect contact.

Differential Diagnosis

Parvovirus infection, pseudorabies, enterovirus infections,
brucellosis, and leptospirosis are among the diseases that
should be considered.

Laboratory Diagnosis

Because this is a new disease with a potential to cause enormous losses, animal health officials should be notified if outbreaks are suspected.

SPECIMENS. These have been detailed under INFECTIOUS
PORCINE ABORTION. Blood for serology and por-
tions of fresh liver and lung for virus isolation and histopathology are submitted from newborn piglets and older pigs
thought to be affected.

PROCEDURES/COMMENTS. The principal means of diagnosis at present is virus isolation and identification, and
the detection of specific viral antibodies in sera. These procedures are only carried out in several specified laboratories.
Microscopic pathologic changes of lung tissue are helpful in
the diagnosis of SIRS.

Treatment

None.

Control

This is carried out by state and federal animal health officials
with measures which may include quarantine and slaughter.

SWINE INFLUENZA / SWINE FLU, HOG FLU

Swine influenza is an acute, highly contagious respiratory
disease, usually of short duration and low mortality, caused
by type A influenza virus and characterized by rapid spread,
fever, coughing, dyspnea, nasal discharge, and occasional
prostration.

It is worldwide in distribution and endemic in temperate

zones. It usually occurs during the colder months, and most pigs recover without complications. The lungworm is no longer thought to be important in its transmission.

Differential Diagnosis

The disease is usually diagnosed clinically. The clinical signs are those of an acute respiratory disease of short duration.

Enzootic pneumonia of pigs, atrophic rhinitis, inclusion body rhinitis, and contagious pleuropneumonia of swine are among the diseases that should be considered.

Laboratory Diagnosis

Because of the usual short duration, a laboratory diagnosis is not usually sought.

SPECIMENS

1. Nasal swabs; portions of affected lungs if available.
2. Paired serum samples.

PROCEDURES/COMMENTS

1. For virus isolation and identification: The virus can be isolated in embryonated eggs. Fluorescent antibody staining of lung tissue.
2. For serology: A hemagglutination inhibition test is carried out in some laboratories.

   Laboratory diagnosis is based on the isolation and identification of the virus or the demonstration of a fourfold rise in titer of paired sera.

Treatment

Treatment is not usually necessary unless complicated by secondary bacteria such as *Haemophilus parasuis, Pasteurella multocida,* and *Streptococcus suis.*

Control

Good management; avoidance of stresses.

The disease is not considered sufficiently important to warrant vaccination.

SWINEPOX

Swinepox is a worldwide, contagious disease caused by a poxvirus (suipoxvirus) and characterized by the formation of papules, followed by vesicles, pustules, and finally scabs. The lesions involve mainly the skin of the abdomen, sides, and back. Lesions with dark hemorrhagic centers are seen on the lower abdomen. The disease is usually mild and runs its course without serious consequences.

The hog louse, *Hematopinus suis,* and direct contact are the principal means of transmission. The incidence in North America is low. Although the disease is seen most frequently in young pigs, all ages may be affected.

Some outbreaks of swinepox have been attributed to vaccinia virus (derived from cowpox virus).

Differential Diagnosis

The typical lesions along with louse infestation make for a highly presumptive clinical diagnosis.

Mange, ringworm, exudative epidermitis, parakeratosis, and pityriasis rosea should be considered.

Laboratory Diagnosis

This is not usually carried out, although it may be advisable to rule out vesicular diseases. The procedures are the same as those described for COWPOX. Electron microscopy of material from lesions will indicate the presence of poxvirus.

Treatment

Treatment is not usually necessary.

Control

Elimination of lice. Recovered pigs are solidly immune.

SWINE PROLIFERATIVE ENTERITIS COMPLEX

Included in this disease complex are several intestinal abnormalities that appear to be etiologically and clinically related. These intestinal abnormalities include intestinal adenomatosis, regional ileitis, proliferative hemorrhagic enteropathy, and necrotic enteritis. *Campylobacter mucosalis* is thought to be the principal causal agent.

Proliferative hemorrhagic enteropathy is an acute to peracute disease of recently weaned pigs and pigs in the age range of 4–9 months. It is characterized by inflammatory, proliferative, and hemorrhagic changes involving the ileum and extending to the large intestine. Occasionally, the lesions are restricted to segments of the ileum (regional ileitis). Sudden onset, inappetence, loss of condition, with diarrhea and absence of fever are also seen with this disease complex.

Intestinal adenomatosis and necrotic enteritis are characterized by thickening and coaggulative necrosis of ileal mucosa. The small intestine becomes very rigid, giving the appearance of garden hose. Recovery is usually within 4–6 weeks in milder cases. Advanced cases result in dysentery and anemia. In some cases, much blood is passed in the feces and death ensues in several days.

Campylobacter hyointestinalis has also been isolated often with *C. mucosalis*. The precise etiology of this disease complex is still in doubt.

Differential Diagnosis

Swine dysentery, esophagogastric ulcers, hemorrhagic bowel syndrome, and infectious necrotic enteritis are among the diseases that should be considered.

Laboratory Diagnosis

The diagnosis of these enteropathies requires necropsy of affected pigs. Gross and microscopic changes are helpful in the differentiation of proliferative hemorrhagic enteropathy and intestinal adenomatosis. Hemorrhage is particularly characteristic of the proliferative hemorrhagic enteropathy. In intestinal adenomatosis, the ileum is thickened and corrugated and has been likened to a garden hose.

SPECIMENS

1. For histopathology: Fixed portions of the affected intestine including the ileum.
2. For culture: Fresh portions of the affected intestine including the ileum. If specimens cannot be cultured within 2 or 3 hours, they should be frozen over dry ice prior to examination.

PROCEDURES/COMMENTS

1. Gross and microscopic changes are useful in the differentiation of this disease complex. The finding of typical campylobacter organisms in sections of lesions stained by the Warthin-Starry method is supportive.
2. *C. mucosalis* is a fragile, fastidious organism that requires special procedures for isolation.

A final diagnosis will depend upon the clinical picture and the results of the pathologic and microbiologic examinations including the isolation and identification of *C. mucosalis* and/or *C. hyointestinalis*.

Treatment

Various antimicrobial drugs including tylosin, furazolidone, and tetracyclines have given variable results.

Control

Specific measures have not yet been developed for the control and prevention of these diseases.

TESCHEN AND TESCHEN-LIKE DISEASES / PORCINE POLIOENCEPHALOMYELITIS, PORCINE ENCEPHALOMYELITIS, TALFAN DISEASE

These encephalitides are caused by several serologically, closely related picornaviruses (enteroviruses). They occur in pigs of all ages and are characterized by a fever and an encephalomyelitis that results in incoordination, convulsions, stiffness, spasms, and paralysis. Mortality is 50–90% in young pigs.

This group of diseases is probably worldwide in distribution. Generally speaking, only mild forms of the disease have been reported from North America. The acute disease has been reported from Central Europe and Africa. The encephalitic manifestation is seen in pigs that lack resistance to the virulent virus.

Both virulent and avirulent viruses occur. They may be carried in the intestine as subclinical infections with virus being shed in the feces. The mode of infection is by ingestion and spread is by direct or indirect contact.

Differential Diagnosis

The disease is similar to human poliomyelitis and the cardinal clinical sign is progressive paralysis. In the acute disease, death may occur 3–4 days after onset of signs.

Hog cholera, pseudorabies, edema disease, and vomiting-and-wasting disease are among the diseases that should be considered.

A laboratory diagnosis is required.

Laboratory Diagnosis
SPECIMENS
1. For virus isolation and histopathology: Fresh brain is halved longitudinally; one half is submitted fresh, while portions of the other half are fixed for histopathology.
2. For serology: Sera from early and late cases, as well as from healthy pigs.

PROCEDURES/COMMENTS
1. The virus can be propagated and identified in porcine cell cultures. The histopathologic changes are not specific for this disease.
2. The sera may be sent to a reference laboratory for virus neutralization and/or complement fixation tests. Fourfold increases in titers of paired sera provide strong evidence of Teschen or Teschen-like disease.

   Definitive diagnosis depends upon the isolation and identification of the virus. Most neurotropic enteroviruses belong to serotype 1.

Treatment
None.

Control
Isolation of infected pigs. In the United States, strict import regulation must be followed for Teschen disease caused by serotype 1.

Live and inactivated vaccines are used in some European countries.

TETANUS
Tetanus is an acute, noncontagious disease of farm and other animals (rare in cat, dog, and fowl) caused by the neurotoxin of *Clostridium tetani,* which is produced in necrotic tissue resulting from a wound. It is characterized by painful tonic and clonic spasms of skeletal muscles.

The disease is worldwide in distribution and is seen in practice most commonly in horses and sheep. In sheep, it occurs occasionally after castration, particularly with rubber bands, docking, and branding. All ages are susceptible. The spores of *C. tetani* can germinate in a variety of wounds if necrosis is present.

As is sometimes thought, the organism is not more prevalent in horse manure, but horses sustain more wounds that allow for the growth of *C. tetani.*

Differential Diagnosis

The disease is almost always diagnosed clinically. Some features of tetanus are wounds (not always found, particularly in horses), gradual onset of stiffness, hyperesthesia, followed by tetanic spasms of all voluntary muscles. In contrast to tetanus, acute strychnine poisoning runs a course of one to several hours.

Laboratory Diagnosis

This disease is so characteristic clinically that a laboratory diagnosis is not required.

If it is desired to attempt isolation and identification of *C. tetani,* material (pus, necrosed tissue) from the wound should be taken so as to minimize exposure to air, preferably in an anaerobic transport system.

Gram-stained smears from a wound may reveal the characteristic drumstick (terminal spore) bacteria; however, their absence does not exclude tetanus.

Treatment

1. Expose, clean, and disinfect wound.
2. Muscle relaxants and sedatives.
3. Penicillin and an adequate dose of tetanus antitoxin; intrathecal administration of antitoxin is used by some clinicians.

Control

To prevent tetanus in a wounded animal, clean and disinfect the wound. Administer antitoxin and toxoid at different locations; a large dose of penicillin may also be given.

For prevention administer toxoid to horses, and in some instances to ewes to provide passive protection of lambs.

TRANSMISSIBLE GASTROENTERITIS OF SWINE

Transmissible gastroenteritis (TGE) of swine is a severe, highly contagious disease of young pigs caused by a coronavirus and manifested clinically by vomiting, diarrhea, and dehydration. The morbidity and mortality are usually high.

It is worldwide in distribution, spreads rapidly, and strikes whole litters of neonatal pigs. Those 10 days of age or less are most susceptible. The disease in adult pigs is mild or inapparent.

Differential Diagnosis

Escherichia coli enteritis, enterotoxemia, diarrhea, vomiting-and-wasting disease, rotavirus and pararotavirus infection, and adenovirus infection are among the diseases that should be considered. Laboratory confirmation should be sought.

Laboratory Diagnosis

SPECIMENS

1. For fluorescent antibody (FA): Portions of affected small intestine, preferably at the onset of the disease.
2. For virus isolation: Portions of affected small intestine (jejunum and ileum).
3. For histopathology: Small portions of affected small intestine, formalized.

PROCEDURES

1. Demonstration of the virus by FA staining is the most effective means of diagnosis. Smears from scrapings, and cryostat sections allow for rapid diagnosis.
2. Difficulty is often experienced in isolating the virus. Electron microscopy reveals virus particles in feces.
3. Demonstration of the characteristic villous atrophy of the mucosa of the small intestine is strongly suggestive of TGE.

Treatment

1. Good nursing.
2. Fluids to cope with the dehydration.
3. The value of antimicrobial drugs is questionable.

Control

Herds can only be kept free of TGE by diligence in preventing introduction of the virus by carrier pigs, contaminated conveyances, and people.

Live attenuated virus vaccines are available for the immunization of sows and/or newborn pigs but they are not always effective. Planned infection of sows in early pregnancy is effective but should only be used if exposure of young pigs is inevitable.

TRICHOSPORONOSIS

This disease is caused by the soil-borne yeast *Trichosporon beigelii,* which has been recovered from a relatively small number of infections in animals including a nasal granuloma in a cat, dermatitis in the horse and monkey, mastitis in cattle and sheep, and bladder infections in cats.

TUBERCULOSIS

The most significant tuberculosis encountered in cattle is due to *Mycobacterium bovis* (see BOVINE TUBERCULOSIS).

In North America, tuberculosis in the other domestic species, except poultry, is not usually a prevalent or economically significant disease. For this reason only a very brief summary is provided below.

Infrequent infections due to mycobacteria other than the classical species occur in all the domestic animals. An example is skin tuberculosis of cattle due to noncultivable mycobacteria.

Swine: Swine are subject to infection by *M. bovis, M. avium,* and *M. tuberculosis.*

M. *avium* (*intracellulare* complex) and *M. tuberculosis:* Lesions are usually confined to the intestinal tract, associated lymph nodes, and particularly the submaxillary and cervical lymph nodes.

M. *bovis:* The infections are frequently generalized and rapidly progressive.

Sheep and Goats: Tuberculosis is rare in sheep and goats because, although quite susceptible, they are seldom exposed.

M. *bovis:* When disease occurs, it is usually caused by *M. bovis* and is similar to that of cattle.

M. *avium:* Has been reported to produce progressive lesions in sheep.

Horses: The most common form of tuberculosis seen in horses involves the cervical vertebra and is caused by *M. bovis.*

Dogs: *M. tuberculosis* and *M. bovis* are capable of causing generalized infections in dogs.

Cats: The cat is resistant to *M. tuberculosis* and *M. avium*

but is susceptible to generalized infection with *M. bovis*.
FELINE LEPROSY is discussed separately.

Laboratory Diagnosis

Tuberculosis in the above species is most often diagnosed at
necropsy. A highly presumptive diagnosis is usually based on
the demonstration of typical acid-fast organisms in acid-fast
stained smears from lesions.

An alternate staining procedure uses fluorescein dyes.
Mycobacteria stained by this procedure stain yellow. This
procedure may not be available in many laboratories.

The tuberculin test (false negatives are common in dogs)
and radiography may be helpful in diagnosis.

Although isolation may be carried out in a local diagnostic laboratory, definitive identification is usually made in a
reference laboratory.

Treatment

This is not usually carried out in animals, mainly because of
public health considerations and the fact that an antemortem
diagnosis is seldom made.

Control

Isoniazid has been used prophylactically to control tuberculosis in zoos and animal parks.

If multiple cases of tuberculosis occur, tuberculin testing
may be helpful with elimination or segregation and treatment
of positive animals.

USDA-licensed mycobacterial antigens are available
commercially for intradermal testing in animals (see 8, Appendix A).

TULAREMIA

Tularemia is a disease of wild rodents and other wild animals,
particularly rabbits, caused by *Francisella tularensis*. It is
characterized by fever, weakness, inappetence, sometimes
dyspnea and diarrhea, followed by prostration and frequently death if untreated. What begins as a localized infection proceeds to a bacteremia with the formation of granulomatous, necrotic foci in the lymph nodes, liver, and spleen.

Francisella tularensis consists of two biotypes: the more
virulent type A, referred to as *tularensis,* and the milder type

B, as *palaeartica*. Both are small, pleomorphic, nonmotile, gram-negative rods and coccobacilli. The biotypes differ in host specificity, biochemical activity, and geographical distribution. *F. tularensis* occurs mainly in the northern hemisphere with biotype A, *tularensis,* predominating in North America and biotype B, *palaeartica,* in Eurasia.

Wild animals are the reservoir of infection, especially rabbits and hares, but also the beaver, muskrat, squirrel, woodchuck, opossum, skunk, deer, and fox. *F. tularensis* is most frequently transmitted by any of a large range of biting arthropods including flies, mites, mosquitoes, lice, and ticks. An appreciable number of infections in farm animals can occur in some regions, especially in sheep. Tularemia is rarely seen in dogs, but cats are more susceptible and there are reports of transmission from cats to humans via bite wounds. Domestic fowl can act as a reservoir of infection.

Differential Diagnosis

A history of previous cases may lead to a suspicion of tularemia. Exposure to biting arthropods, particularly ticks that may have been feeding on infected wild animals, e.g., rabbits, beaver, and muskrats, could suggest the disease.

The clinical signs are similar to those of several bacterial diseases that may give rise to a bacteremia or septicemia, e.g., salmonellosis, pasteurellosis, listeriosis, and erysipelas.

Laboratory Diagnosis

If tularemia is suspected, great care should be taken in performing a necropsy. All work with material from suspected tularemia cases must be carried out in a biologic safety cabinet or alternatively sent to a laboratory equipped to handle this dangerous organism.

SPECIMENS

1. For serology: Serum samples taken in the advanced disease and paired samples if obtainable.
2. For culture and smears: Portions of liver, spleen, and lymph nodes with the characteristic necrotic foci.

PROCEDURES/COMMENTS

1. An agglutination test is usually positive late in the disease. A substantial rise in titer of paired sera is significant. Such

positive reactions along with the characteristic lesions provide a highly presumptive diagnosis of tularemia.

2. This gram-negative organism, which somewhat resembles a *Brucella* species, requires a medium containing cystine for growth. Specimens frequently contain extraneous bacteria. Guinea pig inoculation of such specimens usually makes possible the isolation of *F. tularensis.*

The most rapid means of identifying *F. tularensis* is by the specific fluorescent antibody staining of smears from lesions.

A slide agglutination test using known specific antisera is also available in some diagnostic laboratories to identify colonies of *F. tularensis.*

Treatment

Streptomycin is the drug of choice. Prolonged treatment with tetracyclines.

Control

Prevention of exposure to sources of *F. tularensis,* such as infected ticks, animals, and contaminated water and food.

A live attenuated vaccine is used in people whose risk of infection is high. Animals are not vaccinated.

TYZZER'S DISEASE

Tyzzer's disease is a severe, frequently fatal, necrotizing hepatitis of laboratory mice, rats, hamsters, gerbils, rabbits, nonhuman primates, horses, dogs, cats, and other animals. Disease is caused by *Bacillus piliformis* and is characterized by enteritis (not in all cases); colitis; and focal, necrotic hepatitis.

The disease is probably worldwide. Although known for many years, it has only recently been reported in dogs, cats, and foals. The organism, which has not been cultivated in artificial media, is carried in the intestinal tract, presumably as a commensal. It is not a true *Bacillus* species.

The mode of infection is by ingestion. The disease is thought to result from various stresses, e.g., in laboratory rodents, it may be stresses due to certain testing procedures. Poor sanitation may also be a factor. The age range in foals has been given as mostly between 10 and 30 days. Adult horses may be carriers.

Differential Diagnosis

Most animals are found dead or in a coma, without showing premonitory signs. The clinical signs, if seen, are only apparent for a few hours. Signs include fever, icterus, and sometimes diarrhea.

Acute salmonellosis, sleepy foal disease, and *Rhodococcus equi* septicemia and other acute microbial infections are among the diseases that should be considered.

Laboratory Diagnosis

SPECIMENS. For pathology and smears: It is best to submit a sick or recently dead animal; failing this, portions of the liver, fresh and fixed.

PROCEDURES/COMMENTS. The disease is usually diagnosed on the basis of finding the typical liver lesions (multifocal necrosis) and demonstrating the characteristic organisms in hepatocytes in stained smears. Liver sections stained by the silver impregnation method are also useful for the demonstration of the organism.

Treatment

Treatment is not considered effective. Erythromycin and tetracyclines have been used prophylactically, particularly in rodents.

Control

Improvement of sanitation; removal of stresses. Tetracycline administered in the drinking water is thought to be effective in preventing additional deaths during outbreaks in laboratory rodents.

Bacillus piliformis produces spores that require a temperature of 80°C for 30 minutes for killing.

ULCERATIVE DERMATOSIS / LIP AND LEG ULCERATION, VENEREAL VULVITIS AND BALANOPOSTHITIS

Ulcerative dermatosis is an acute, contagious disease of sheep caused by a poxvirus and manifested in two different clinical forms. One is characterized by the formation of ulcerative lesions involving the lips, mouth, face, and legs. The other is transmitted venereally and is characterized by ulceration involving the vulva, prepuce, and penis.

It is probably worldwide (except in Australia) in distribution but is not as frequent in occurrence or as important as contagious ecthyma. The morbidity and mortality rates are usually low.

Differential Diagnosis

The lesions of this disease are ulcerative rather than proliferative as in contagious ecthyma. Photosensitization, mycotic dermatitis (dermatophilosis), bluetongue, and bacterial balanoposthitis should be considered. Contagious ecthyma does not cause genital lesions.

Laboratory diagnosis should be sought.

Laboratory Diagnosis

SPECIMENS. For virus isolation: Scrapings from early lesions.

PROCEDURES/COMMENTS. The virus can be grown and identified in cell cultures and demonstrated in scrapings by electron microscopy.

Treatment

Only if secondary bacterial infections become serious.

Control

Isolation of infected animals. Those with genital lesions should not be bred.

ULCERATIVE LYMPHANGITIS

Ulcerative lymphangitis is a contagious disease of horses and mules caused by *Corynebacterium pseudotuberculosis* (*C. ovis*) and characterized by the development of nodules that may ulcerate in the skin, lymph vessels, and nodes in the region of the fetlock.

The nodules, which may extend upward on the leg, eventually rupture and exude a greenish-tinged pus. A form is also described involving inflammation of the lymphatics without abscessation. Systemic involvement is rare.

The disease occurs most commonly in tropical and subtropical countries and is rarely seen in the United States and Canada. The organisms gain entrance via wounds usually in the fetlock area.

Occasionally *C. pseudotuberculosis* causes pectoral abscesses in horses.

Differential Diagnosis

Cutaneous glanders, farcy (caused by *Nocardia asteroides*), epizootic lymphangitis, and sporotrichosis are among the diseases that should be considered.

Laboratory Diagnosis

SPECIMENS/PROCEDURES. For culture: Pus is collected on a swab, preferably from an excised developing nodule. Discharging nodules may have considerable extraneous bacteria.

The isolation and identification of *C. pseudotuberculosis* constitutes a definitive diagnosis.

Treatment

Broad-spectrum antibiotics are of value in the early disease and in the lymphangitis form. When suppurative abscesses are present, antimicrobial therapy is of less value. Efforts may be directed toward treating the nodules surgically, by heat, irrigation, and the application of ointments.

Control

Infected animals should be isolated.

Avoid crowding and circumstances that contribute to injuries.

VESICULAR STOMATITIS

Vesicular stomatitis is a contagious disease of cattle, horses, and pigs caused by a rhabdovirus. It is characterized by the formation of vesicles, followed by erosions, involving the mucous membrane of the mouth and the skin of the feet.

The disease occurs periodically in south, central, and northern regions of the United States and in Central and South America. The incubation period is usually 24 hours, and the disease is spread rapidly by direct contact, biting insects, and fomites. The two important serotypes are designated New Jersey and Indiana. The latter type has three subtypes that occur in South America. Sheep and goats are resistant to infection.

Differential Diagnosis

The precise diagnosis of this disease is of paramount importance because of its close resemblance to foot-and-mouth disease. The susceptibility of cattle, horses, and swine to experimental infection with viruses of the four principal vesicular diseases varies (Table 2.13).

Table 2.13. Susceptibility to the four principal vesicular diseases

Disease	Cattle	Swine	Horses
Foot-and-mouth disease	+	+	−
Vesicular stomatitis	+	+	+
Vesicular exanthema	−	+	±[a]
Swine vesicular disease	−	+	−

[a]Some strains produce vesicles, others do not.

When a vesicular disease occurs, it should be reported immediately to the state and federal officials in charge of animal health.

Laboratory Diagnosis

SPECIMENS. In many countries these will be collected by state, provincial, or federal animal health officials.

Epithelial tissue covering the vesicles in the mouth, or on the feet or teats should be collected and placed in buffered glycerol or frozen for shipment. If available, vesicular fluid should be collected aseptically in a sterile vial and frozen. Esophageal-pharyngeal fluid obtained with a probang should be deposited in sterile tissue culture medium containing an antibiotic, and frozen.

Paired serum samples, acute and convalescent, can be used for complement fixation (CF) or virus neutralization (VN) tests to show a rise in vesicular stomatitis antibodies.

PROCEDURES. Among the tests performed are virus isolation from lesions, and CF and VN tests for specific antibodies.

Horse, cattle, and swine are sometimes inoculated. Foot-and-mouth disease does not affect the horse.

Treatment

None except the use of mild antiseptics and astringents on the mucosa of the mouth.

Control

Quarantine. Vaccine available in some countries.

VOMITING-AND-WASTING DISEASE OF SWINE /
HEMAGGLUTINATING ENCEPHALOMYELITIS VIRUS (HEV) INFECTION
OF PIGS

This is an acute disease of nursing pigs (5–21 days of age) caused by a coronavirus and characterized by vomiting, anorexia, constipation, chronic emaciation, and in some instances acute encephalomyelitis.

Clinical disease is seen when fully susceptible pigs are exposed to virulent strains of the virus. When herd immunity develops, clinical cases no longer occur. There is evidence that the so-called "vomiting-and-wasting disease" and the encephalitis are caused by two different strains of the coronavirus.

Differential Diagnosis

Vomiting and neurologic signs in young pigs are suggestive. Because neurologic signs are seen in a number of other diseases, laboratory confirmation is recommended.

Transmissible gastroenteritis, Teschen and Teschen-like diseases, pseudorabies, and clostridial enterotoxemia should be considered.

Laboratory Diagnosis

SPECIMENS. For histopathology, fluorescent antibody test, and virus isolation: Submit a pig with clinical signs, or brain (halved lengthwise, fresh and fixed) and portions of the cervical cord, both fresh and formalized. Nasal washings, lung, tonsils, stomach, and duodenum for virus isolation.

PROCEDURES/COMMENTS. Histopathologic lesions characteristic of a viral encephalitis may be found in the brain stem, cervical cord, and paravertebral ganglia. Infected cells can be demonstrated in frozen sections by fluorescent antibody. The virus is difficult to culture.

The isolation and identification of this hemagglutinating coronavirus from brain, cord, and other tissues along with characteristic lesions and clinical signs is definitive.

Treatment

None.

Control

No practicable measures available.

WEEKSELLA

Bacteria that were earlier called *Flavobacterium* sp. group IIj have now been named *Weeksella zoohelcum*. These aerobic, gram-negative rods are of interest because they are part of the normal flora of the mouth and paws of dogs and cats, and may cause bite or scratch infections in humans. They do not appear to cause significant infections in dogs and cats.

WINTER DYSENTERY / WINTER SCOURS, BLACK SCOURS

Winter dysentery is an acute, contagious disease of cattle characterized by the sudden onset of enteritis leading to diarrhea and/or dysentery. The disease, which runs a short course, spreads rapidly within a herd and the morbidity ranges from 10 to almost 100%. Although the mortality is low, there is serious loss of condition and milk production.

The precise cause is still in doubt; however, *Campylobacter jejuni* or coronavirus is thought to be causally associated with the disease. Several viruses have been postulated as primary agents.

The disease is prevalent in North America, Europe, Middle East, and Australia.

Differential Diagnosis

A number of bacteria, viruses, and parasites can cause diarrhea in cattle. Salmonellosis, bovine virus diarrhea, coccidiosis, enterotoxemia, rinderpest, Johne's disease, and various toxic agents should be considered.

Laboratory Diagnosis

A clinical diagnosis is made on the basis of the occurrence of an explosive diarrhea in winter months, with high morbidity and short course.

SPECIMENS/PROCEDURES. Attempts are made to isolate and identify putative causal agent(s) from fecal specimens.

Treatment

Supportive therapy is recommended as there is no specific treatment.

Antimicrobial agents are sometimes used for possible secondary bacterial infection.

Control

Efforts should be directed to minimizing spread of infection by contact and various fomites.

YERSINIA ENTEROCOLITICA INFECTION

Yersinia enterocolitica causes a disease that has a number of similarities with the disease caused by the closely related organism, *Y. pseudotuberculosis*. The infection has received most attention in humans, in which it is characterized mainly by gastroenteritis and mesenteric lymphadenitis. Other less frequent manifestations are septicemia, and splenic and colonic abscesses. The same manifestations are seen in animals.

Infections have been reported in chinchilla, mink, laboratory animals, raccoon, fox, deer, elk, many avian species, other wild animals, and some fish. Among the domestic animals, infections have been reported from cattle, sheep, horse, goat, camel, dog, and swine.

Many animals develop an asymptomatic carrier state in which the organism is shed in their feces, thus constituting a source of infection for other animals and humans. As a result of the large reservoir of infection, there are many inanimate sources of *Y. enterocolitica* resulting from fecal contamination; e.g., rivers, streams, ponds, milk, drinking water, ice cream, meat products, etc. The epidemiology of yersiniosis resembles somewhat that of salmonellosis.

Both *Y. pseudotuberculosis* and *Y. enterocolitica* have been incriminated in outbreaks of diarrhea in captive deer. The latter has been isolated frequently from the tonsils, tongues, and mesenteric nodes of as many as 25% of pigs.

This infection, like that caused by *Y. pseudotuberculosis,* is usually diagnosed after a bacteriological examination.

Laboratory Diagnosis

The laboratory diagnosis is essentially the same as that for *Y. pseudotuberculosis* (q.v.) except that, in addition to using primary media, a cold enrichment procedure should also be used.

It should be kept in mind that serotype O9 of *Y. enterocolitica* serologically cross-reacts with *Brucella abortus*.

Treatment

Treatment is the same as for *Y. PSEUDOTUBERCULOSIS* INFECTION (q.v.).

YERSINIA PSEUDOTUBERCULOSIS INFECTION /
PSEUDOTUBERCULOSIS

Yersinia pseudotuberculosis causes a disease principally of guinea pigs, rats, mice, rabbits, hares, turkeys, and deer. Two forms of the disease are seen: The acute is characterized by a septicemia with death usually within 48 hours; and the classical form is manifested by enteritis with numerous necrotic and caseous lesions in the mesenteric lymph nodes, liver, spleen, and lungs.

The organism has been isolated frequently from the feces of cattle, sheep, goats, pigs, and cats, but clinical disease is rarely seen in these animals. It has been incriminated as a cause of diarrhea in captive deer.

Humans occasionally contract the disease and the source is usually carrier animals. There is an acute typhoidal disease that occurs in humans, as well as a less serious form, which is characterized by a mesenteric lymphadenitis that simulates appendicitis.

Laboratory Diagnosis

SPECIMENS. For culture: Feces and portions of tissues with necrotic and caseous lesions.

PROCEDURES. This organism, which is gram-negative and belongs in the Enterobacteriaceae, can be isolated and identified by conventional methods. Antimicrobial susceptibility tests should be performed.

Treatment

Among the antimicrobial drugs that have been effective are chloramphenicol, tetracyclines, ampicillin, gentamycin, neomycin, and kanamycin.

ZYGOMYCOSIS / MUCORMYCOSIS, PHYCOMYCOSIS

Zygomycosis denotes a usually chronic fungous infection occurring infrequently in cattle, pigs, horses, dogs, cats, and other animals caused by widespread fungi of the genera *Mucor, Absidia, Rhizopus,* and *Mortierella.* Infection is by inhalation or ingestion with the production of focal granulomatous lesions in lymph nodes associated with the lungs or the intestinal tract.

The fungi just listed are sometimes associated with ulceration of the rumen, abomasum, and stomach of cattle and pigs. They have also been implicated in abortion in cattle on several continents. Abortion in cattle due to *Mortierella* may be followed by an acute pneumonia.

Basidiobolomycosis (entomophthoromycosis), which affects many animals, is a zygomycosis caused by fungi in the genera *Basidiobolus* and *Conidiobolus. B. ranarum* and *C. coronatus* cause ulcerative granulomas involving subcutaneous tissues and oral and nasal mucous membranes of the mouth and nasal passages. Lesions caused by *B. ranarum* may be large and involve the skin of the head, neck, and chest.

Unless there is an immune deficiency, prolonged administration of antibiotics, a malignancy, or other predisposing factor, the disease is usually mild. Most cases are diagnosed at postmortem, and the lesions seen may not always have been the cause of death.

Laboratory Diagnosis

SPECIMENS

1. For culture: Portions of lymph nodes with lesions and other tissues, if affected.
2. For histopathology: Same portions as above, but fixed.

PROCEDURES/COMMENTS. Prior to culturing, material from lesions should be examined in wet mounts for fungal elements.

Stained sections of tissue are examined for fungal elements, which will be nonseptate hyphae in zygomycosis.

Because these fungi are widespread in nature and are often contaminants in specimens and on media, the finding of the fungal elements in tissue sections is especially significant.

In suspected mycotic abortion, attempts are made to demonstrate and culture fungi from the necrotic placental lesions and from the fetal skin lesions if present. A diagnosis of mycotic abortion is based upon the demonstration, in the case of zygomycosis, of nonseptate hyphae in tissue sections. Recovery of a fungus may enable the precise cause to be determined.

Treatment
1. Amphotericin B is the drug of choice.
2. Surgical excision and treatment with ketoconozole have been effective.

Control
Not usually feasible.

SECTION 3 | Microbial Diseases Foreign to North America

Listed in this section are most of the animal diseases that ordinarily do not occur in North America. Many of them are of such significance to the livestock industry that major efforts are directed toward preventing their introduction, and should they be introduced and detected, efforts are directed toward control and eradication.

Most of the diseases in this section are "notifiable," that is, if they are suspected by the practicing veterinarian, then state/provincial and federal veterinary officials are informed. They then take charge of the diagnosis and, if indicated, implement what control measures are mandated.

Some of the diseases in this section are of great economic importance and, consequently, have been given the most attention. The descriptions of the diseases of lesser importance are brief and they are included mainly because the practitioner should at least be aware that they occur.

Because the laboratory diagnosis of all of these diseases is often quite involved and is carried out usually in federal laboratories, it has not been dealt with fully in this section. For details of the laboratory diagnosis of these diseases, readers are referred to Appendix B, Sources for Additional Information.

AFRICAN HORSE SICKNESS

African horse sickness is a usually highly fatal, arthropod-borne disease of equidae caused by an orbivirus and manifested in acute pulmonary, cardiac, mixed cardiac and pulmonary, and subclinical forms.

This disease, which is endemic in Africa, has spread to a

number of Middle Eastern countries, Portugal, Spain, Pakistan, and India. This orbivirus occurs as nine different serotypes and is transmitted by biting arthropods, particularly members of the *Culicoides*. It is thought that there may be an invertebrate reservoir.

The fatality rate may be as high as 90% in fully susceptible horses.

Differential Diagnosis

Some of the clinical signs are as follows:

Pulmonary form: Fever; signs of severe pulmonary infection; coughing, choking, and frothy fluid from the nostrils. Rapid course.

Cardiac form: Slower course; swelling of head, neck, eyelids, brisket, and ventral aspect of thorax and abdomen.

Subclinical form: Fever for several days; mild malaise with recovery.

Anthrax, equine viral arteritis, equine influenza, equine infectious anemia, and trypanosomiasis are among the diseases to be considered.

Laboratory Diagnosis

SPECIMENS

1. Unclotted blood at or before the febrile period. Portions of spleen, brain, heart, lung, liver, and kidney.
2. Clotted blood collected 5–6 days after the highest temperature.

PROCEDURES

1. Horse and mouse inoculation for virus isolation. Mouse passages may be necessary. Serotype identification by the complement fixation (CF) test.
2. CF test for specific antibodies. Other procedures used are enzyme-linked immunosorbent assay, virus neutralization, and agar gel immunodiffusion.

Treatment

None.

Control

1. Polyvalent attenuated vaccine of mouse brain origin.
2. Prevent introduction of infected animals to disease-free areas.

3. Control of biting insects is important.

AFRICAN SWINE FEVER / WARTHOG DISEASE

African swine fever is a highly contagious disease of swine caused by an iridovirus and characterized by an acute or peracute viremia with hemorrhages of internal organs, cyanosis of the skin, and a mortality rate that may reach 100%. The endemic form of the disease has a lower mortality and resembles the endemic form of hog cholera, including the production of similar lesions.

It occurs in Africa, Spain, and Portugal. There have been outbreaks in France, Italy, Cuba, Haiti, Dominican Republic, and Brazil.

The disease is transmitted by direct and indirect contact with carrier pigs. Warthogs and forest and bush pigs also serve as a reservoir of the virus. Ticks and lice may be biologic vectors.

Differential Diagnosis

Among the diseases to consider are hog cholera, erysipelas, and salmonellosis.

Laboratory Diagnosis
SPECIMENS

1. For virus isolation and identification: Blood, portions of spleen, lung, and a variety of lymph nodes.
2. For serology: Serum samples from a number of affected pigs, including those infected for the longest period of time.

PROCEDURES

1. Inoculation of blood and tissues into cell cultures, and into susceptible and immune pigs.

    FA identification of the virus in frozen sections of tissues and in cell cultures. Hemadsorption test in pig buffy coat cultures.
2. Agar gel immunodiffusion test, virus neutralization test, electroosmophoresis, and enzyme-linked immunosorbent assay.

Treatment

None.

Control

The disease has only been effectively controlled by a policy of strict quarantine and slaughter. Although various vaccines have been used, none have been found to be satisfactory and safe.

AKABANE DISEASE / ENZOOTIC BOVINE ARTHROGRYPOSIS, HYDRANENCEPHALY

Akabane disease of cattle, sheep, and goats is caused by the gnat- or mosquito-transmitted Akabane virus (*Bunyavirus*). It is characterized by fetal infections resulting in stillbirths, abortion, premature births, mummified fetuses, and various deformities and abnormalities of live-born calves and fetuses.

Akabane virus is widely distributed among cattle, sheep, and goats in both tropical and temperate regions. The disease has been reported from Australia, Japan, South Africa, Zimbabwe, Israel, the Middle East, and Argentina. There is a report of an outbreak in sheep in Texas.

Definitive diagnosis is based upon the isolation and identification of the virus. A number of serologic tests are useful for detecting and measuring the antibody response.

BORNA DISEASE

Borna disease is primarily a meningoencephalomyelitis of horses and sheep caused by an, as yet, unclassified virus. The disease, which has a low morbidity but high mortality, occurs in Germany and neighboring countries. It resembles equine encephalomyelitis clinically. Although both sheep and horses can be infected by aerosol, the natural means of transmission is still in doubt. The disease is not transmissible to humans.

Laboratory diagnosis involves virus isolation, detection of virus in tissues, and an indirect fluorescent antibody procedure to detect antibody.

BOVINE PETECHIAL FEVER / ONDIRI DISEASE

Bovine petechial fever is a noncontagious disease caused by the rickettsia *Ehrlichia ondiri* and characterized by fever, petechial hemorrhages of mucous membranes, edema of the conjunctiva, with collapse followed by death in acute cases.

The disease has occurred only in the highlands of Kenya and in neighboring countries at similar altitudes. Some wild ruminants serve as a reservoir of the rickettsia and although biting arthopods are suspected as vectors, their role in transmission has not been proven.

Laboratory Diagnosis

The disease, which is sporadic in occurrence, is diagnosed by the demonstration of the rickettsia in Geimsa-stained blood and spleenic smears.The organisms are found in monocytes and granulocytes. Blood smears may have to be examined on several successive days in order to detect organisms.

BOVINE SPONGIFORM ENCEPHALOPATHY

Bovine spongiform encephalopathy (BSE) is a chronic, insidious, degenerative disease of the central nervous system of adult cattle, probably caused by a prion (small particle of protein). It is characterized by a long incubation period (2–8 years), slow progress, and fatal outcome. The disease resembles scrapie, and clinical signs include loss of weight and condition, apprehension, aggression, gait ataxia, tremors, excitability, and eventually generalized paresis and death.

BSE has been reported from Great Britain, Ireland, France, Switzerland, and Oman. Fibrils similar to those found in the brains of sheep with scrapie have been demonstrated in the brains of cattle with BSE. Brain homogenates from BSE cases produced a scrapie-like disease when inoculated into mice. There is no evidence of cattle-to-cattle transmission and it is thought that animal proteins, e.g., in meat and bone meal, are the most likely source for the agent of BSE. The feeding of rations containing protein of ruminant origin to cattle has been suspended in Great Britain.

Differential Diagnosis

Rabies, particularly the furious form; hypomagnesemia; listeriosis; and other neurologic diseases may evince clinical signs resembling early BSE.

Laboratory Diagnosis
SPECIMENS/PROCEDURES

1. For animal inoculation: Portions of brain and cord, fresh.
2. For histopathology: Portions of brain and cord, fixed.

COMMENTS. Diagnosis is based on the characteristic clinical signs and histopathologic changes in the brain and cord. The characteristic histologic changes in BSE and scrapie are widespread neuronal vaculation, gliosis, and varying amounts of neuronal loss.

For confirmatory purposes, mice and possibly other animals are inoculated with fresh brain and cord.

Treatment
None.

Control
This involves slaughter of all affected cattle.

CHUZAN DISEASE
Chuzan disease (CD) affects calves and is characterized by an hydranencephaly-cerebellar hypoplasia syndrome resulting in congenital anomalies. CD has only occurred in Japan and is thought to be caused by an arthropod-borne virus belonging in a subgroup of orbivirus.

The disease affects mainly beef cows. The most common clinical signs in calves are epileptiform seizures, opisthotonus, blindness, and failure to nurse. Viremia in cows may last for several weeks as in other orbivirus infections, e.g., bluetongue and Akabane disease. The midge, *Culicoides oxystoma,* is thought to be the principal vector.

Laboratory diagnosis involves tests for antibodies to the Chuzan virus and attempts to recover the virus from the blood of cows. The principal histologic lesions seen are hydranencephaly and cerebellar hypoplasia. Arthrogryposis has not been reported.

Although an inactivated virus vaccine is being studied, there is as yet no vaccine available for cattle at risk.

CONTAGIOUS BOVINE PLEUROPNEUMONIA
Contagious bovine pleuropneumonia is caused by the small bacterium *Mycoplasma mycoides* ssp. *mycoides* and is characterized by a septicemia or bacteremia resulting in acute, subacute, and chronic forms. The localization in the lungs and pleura often results in a fibrinous bronchopneumonia with extensive pulmonary consolidation.

The disease occurs in Africa; some regions of Asia including China, Nepal, and Sri Lanka; and India. There are occasional outbreaks in the Middle East.

It is mainly a disease of cattle and occurs much less frequently in other ruminants, including water buffaloes. The infection is derived from infected and carrier animals and the principal mode of infection is by inhalation. The organism, which is fragile (no cell wall), does not survive long outside the host.

Differential Diagnosis

The clinical signs are those of pneumonia and pleurisy. Other bovine respiratory diseases (see BOVINE RESPIRATORY DISEASE) should be considered. The marbling seen in the lungs is like that of bovine pneumonic pasteurellosis.

Laboratory Diagnosis

Definitive diagnosis depends on isolation and identification of the causal organism.

SPECIMENS

1. Acute and convalescent sera if possible.
2. Tissues and fluids from affected lungs.
3. Sick or dead animals for necropsy.

PROCEDURES/COMMENTS

1. Complement fixation test; an enzyme-linked immunosorbent assay. Early and incubating cases may be seronegative.
2. Isolation and identification of the organism: Agar gel precipitin test to detect antigen in tissue. Fluorescent antibody procedure for identification of the organism in tissues.
3. Gross pathology: Bronchopneumonia with varying degrees of consolidation resulting in a marbled appearance. Thickened, inflamed pleura with sometimes large amounts of turbid fluid containing fibrin flakes. In the chronic form, there are walled-off capsulated necrotic areas (sequestrae).

Treatment

Ineffective.

Control

Notifiable disease in most countries. A live attenuated vaccine is employed in areas where eradication is not feasible.

EPHEMERAL FEVER /
THREE DAY SICKNESS, BOVINE ENZOOTIC FEVER

This is an arthropod-transmitted disease of cattle, buffaloes, and some wild ruminants caused by a rhabdovirus and characterized by high fever, lacrimation, lameness, stiffness, muscular tremors, enlargement of superficial lymph nodes, and a short course with a rapid spontaneous recovery.

This disease, which is of minor significance, has been reported from Australia, Asia, the East Indies, and Africa. The mortality rate is less than 1%.

Differential Diagnosis

Because infections are often mild and the clinical signs are not distinctive, the disease can only be diagnosed with certainty by laboratory means.

Laboratory Diagnosis

SPECIMENS. For virus isolation and animal inoculation: Unclotted blood taken during the acute phase of the disease.

PROCEDURES/COMMENTS. Susceptible and immune cattle are sometimes inoculated.

Weanling mice and hamsters are susceptible to experimental infection and are inoculated intracerebrally. The virus is identified by neutralization procedures.

Treatment

None.

Control

Little can be done other than protection of cattle from biting arthropods.

EPIZOOTIC LYMPHANGITIS /
EQUINE PSEUDOGLANDERS, AFRICAN GLANDERS

Epizootic lymphangitis is a chronic, contagious disease of horses (rarely cattle) caused by the dimorphic fungus *Histoplasma farciminosum* and characterized by the development of suppurative nodules involving the skin, mucous membranes, superficial lymph vessels and nodes. Most lesions develop on the limbs but they may also be present on the sides, back, and neck. A pulmonary form has been reported.

The disease occurs in Asia, Africa, and some Mediterranean countries. Outbreaks occur when numbers of horses from different sources are collected in one place. The mortality can be as high as 15% in fully susceptible animals. Although the organism may occur in nature, most cases are considered to derive from other infected animals. The organism gains entrance via wounds and abrasions. The natural habitat, other than horses, is not known.

The organism has been placed in the genus *Histoplasma*, although it will be eventually reclassified.

Differential Diagnosis

Ulcerative lymphangitis, cutaneous glanders, and sporotrichosis should be considered.

Definitive diagnosis is dependent on isolation and identification of the fungus.

Laboratory Diagnosis

SPECIMENS. Fresh pus is collected from incised nodules to reduce extraneous organisms.

PROCEDURES
1. For direct examination: A diagnosis is usually based upon the demonstration of the typical yeast-like cells of *H. farciminosum* in wet mounts of pus.
2. For culture: Appropriate media are inoculated and incubated at 37°C and 25°C to obtain the yeast phase and the mycelial phase, respectively. These are necessary for identification.

Treatment

In general, treatment has not been satisfactory. Iodides orally; local application of iodine and silver nitrate. Modern antifungal drugs do not appear to have been adequately applied.

Control

Isolation of clinical cases and elimination of those that do not respond to treatment.

An alum-precipitated type of vaccine has been used where the disease is a continuing problem.

FOOT-AND-MOUTH DISEASE

Foot-and-mouth disease (FMD) is a highly contagious disease of cloven-footed domestic and wild animals caused by a picornavirus (aphthovirus). It is characterized by vesicular lesions, followed by erosions of the epithelium of the mouth, nares, muzzle, feet, udder, and teats.

The morbidity is high, and although the mortality is low, great economic loss results from the effects of the disease, which include lameness, loss of milk production, weight loss, mastitis, debilitation, and abortion.

FMD occurs in many major livestock-producing countries with the exception of North America, Australia, New Zealand, and Ireland. Great Britain and several countries of Europe are usually free.

There are 7 immunologically distinct types of FMD virus, viz., types O, A, C, SAT-1, SAT-2, SAT-3, and Asia-1. Within the 7 types there are more than 60 subtypes.

Differential Diagnosis

Bovine virus diarrhea, rinderpest, bovine papular stomatitis, vesicular stomatitis, and swine vesicular disease are among the diseases that should be considered. Any disease characterized by the formation of vesicles or erosions of the mouth, muzzle, nares, feet, udder, and teats is suspect.

Laboratory Diagnosis

This is a notifiable disease in almost all countries where it is not established. If the disease is suspected, state/provincial and federal veterinarians should be contacted. Ordinarily they arrange for the laboratory diagnosis and the specimens collected will depend upon the tests and procedures available. The procedures given below have been taken from literature provided by the U.S. Department of Agriculture.

SPECIMENS. Esophageal-pharyngeal fluid, obtained with a probang, deposited in sterile tissue culture medium containing antibiotic; vesicle fluid collected with aseptic technique in a sterile vial; lesion scrapings or epithelial flaps placed in tissue culture medium containing antibiotic; paired sera from individual animals or sera from separate animals taken at early and later stages.

All specimens are immediately frozen for shipment

(preferable) or placed in glycerol. Specimens packed in dry ice must be completely sealed to prevent the introduction of CO_2 gas and a subsequent drop in pH, which can destroy the infectivity of the virus.

PROCEDURES. These will vary from one laboratory to another.

Virus identification: Virus antigen can often be identified in tissues by complement fixation, agar gel immunodiffusion (AGID), enzyme-linked immunosorbent assay (ELISA), and fluorescent antibody (FA). The virus can be propagated in cell cultures and identified by virus neutralization, complement fixation, AGID, FA, and ELISA. Electron microscopy can contribute to a rapid diagnosis. Inoculation of unweaned mice and guinea pigs with infected materials produces characteristic lesions. Differentiation of FMD, vesicular stomatitis, and vesicular exanthema can be accomplished by the inoculation of horses, cattle, and swine (see VESICULAR STOMATITIS, Section 2).

Treatment
Mainly local treatment to prevent and cope with secondary bacteria.

Control
In countries free of FMD a policy of quarantine and slaughter is usually practiced with the goal of complete eradication.

A number of inactivated vaccines, including those prepared in cell culture, containing the appropriate type(s) or subtypes, are used in countries where the disease is endemic. The duration of immunity may be as short as 4 months. Genetically engineered and other vaccines are under development.

GETAH DISEASE OF HORSES
Getah disease in horses is an acute or subacute, viral infection characterized principally by fever, edema of the hind limbs, and an urticarial rash on various regions of the body. The causal alphavirus is transmitted by mosquitoes and is capable of producing a peracute, fatal disease in neonatal piglets.

The disease has been reported from Japan and several other Asian countries. Although a variety of animals can become infected, clinical disease has only been seen in horses and neonatal piglets. The Getah virus is in the same genus, *Alphavirus,* as the agents of the common viral equine encephalitides (Eastern, Western, and Venezuelan).

Differential Diagnosis

The clinical signs of Getah disease in horses resemble those of EQUINE VIRUS ARTERITIS (Section 2) and mild AFRICAN HORSE SICKNESS.

Laboratory Diagnosis

This is essentially the same as for the equine encephalitides.

Treatment

None.

Control

Mosquito control. An inactivated vaccine is used annually in Japan.

GLANDERS / FARCY

Glanders is a contagious disease of solipeds (horses, mules, donkeys) caused by the gram-negative rod *Pseudomonas mallei* and characterized usually by acute and chronic manifestations resulting from a septicemia or bacteremia. In the latter chronic type, tubercles or nodules eventually ulcerate involving the nasal mucosa (nasal form), the lungs (pulmonary form), or the skin (cutaneous form). The course in the acute form is several days, whereas chronic cases may persist for weeks.

This infrequent disease, which has been eradicated from North America, occurs in North Africa, Asia, Eastern Europe, and some countries of the Middle East.

In addition to solipeds, humans and members of the cat family may be infected, usually fatally, in the absence of treatment. The source of the agent is always infected animals, usually horses. The mode of infection is by ingestion and possibly inhalation.

Differential Diagnosis

The incubation period is about 2 weeks. In the acute form, signs include fever, cough, nasal discharge, ulceration of nasal mucosa and skin, with nodules appearing on the skin of the lower limbs. Death follows within several days as a result of a septicemia. In the chronic form, signs include cough, dyspnea, and epistaxis when localization involves the lung. The skin and nasal form is characterized by the formation of ulcers and subcutaneous nodules. Some chronic cases recover and are sources of infection.

Epizootic lymphangitis, ulcerative lymphangitis, sporotrichosis, farcy (caused by *Nocardia asteroides*), zygomycosis, and pneumonias due to various agents are among the diseases that should be considered.

Laboratory Diagnosis

A definitive diagnosis is based on the isolation and identification of *P. mallei*. In some situations a mallein test is used to screen horses for possible glanders.

SPECIMENS

1. Swabs are taken from ulcers and incised nodules. Pus may also be aspirated by syringe from nodules. Skin biopsies.
2. If a necropsy is performed, portions of nodules and affected lung, fresh and fixed, should be submitted.

PROCEDURES

1. Isolation and identification of *P. mallei*.
2. Histopathologic examination.

Treatment

Treatment is only employed in endemic areas. Sulfadiazine for 3 weeks has been used successfully.

Control

Vaccination is not practiced. Ordinarily if glanders is detected, the premises are quarantined. Clinical cases and reactors to the mallein test are slaughtered.

HEARTWATER / COWDRIOSIS

Heartwater is a disease of ruminants caused by the rickettsia *Cowdria ruminantium* and transmitted by ticks of the *Amblyoma* spp. It occurs in peracute, acute, and subacute forms and is characterized by septicemia, hydropericardium, pyrexia, and neurologic signs.

Heartwater occurs in Africa, Madagascar, Guadeloupe, and other islands of the Caribbean. It has been reported occasionally from Europe. Cattle, sheep, and goats are affected and indigenous breeds are more resistant than imported ones. Wild ruminants including antelope, blesbok, and wildebeest are susceptible.

The source of this intracellular parasite, which colonizes endothelial cells, is infected animals and it is transmitted by the three-host *Amblyoma* ticks.

Differential Diagnosis

Peracute: High fever, hyperesthesia, convulsions, and death.

Acute and subacute: Neurologic signs including circling, high-stepping, convulsions followed by prostration and death.

Cerebral babesiosis, anthrax, and hypomagnesemia should be considered.

Laboratory Diagnosis

SPECIMENS

1. Brain: Fresh and in 10% formalin. Portions of aorta and jugular vein, fresh and formalized.
2. Serum.

PROCEDURES/COMMENTS

1. Squash and crush smears are made from the hippocampus or cerebral cortex and stained for rickettsiae by the Giemsa method. Smears from the endothelium of the aorta and jugular vessels are similarly stained.
2. An indirect fluorescent antibody (FA) test is used to detect antibodies.

   The indirect FA test is used to determine the immune status rather than for diagnosis.

Treatment

Tetracyclines administered early.

Control

Control of ticks.

Simultaneous infection with infectious blood and treatment with tetracyclines provides protection against homologous strains, but little protection against heterologous strains.

Very young animals are resistant to natural and experimental infection.

HEMORRHAGIC SEPTICEMIA

Hemorrhagic septicemia (HS) is an acute pasteurellosis, principally of cattle and water buffaloes caused by two serotypes (B:2 and E:2) of *Pasteurella multocida* and characterized by a rapid course, edematous swelling in the head-throat-brisket region, swollen and hemorrhagic lymph nodes, and the presence of numerous subserous petechial hemorrhages.

HS caused by the type B:2 strains occurs in southern Europe, North Africa, countries surrounding the Mediterranean, the Near East, and South and Southeast Asia including Indonesia and the Philippines. It does not occur in North America (except in bison), Australia, Oceania, Japan, and South America as far as is known. HS caused by type E:2 strains has only been reported from African countries. Some African countries have both serotypes.

The disease occurs most frequently at the beginning and during the monsoon or rainy season. The morbidity rate varies greatly but the mortality is always high. A small percentage of animals are carriers; a larger percentage are carriers after an outbreak.

Differential Diagnosis

There is often a history of previous outbreaks in the herd or region.

Highly suggestive is the occurrence at the beginning of the rainy season, of high fever, edematous swellings, and a short fatal course.

Anthrax, pneumonic pasteurellosis, acute salmonellosis, and rinderpest are among the diseases that should be considered.

Laboratory Diagnosis

SPECIMENS. For culture: Swabs from heart blood, liver, spleen, and lymph nodes. Portions of the aforementioned tissues may also be submitted. A rib or long bone may be submitted if refrigeration is a special problem.

PROCEDURES/COMMENTS. Definitive diagnosis can only be made on the basis of the isolation and identification of *P. multocida* with subsequent serotype identification (B:2

or E:2) by serologic or immunologic (serum protection in mice) means.

Mice or rabbits are often useful in the recovery of *P. multocida* from swabs or tissues containing postmortem contaminants.

Treatment

Penicillin and streptomycin, tetracyclines, chloramphenicol, and sulfonamides are effective although treatment is not usually practicable.

Control

Annual administration of oil-adjuvant bacterin or more frequent administration of alum precipitated–type bacterin. An experimental live vaccine has shown promise.

HOG CHOLERA / SWINE FEVER

Hog cholera, a highly contagious disease, is caused by a pestivirus (togavirus) and is characterized in fully susceptible pigs by an acute form with a viremia, high temperature, and high mortality. When the disease becomes endemic, a chronic form is seen that includes infection of the fetus resulting in congenital defects.

The disease occurs in many countries of Europe, Africa, and Asia. Australia, New Zealand, the United Kingdom, and North America are free of the disease. The disease is spread by direct and indirect contact. Recovered carrier pigs serve as a source of the disease.

Differential Diagnosis

African swine fever, salmonellosis, and erysipelas should be considered.

Laboratory Diagnosis

SPECIMENS. Blood samples. The brain, sections of intestine, and other internal organs should be preserved in 10% formalin. Fresh, unfixed pancreas, lymph node, the entire tonsil, and large pieces of spleen should be shipped in sealed containers under refrigeration.

PROCEDURES. Fluorescent antibody (FA) techniques allow rapid detection of antigen in frozen tissue sections or impression smears, and in infected cell cultures. The agar gel precipitin test detects antigen in tissues with immune sera, preferably using pancreas from suspect pigs as the source of the antigen. Antibody can be detected by the FA neutralization test, or an indirect enzyme-labelled antibody test that uses enzyme-labelled anti-porcine gammaglobulin to detect antigen-antibody complex.

Treatment
None.

Control
In countries free of the disease, eradication is accomplished by a policy of strict quarantine and slaughter.

Inactivated tissue vaccines such as the crystal violet vaccine are only partially effective. Attenuated virus vaccines, such as the lapinized (rabbit) vaccine, are used in some countries. Among the live attenuated vaccines, the so-called "Chinese strain" has found wide acceptance.

HORSEPOX
Horsepox, caused by a poxvirus, is a rare disease, reported from several European countries. It is characterized by the development of papules, followed by vesicles and pustules on the skin of the lips, nares, back, pastern, fetlock regions, and the buccal mucous membrane. Transmission is by contact and such fomites as saddles, combs, brushes, and harnesses.

If laboratory diagnosis is sought, the characteristic morphology of the virus can be seen in sections examined with the electron microscope. The virus can be cultivated in cell cultures of equine origin.

Control involves elimination of this rather resistant virus by isolation of infected horses until they fully recover and implementation of strict sanitary measures.

JAPANESE ENCEPHALITIS
Japanese encephalitis is an arthropod-borne disease of horses, swine, and humans, caused by a flavivirus and characterized by an encephalitis in horses that is usually milder than that caused by the viruses of the three well-known equine encephalitides. Pregnant sows may abort and neonatal swine may die.

The reservoir of the virus is in birds and mammals, and the distribution is mainly in the Far East. Mosquitoes (*Culex*) are the principal vector.

Laboratory diagnosis is similar to that of the three important equine encephalitides; i.e., serologic tests, isolation, and identification of the virus.

JEMBRANA DISEASE

Jembrana disease is an infectious malady of Balinese cattle (*Bos sondaicus*) and water buffaloes. It is thought to be caused by a rickettsia. The disease, as originally described, had high morbidity and mortality rates both in Balinese cattle and buffaloes. Among the clinical signs are fever, inappetence, swollen superficial lymph nodes, nasal discharge, lacrimation, and anemia. Gross lesions include generalized lymphadenopathy, widespread hemorrhages, splenomegaly, and catarrhal enteritis.

The disease has only been reported from Bali and South Sumatra in Indonesia. The mode of transmission is not known, although ticks are suspected.

Differential Diagnosis

Rinderpest, babesiosis, bovine malignant catarrh, East Coast fever, and bovine petechial fever are among the diseases that should be considered.

Laboratory Diagnosis

The disease has been diagnosed on the basis of demonstrating rickettsia-like organisms in smears from lymph nodes.

LECHIGUANA

Lechiguana is a recently described, sporadic, chronic disease of cattle characterized by a progressive fibrogranulomatous process involving the subcutis and regional lymph nodes of mainly the neck and shoulder region. The course of the natural disease ranges from 3 to 8 months, and the subcutaneous tumorous mass produced may attain a size as great as 20 × 50 cm. A proposed new species, *Pasteurella granulomatis,* has been recovered from lesions and is thought to have causal significance. This infrequent disease, which does not appear to be contagious, has thus far only been described in Southern Brazil. It is thought that lesions due to *Dermatobia hominis* (human botfly) may initiate the disease process.

When well established, the disease is clinically obvious. Diagnosis is confirmed by recovery of *P. granulomatis* and the finding of the characteristic histopathologic changes in tissues from lesions.

Affected animals respond and survive if treated with chloramphenicol. Based on the results of susceptibility tests, other broad-spectrum antibiotics may be effective.

LOUPING ILL

Louping ill is an acute, noncontagious encephalomyelitis, principally of sheep and less commonly of cattle, caused by a flavivirus (togavirus) and characterized by diphasic fever, locomotor incoordination, trembling, salivation, coma, and death. It is transmitted by the sheep tick, *Ixodes ricinus,* and is endemic in the British Isles and Russia.

In humans it causes a serious but not fatal encephalitis.

Definitive diagnosis is based upon the isolation and identification of the virus.

LUMPY SKIN DISEASE

Lumpy skin disease is an infection of cattle and African buffaloes caused by a poxvirus (Neethling virus) and characterized by an initial fever with, in the nonsystemic form, the sudden appearance of multiple lumps or nodules involving the skin; in the systemic form, nodules develop in other tissues and organs. In both forms, there is edema of one or more limbs and swelling of superficial lymph nodes.

This disease, which is thought to be mainly transmitted mechanically by biting arthropods, is confined to the African continent in regions east and south of the Sahara desert. The Neethling virus is closely related to the Allerton virus (pseudo–lumpy skin disease) and the viruses of sheep- and goatpox.

Differential Diagnosis

Bovine ulcerative mammallitis (Allerton virus), skin tuberculosis, insect and tick bites, photosensitization, and warble and screwworm infestation are among the diseases that should be considered.

Laboratory Diagnosis

Definitive diagnosis is based upon the isolation and identification of the virus. The finding of the characteristic inclusion bodies in typical lesions is presumptive evidence of the disease.

Control

Affected animals are slaughtered. Sheeppox vaccine and other attenuated poxvirus vaccines are used.

MALIGNANT CATARRHAL FEVER (AFRICAN)

Two manifestations of malignant catarrhal fever (MCF) are seen. The well-known disease occurs worldwide and has been described with the diseases occurring in North America. The other manifestation of the disease is African MCF, which is caused by alcephaline herpesvirus-1. This virus is carried by the wildebeest, and MCF may develop when these animals graze with cattle. The clinical and pathologic characteristics of the two infections are similar.

Laboratory Diagnosis

(See MALIGNANT CATARRHAL FEVER, Section 2). The alcephaline herpesvirus-1 has been propagated and identified in cell cultures.

MELIOIDOSIS

Melioidosis is a sporadic acute or chronic disease of animals and humans caused by *Pseudomonas pseudomallei* and characterized by a septicemia in the acute form, and the presence of multiple, suppurative abscesses or nodules in the lymph nodes and viscera in the less severe but often progressive chronic form.

Melioidosis occurs in Southeast Asia and Australia. It has been reported from the Caribbean. The disease has occurred in all domestic animal species, some wild animals, rodents, humans, and also animals in zoos, including primates. Some infections are clinically inapparent.

This gram-negative organism lives freely in tropical soil and water and is acquired via wounds, ingestion, and inhalation.

Two principal forms of the disease are seen:

Acute form: Less common in animals than humans. Rapidly

fatal, febrile disease due to a septicemia.

Chronic form: The chronic disease may be progressive and the signs depend upon the location of the suppurative lesions. Pneumonic signs due to pulmonary lesions are seen in sheep and goats more frequently than in other species. Lameness is seen with joint involvement, and neurologic signs occur if the brain is involved.

Differential Diagnosis

A presumptive diagnosis is made in the abattoir and at necropsy on the basis of multiple abscesses seen in various organs and tissues including the liver, spleen, lungs, subcutis, and lymph nodes. The extent and character of the abscesses depend on the age of the host and the severity of the disease. The abscesses in sheep resemble those of pseudotuberculosis and contain thick or caseous greenish-colored pus.

Caseous lymphadenitis, cervical abscesses in swine, actinobacillosis, glanders, strangles, and multiple abscesses due to other bacteria are among the diseases that should be considered.

Laboratory Diagnosis

Diagnosis is based upon the isolation and identification of *P. pseudomallei*. This disease has occurred in North America in animals that have been infected prior to importation, most frequently dogs and primates.

SPECIMENS. Material from fresh abscesses; portions of organs or tissues containing abscesses, fresh and fixed.

PROCEDURES. Isolation and identification of the organism.

Histopathologic examination of tissues. Although serologic procedures have been developed for this disease, e.g., complement fixation and hemagglutination, they are not routinely available for animals.

Treatment

Treatment is not always successful when the disease is well established. Sulfonamides, trimethoprim-sulfamethoxazole, tetracyclines, and chloramphenicol have been used.

Control

Isolation of infected animals. Vaccination is not practiced.

NAIROBI SHEEP DISEASE

Nairobi sheep disease is an acute, noncontagious infection, thought to be caused by a bunyavirus, and characterized by fever, hemorrhagic gastroenteritis, and diarrhea. It is transmitted by the brown dog tick, *Rhipicephalus appendiculatus,* and is endemic in central Africa where it causes significant losses in sheep.

PESTE DES PETITS RUMINANTS /
PEST OF SMALL RUMINANTS

Peste des petits ruminants is an acute, subacute, or chronic rinderpest-like disease of sheep and goats caused by a morbillivirus that is closely related antigenically to that causing rinderpest. The disease is transmitted by direct and indirect contact, and the clinical signs, which resemble those of rinderpest, include fever, nasal discharge with encrustation, oral mucosal erosions, diarrhea, and emaciation. The mortality, depending on the form, varies from 10 to 90%.

The disease has been reported from west and central Africa and the Middle East. It can be prevented by immunization with rinderpest vaccines.

Definitive laboratory diagnosis involves isolation and identification of the virus.

RIFT VALLEY FEVER

Rift Valley fever is an acute, febrile malady of cattle, sheep, goats, camels, and humans caused by a mosquito-borne bunyavirus (phlebovirus) and characterized by hepatic necrosis and high mortality in young animals and abortion in pregnant animals. The virus causes an influenza-like disease in humans.

This disease occurs in most regions of sub-Saharan Africa. It is transmitted principally by species of *Aedes* and *Culex* mosquitoes. Humans usually become infected from direct contact with infected tissues.

Laboratory diagnosis involves isolation and identification of the virus.

RINDERPEST

Rinderpest is an acute or subacute, highly contagious, febrile disease primarily of cattle but also of sheep, goats, swine,

and wild ruminants caused by a morbillivirus and characterized by severe congestion, hemorrhages and erosions of the
mucous membranes of the alimentary tract, with diarrhea.

The disease is only found in parts of Asia and Africa.
Transmission is by direct contact and fomites. In fully susceptible cattle, the mortality may approach 100% with some virulent strains.

Differential Diagnosis

This is a notifiable, major animal plague.

Malignant catarrhal fever, bovine virus diarrhea, Jembrana disease and other diseases characterized by the production of erosions of mucous membranes and diarrhea should
be considered. If rinderpest were to appear in fully susceptible cattle, the high mortality rate and rapid spread would set
it apart from most other infectious diseases.

Laboratory Diagnosis

If rinderpest is suspected, animal health officials will arrange
for laboratory examinations.

SPECIMENS/PROCEDURES

1. For virus isolation: Heparinized blood, mesenteric lymph
   nodes, and spleen are collected early in the acute phase of
   the disease. One portion of the heparinized blood should
   be shipped refrigerated; other specimens should be frozen.
   Blood should also be collected from animals that have
   been ill for the longest period of time during the outbreak.
2. For histopathology: Specimens of tonsils, liver, spleen,
   kidney, and portions of intestines showing lesions should
   be collected in 10% neutral, buffered formalin.
3. Attempts to isolate the virus are carried out in tissue culture or animals.
4. The complement fixation, immunodiffusion, and counter
   immunoelectrophoresis tests with rabbit hyperimmune serum can be used to detect viral antigen in extracts of
   lymph nodes from infected animals. Agar gel immunodiffusion is the most extensively used diagnostic procedure.
   Enzyme-linked immunosorbent assay and virus neutralization tests in cell cultures may be carried out with the
   sera of animals that were sick long enough to develop
   antibodies.

A definitive diagnosis may be obtained by cross-protection tests using immune and susceptible cattle.

Treatment
None.

Control
Quarantine and slaughter.

Inactivated tissue and cell culture vaccines and attenuated live virus vaccines are employed where the disease occurs.

SHEEPPOX AND GOATPOX
Sheeppox and goatpox, in fully susceptible animals, is an acute, highly contagious, and often fatal disease caused by a poxvirus (capripoxvirus) and characterized by fever and pox on the unwooled skin and buccal, digestive, and respiratory tract mucous membranes. As in other pox diseases, papules progress to pustules, then to scabs.

The disease occurs in some European countries, Asia, and Africa. Transmission is by direct and indirect contact, and the virus can survive on contaminated premises for as long as 6 months.

Laboratory Diagnosis
The laboratory diagnosis involves the demonstration and identification of the specific poxvirus in tissues using smears and sections with the light microscope, the electron microscope, and specific fluorescent antibody (FA) staining. The virus can be cultivated in cell cultures and chicken embryos. Specific antibodies in the sera of sheep are detected by virus neutralization, complement fixation, indirect FA, and agar gel immunodiffusion tests.

Treatment
None.

Control
Import restrictions. Quarantine and slaughter in countries where the disease does not occur. Attenuated and inactivated vaccines are used where the disease is endemic.

SWINE VESICULAR DISEASE

Swine vesicular disease (SVD) is a contagious disease of swine caused by a picornavirus and characterized by vesicular lesions on the mouth, tongue, nares, lips, and feet leading to erosions.

This disease, which does not affect other animal species except humans, produces lesions that are grossly indistinguishable from those of foot-and-mouth disease, vesicular exanthema, and vesicular stomatitis. In the natural disease the prognosis is favorable; however, in most countries as soon as it is recognized the pigs are slaughtered.

This disease, which has been reported from several European countries and Asia, does not occur in North America.

Differential Diagnosis

Foot-and-mouth disease, vesicular stomatitis, and vesicular exanthema should be considered. The susceptibility of SVD for cattle, swine, and horses is shown in Table 2.13 (Section 2). Definitive diagnosis is dependent on laboratory procedures.

Laboratory Diagnosis

The procedures used for the laboratory diagnosis of swine vesicular disease are essentially those outlined under FOOT-AND-MOUTH DISEASE. They involve identification of the virus in specimens, virus isolation, and serologic tests to detect specific antibody.

Treatment

None.

Control

Quarantine and slaughter are carried out in countries where the disease does not occur.

TICK-BORNE FEVER / PASTURE FEVER

Tick-borne fever is a disease of cattle, sheep, and goats caused by the rickettsia *Ehrlichia phagocytophilia* and transmitted by *Ixodes* and *Rhipicephalus* ticks. It is characterized by fever, depression, reduced milk production, respiratory distress, and occasionally by abortion.

There are recurring febrile periods and animals may remain infected for months and even years. Parasitized neutrophils and a leukopenia predispose animals to serious secondary infections.

The disease has been reported from the United Kingdom, Scandinavia, and India.

Laboratory Diagnosis

Diagnosis is accomplished by demonstration of rickettsiae in Giemsa-stained blood smears. Granulocytes and monocytes are infected in large numbers during the initial febrile period. A reliable complement fixation test has been developed.

Treatment

Tetracyclines are effective.

Control

This mainly involves control of the tick population.

VESICULAR EXANTHEMA OF SWINE

Vesicular exanthema (VE) of swine is an acute, contagious, febrile disease caused by a calicivirus and characterized by the formation of vesicles on the feet, snout, lips, and mouth with subsequent erosion.

VE is clinically indistinguishable from foot-and-mouth disease, vesicular stomatitis, and swine vesicular disease. Some strains of VE virus will produce vesicles when inoculated into horses but not when injected into cattle (see Table 2.13, Section 2).

VE has not been reported in swine since its last occurrence in the United States in 1955. A virus that was isolated from pinnipeds (San Miguel sea lion) is identical or closely related to the VE virus and experimentally results in a disease that is clinically indistinguishable from VE. It has been concluded that the disease in swine does not occur at present.

Differential Diagnosis

Swine vesicular disease, vesicular stomatitis, and foot-and-mouth disease are the principal diseases that should be considered.

Laboratory Diagnosis

The same specimens and procedures are employed as are used for foot-and-mouth disease, vesicular stomatitis, and swine vesicular disease. The susceptibility of VE to cattle, swine, and horses is shown in Table 2.13 (Section 2).

WESSELSBRON DISEASE

Wesselsbron disease is an acute infection of sheep and occasionally of cattle in South Africa. It is caused by a mosquito-borne flavivirus (togavirus). It is characterized by a high mortality in neonatal lambs and abortion in ewes. In cattle there may be abortion, and in calves porencephaly and cerebellar hypoplasia may occur. Human infections with fever and muscular pains have been reported. The disease resembles Rift Valley fever clinically and epidemiologically, but the viruses are immunologically distinct. An attenuated vaccine is used in nonpregnant sheep and cattle.

Laboratory diagnosis depends upon isolation and identification of the virus.

APPENDICES

APPENDIX A. Commercial Sources of Transport Media, Swab Systems, and Diagnostic Reagents and Kits

1. Abbott Laboratories
   1 Abbott Park Road
   Abbott Park, IL 60064
2. Accu-Med Corporation
   Medical Laboratory Automation, Inc.
   270 Marble Avenue
   Pleasantville, NY 10570
3. AGDIA, Inc.
   30380 Country Road 6
   Elkhart, IN 46514
4. Animal Biotech Corp.
   1531 Monrovia Avenue
   Newport Beach, CA 92663
5. Becton Dickinson Microbiology Systems
   Box 243
   Cockeysville, MD 21030
6. Binax, Inc.
   95 Darling Avenue
   South Portland, ME 04106
7. Cambridge BioScience Corp.
   365 Plantation Street
   Worcester, MA 01605
8. Cooper Animal Health, Inc.
   2000 South 11th Street
   Kansas City, KS 66103
9. Fermenta Animal Health Co.
   10150 North Executive Hills Boulevard
   P.O. Box 901350
   Kansas City, MO 64190
10. Fisher Scientific
    711 Forbes Avenue
    Pittsburgh, PA 15219
11. Fort Dodge Laboratories, Inc.
    P.O. Box 518
    Fort Dodge, IA 50501
12. IDEXX Corp.
    100 Fore Street
    Portland, ME 04101
13. Immucell Corporation
    966 Riverside Street
    Portland, ME 04103
14. Medical Wire & Equipment Co.
    4650 W. 160th Street
    Cleveland, OH 44135
15. Microbiological Associates, Inc.
    5221 River Road
    Bethesda, MD 20816
16. Pitman-Moore, Inc.
    421 E. Hawley St.
    Mundelein, IL 60060
17. ProScience Corporation
    107 Carpenter Drive
    Suite 100
    Sterling, VA 22170
18. Rhone Merieux Laboratories, Inc.
    115 Transtech Drive
    Athens, GA 30601

19. SmithKline Beecham Animal
    Health
    812 Springdale Dr.
    Exton, PA 19341
20. Synbiotics Corporation
    11011 Via Frontera
    San Diego, CA 92127

21. Veterinary Diagnostic Technology
    4890 Van Gordon Street
    Suite 101
    Wheat Ridge, CO 80033
22. VMRD, Inc.
    P.O. Box 502
    Pullman, WA 99163

APPENDIX B. Sources for Further Information

Adlam, C., and Rutter, J.M. (eds.): *Pasteurella and Pasteurellosis,* London, Academic Press, 1989.

Aitkin, I.D., and Martin, W.B. (eds.): *Diseases of Sheep,* 2d ed., London, Blackwell Scientific Publications, 1990.

Ballows, A. (ed.-in-chief): *Manual of Clinical Microbiology,* 5th ed., Washington, D.C., American Society for Microbiology, 1991.

Benson, A.S. (ed.): *Control of Communicable Diseases in Man,* 15th ed., Washington, D.C., American Public Health Association, 1990.

Biberstein, E.L., and Zee, Y.C.: *Review of Veterinary Microbiology,* Boston, Blackwell Scientific Publications, 1990.

Blood, D.C., and Radostits, O.M.: *Veterinary Medicine,* 7th ed., London, Bailliere Tindall, 1989.

Callis, J.J.; Dardiri, A.H.; Ferris, D.H.; Gay, J.; Mason, J.; and Wilder, F.W.: *Illustrated Manual for the Recognition and Diagnosis of Certain Animal Diseases,* Vol. 1 and 2, Greenport, Long Island, N.Y., Plum Island Animal Disease Center, 1982, 1988.

Carter, G.R., and Chengappa, M.M.: *Essentials of Veterinary Bacteriology and Mycology,* 4th ed., Malvern, Pa., Lea and Febiger, 1991.

Carter, G.R., and Cole, J.R., Jr.: *Diagnostic Procedures in Veterinary Bacteriology and Mycology,* 5th ed., New York, Academic Press, 1990.

Fenner, F.; Bachmann, P.A.; Gibbs, E.P.J.; Murphy, F.A.; Studdert, M.J.; and White, D.O.: *Veterinary Virology,* New York, Academic Press, 1987.

Fraser, C.M. (ed.): *The Merck Veterinary Manual,* 7th ed., Rahway, N.J., Merck and Co., Inc., 1991.

Geering, W.A., and Forman, A.J.: *Animal Health in Australia,* Vol. 9, *Exotic Diseases,* Canberra, Australian Government Publishing Service, 1987.

Gibbs, E.P.J. (ed.): *Virus Diseases of Food Animals,* Vol. 2, New York, Academic Press, 1981.

Green, C.E. (ed.): *Infectious Diseases of the Dog and Cat,* Philadelphia, W.B. Saunders Co., 1990.

Jones, J.C., and Hunt, R.D.: *Veterinary Pathology,* 5th ed., Malvern, Pa., Lea and Febiger, 1983.

Jungerman, P.F., and Schwartzman, R.M.: *Veterinary Medical Mycology,* Philadelphia, Lea and Febiger, 1972.

Kahrs, R.F.: *Virus Diseases of Cattle,* Ames, Iowa State University Press, 1981.

Leman, A.D.; Straw, B.E.; Mengeling, W.L.; D'Allaire, S.; and Taylor, D.J. (eds.): *Diseases of Swine,* 7th ed., Ames, Iowa State University Press, 1992.

Losos, G.L.: *Infectious Diseases of Domestic Animals,* Essex, Longman Scientific and Technical, 1986.

Mohanty, S.B., and Dutta, S.K.: *Veterinary Virology,* Philadelphia, Lea and Febiger, 1981.

Pilchard, E.L.: *Foreign Animal Report,* Hyattsville, Md., U.S. Department of Agriculture (issued quarterly).

Rippon, J.W.: *Medical Mycology,* 3d ed., Philadelphia, W.B. Saunders Co., 1988.

Rose, N.R.; Friedman, H.; and Fahey, J.L. (eds.): *Manual of Clinical Laboratory Immunology,* 3d ed., Washington, D.C., American Society for Microbiology, 1986.

Russell, P.H., and Edington, N.: *Veterinary Viruses,* Foxton, Cambridge, The Burlington Press Ltd., 1985.

Thompson, R.G.: *Special Veterinary Pathology,* Toronto, Can., B.C. Decker Publishing Co., 1988.

Timoney, J.F.; Gillespie, J.H.; Scott, F.W.; and Barlough, J.E.: *Hagan and Bruner's Microbiology and Infectious Diseases of Animals,* 8th ed., Ithaca, N.Y., Cornell University Press, 1988.

Tizard, I.: *Introduction to Veterinary Immunology,* 3d ed., Philadelphia, W.B. Saunders Co., 1987.

Trevino, G.S., and Hyde, J.L. (coords.): *Foreign Animal Diseases,* Richmond, Va., U.S. Animal Health Association, 1984.

INDEX

Page numbers in **boldface** indicate principal references; numbers followed by "t" indicate tables.

DATE DUE

POLITICAL THINKERS
edited by Geraint Parry
University of Manchester

2

EDMUND BURKE

EDMUND BURKE
His Political Philosophy

Frank O'Gorman

*Lecturer in Modern History at
the University of Manchester*

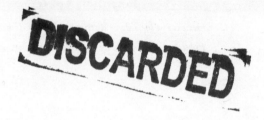

London
George Allen & Unwin Ltd
Ruskin House   Museum Street

First published in 1973

© Frank O'Gorman 1973

ISBN 0 04 921018 1 hardback
0 04 921019 X paper

This edition is not for sale or distribution in the United States.

Published in U.S.A. by Indiana University Press

Printed in Great Britain
in 10 pt Plantin type
by Unwin Brothers Limited
Old Woking Surrey England

To My Mother

CONTENTS

INTRODUCTION

Edmund Burke enjoyed a remarkable historical reputation in nineteenth-century Britain. Although his contemporaries had recognized him as a philosopher, politician and statesman the Victorians saw Burke as a towering hero who had rallied his countrymen to the cause of counter-revolution, saved the constitution of Britain and the empire and moulded the Victorian system of government. They believed that his campaign against the corrupting effects of royal influence inaugurated the constitutional monarchy of the mid-nineteenth century. They admired his endeavours to establish government by party as an anti-cipation of the two party system of that period. In these, and in many other ways, too, Burke appeared to possess a certain prophetic quality of mind, an almost superhuman instinct for perceiving the direction in which history was about to move.

Some reaction against the fulsome praise of the Victorians, was inevitable. In the first half of this century it came and with it, the waning of Burke's reputation. Detailed examination of his career and minute analysis of the political system of the second half of the eighteenth century revealed that Burke was very much a man of his time in his ready acceptance of the political assumptions and institutions of his contemporaries. Far from being a prophet of the liberal con-stitution of the next century Burke sought to *restore* the old Whig constitution established at the Glorious Revolution, and which he accused George III and some of his advisors of violating. It was never Burke's intention to fashion novel political forms which anticipated the future development of the constitution. He wished to defend and protect the aristocratic world of eighteenth-century politics, an objective towards which his reforms were uniformly directed. He was too much involved in the political struggles of his own day to concern himself with the future development of the British constitution. Indeed, Edmund Burke was not a philosopher at all. He was essentially a practical politician and a propagandist rather than a thinker with a systematic philosophy to expound. His political objectives had their origin less in his own thought than in his membership of the Rocking-ham Whig party and his close personal relationship with the Marquis of Rockingham himself.[1] Partisanship and prejudice were evidently

[1] Charles, 2nd Marquis of Rockingham (1739–82) was one of the greatest Whig politicians of the age. He was Prime Minister and First Lord of the Treasury in the two short ministries of 1765–66 and 1782. He was a great Yorkshire landowner and one of the foremost electoral patrons of the day.

just as important in shaping Burke's thought as a concern for justice or impartial inquiry.[2] The awe-inspiring figure of the nineteenth century had become the party hack of the twentieth.

The pendulum of reputation soon swung over to the opposite extreme. After the Second World War there took place both a revival of interest in his work and a considerable shift in the interpretation of his thought. The revival was caused by the opening to scholars of Burke's private papers; the shift was accomplished by the American 'new conservatives' of the 1950s, upon whom Burke's influence was considerable. They saw Burke as a christian philosopher, striving to combat the evils of atheistic Jacobinism by reaffirming the traditional religious and social principles of European civilization. Regarding themselves similarly, as the Christian philosophers of the mid-twentieth century, striving to preserve the west from the infection of atheistic communism, the 'new conservatives' believed that Burke's philosophy was rooted in the christian ethic. They pointed to the central and unifying principle of his philosophy, the Natural Law, which rendered his thought both intelligible and coherent and from which it logically flowed.[3] The Natural Law does indeed enjoy a place in Burke's thought.

Rockingham was not only one of Burke's closest friends. He was his protector and patron. Burke owed his political career to the Marquis.

[2] This is *not* to say that Burke deliberately falsified facts, still less that he was consciously and deliberately self-interested. Edmund Burke hated cruelty, injustice and oppression and his whole career manifested an extraordinary elevation of the human spirit. Nevertheless, it is idle to ignore the simple fact that Burke was a politician and thus involved in the political controversies of his day. Impartial detachment could scarcely be expected from a man in Burke's position. Furthermore, Burke was a man whose entire personality inclined towards commitment rather than towards detachment. He was a man of considerable passion, trained in the law, enjoying extensive knowledge of economics, history, aesthetics, philosophy, languages and the arts. Edmund Burke was immensely fertile in ideas which flowed from him almost uncontrollably. Such a man was not inclined to abstract, rational philosophy.

[3] The Natural Law school makes at least two sorts of statement about Burke which require the exercise of caution. The first is that his thought 'developed, deepened and found new applications' (R. Hoffman and B. Levack, eds. *Burke's Politics* (New York, 1949), xiii). The second assumes that 'it seems now to have become generally recognized that Burke grounded his conception (of law) on the ancient principle of the Law of Nature, that he believed in eternal principles of law of which right legislation is merely declaratory'. (P. J. Stanlis, ed. *The Relevance of Edmund Burke* (Washington, 1964), 16–17). Many scholars no longer accept these assumptions. The first suggests a development, an evolution in Burke's thought which is by no means self-evident. The second presupposes that his thought is 'systematic'; as is argued above, this is unlikely when the context of Burke's thought and career have been considered.

Although it is becoming increasingly fashionable to attack the 'new conservatives', there is some danger that in doing so the baby will be thrown out with the bath water and the moral and religious aspects of Burke's philosophy neglected. Nevertheless, scholars have noticed insurmountable objections to the Natural Law interpretation of Burke's thought. First, it is based upon serious misunderstandings of the conception of the Natural Law itself.[4] Second, Burke rarely refers to the Natural Law, suspicious as he was of such abstract ideas. It is strange that a conception which Burke alludes to only on a few occasions should be credited with such significance.[5] Third, Burke's thought was not systematic. It was articulated as a series of responses to a set of political issues. He developed his ideas whenever the occasion required him to do so but at no time did he outline a detailed and systematic political philosophy, still less, one which was not immediately related to public affairs. Those who seek a system in Burke seek in vain.

Commentators who alternatively embark upon a voyage of discovery for some 'key notions' or 'fundamental concepts' fare no better. Burke was frustratingly ambiguous in his discussions of such ideas as contract, divine providence, and, of course, the law of nature. It is equally

---

[4] Its adherents fail to realize the complexity and the subtlety of competing Natural Law traditions within the framework of Medieval Catholicism and early modern Protestantism. Thus, such statements as the following, which attempt to relate Burke's thought to a single Natural Law tradition, need careful qualification. 'The grand Natural Law tradition of Cicero and the Schoolmen, though battered by Hobbes and confused by Locke, re-emerges in all its strength in Burke's reply to the French revolutionaries.' (Russell Kirk's Introduction to P. J. Stanlis, *Edmund Burke and the Natural Law* (Ann Arbor, 1958), vi.) For a fuller discussion of this point than is possible here, see the comments of P. Lucas, 'Edmund Burke's Doctrine of Prescription; or an Appeal from the New to the Old Lawyers', *Historical Journal*, XI (1968), 35–9. It would be interesting to explore the connection between the decline of belief in the Great Chain of Being and the growing rejection in the eighteenth century of the automatic acceptance of a mysterious harmony in the universe and the location of moral duties in the natural order.

[5] Stanlis concedes that Burke's appeals to the Natural Law 'were almost always indirect, through the British constitution, which was for him merely the practical means of guaranteeing the "rights" of Natural Law' (*Edmund Burke and the Natural Law*, 48). The present writer has always found it unusual that Burke rarely refers, either explicitly or even implicitly, to the principles that are supposed to have been the foundations of his thought. Burke was, indeed, uninterested in the workings of the Divine power. 'The instruments which give rise to this mysterious process of nature are not of our making. But out of physical causes unknown to us, perhaps unknowable, arise moral duties which, as we are able perfectly to comprehend, we are bound indispensably to perform.' *The Works of Edmund Burke* (16 vols, 1815–27) VI, 206. (*Appeal from the New to the Old Whigs, 1791*).

unwise to extract a theme or topic from the corpus of his speeches, writings and letters. Such a proceeding fails to relate Burke's thought to the political circumstances which provoked its expression. Burke's thought, indeed, is not as consistent as some of his commentators would like it to be. Morley's famous comment about Burke, that 'He changed his front but he never changed his ground' has been a favourite quotation for too long. Burke *did* change his ground with regard to several important philosophical matters and to obscure the fact does not help us to understand his philosophy. We should emphasize the *absence* of system in Burke's political ideas and underline his characteristic lapses into inconsistency. Only through understanding the flexibility of his thought can we appreciate its richness, its variety and its humanity.

We will not, therefore, attempt to show that Burke was a member of any particular 'school' or 'tradition'. We will not attempt to 'locate' him in the history of political thought. We will not assume that everything which Burke wrote can be treated upon the same level of abstraction. We will not attempt to collect quotations as though they were 'data', from which we may generalize when we have collected a scholarly number. We will not assume that his ideas developed and deepened in a beautiful, logical progression. We will not even assume that Burke's political actions were invariably prompted by political theory. Rather, we will relate his thought to his career and to the political or social situation which evoked it. In doing so, it will be necessary constantly to consider the extent to which the content of Burke's philosophy was affected by the pressures of propaganda. Only through taking these precautions will it be possible to overcome the danger of extracting isolated quotations from Burke and of using them without reference to the attendant circumstances.

The circumstances which provide a framework for considering Burke's political philosophy are those, of course, of his political career. His initial concern was for the welfare of his party, whose history and whose objectives he chose to define in terms of a Whig theory of the British constitution. Then Burke widened his horizons, fastening his attention upon the great imperial problems of America, Ireland and India. Thereafter, he widened his horizons still further, enunciating a theory of politics and of society which he adduced in response to the challenge of the French revolution. We may detect from the most cursory glimpse of Burke's career, therefore, a gathering universality in his concerns. This universality was part of a wider aspect of Burke's thought, one which has not received the consideration which its importance warrants, his originality. Indeed, originality was almost thrust upon Burke for, by the time that he began to write, the language of political thought was no longer suited to the realities of the political situation in Britain.

The Whiggism that Burke inherited from the seventeenth century had become sterile and largely irrelevant to the politics of the reign of George III. John Locke had defended liberty and the ideal of government arising from the consent of the governed within the framework of the laws, for 'where there is no Law, there is no Freedom'.[6] But by 1760 the Whigs had been in power for nearly fifty years. Whiggism had become the ideology of government by the landed aristocracy whose hereditary function it was to mediate between the claims of the prerogative and the rights of the people. Locke had believed, furthermore, that the pursuit of self-interest was a more potent social force than the pursuit of the public interest but he had assumed that the pursuit of individual liberty and the protection of individual rights (to life, liberty and estates) were consistent with the common good. To the Whigs of 1760, however, the connection between the pursuit of the public interest and the pursuit of individual liberty was much weaker than it had been some two generations earlier. In other ways, too, Lockian Whiggism had undergone a transformation of meaning. Locke had equated political power with property. It was left to the Whigs of early Hanoverian England to equate political power with *landed* property. Although, for Locke, the king remained the head of the executive, he remained accountable to the people as represented in parliament. After 1714, however, the realities were very different. The Whigs dominated both houses of parliament and the people's voice could scarcely be heard. In short, Locke's philosophy was much less relevant to the political situation in England in the 1760s than it had been eighty years earlier. In the late seventeenth century Whiggism had been the ideology of opposition, of limited government, of popular rights. In the 1760s it had become the ideology of power.[7] It was to be one of Burke's earliest achievements to cast Whiggism into a fresh mould and to endow it with new purpose and new meaning.

[6] John Locke, *Second Treatise on Government*, P. Laslett, ed. (Cambridge, 1960), 324.

[7] Although this is not the place to plunge into controversial matter, it is worth remarking that if Whiggism had ever acquired a 'possessive' or a proto-capitalistic aspect in the seventeenth century (even though the extent to which MacPherson and others undervalue the strictures placed upon acquisitiveness by writers like Locke is surprising) it had largely lost it during the eighteenth century. That tradition must be sought less in the writings of the English philosophers than in those of Montesquieu, Franklin and the Scottish school.

His Whiggery did not prevent Burke from taking over such ideas and notions as suited him from Bolingbroke and the neo-Harringtonians, the prevalent (and possibly the only) alternative coherent system of political ideas which was current in the second half of the eighteenth century.[8] The classical and humanist ideal of the neo-Harringtonians of the later seventeenth century glorified a polity in which men of property remained independent of the court. They believed that the corruption of the state would result from property becoming dependent upon the government. Bolingbroke thought of politics in terms of property. He regarded the British constitution as a balance of property between the crown and parliament.[9] Through Walpole's 'corrupt' government, and, especially, through his manipulation of royal 'influence', that balance, in Bolingbroke's opinion, was being upset and the constitution endangered. He sought to restore the independence of parliament and to liberate the monarchy from the shackles of oligarchic domination. To this end, Bolingbroke thought it necessary to appeal to the gentry, the traditional governors of the country, men of breeding and manners, and to displace the new monied men whom Walpole was busily attaching to the service of the Whigs. Bolingbroke's attack on Walpole and the Whig system of government was far more than the irate squeals of the 'outs' against the 'ins', more even, than the traditional distinction in British political life between 'court' and 'country'. He was using the language and the concepts of an ideal of society and politics which were quite different in many of their assumptions from the politics of administration and the rule of the aristocracy associated with Walpole and the Whigs. It is not our intention to pursue the subject of Bolingbroke's motivations. It is quite sufficient, for the present, to establish that there existed in the middle of the eighteenth century an ideal and a vocabulary of politics removed from and opposed to that of Walpole and the Whigs.

Burke was a partisan of neither side (of Locke nor of Bolingbroke) but he drew heavily on both of them, fusing elements from each into an ideological synthesis which was purely his own. From Locke he derived his fundamental assumptions about the British constitution,

[8] For a provocative discussion of the neo-Harringtonian tradition in British thought, see J. G. A. Pocock, 'Machiavelli, Harrington and English Political Ideologies in the Eighteenth Century', *William and Mary Quarterly*, XXII (1965).

[9] Recent discussions of Bolingbroke which enlarge upon the notions discussed above include J. Hart, *Viscount Bolingbroke, Tory Humanist* (Toronto, 1965) and I. Kramnick, *The Politics of Nostalgia: Bolingbroke and his Circle* (Harvard, 1968).

from the post-Lockian Whigs his view of a balanced constitution in which an hereditary nobility played a dominant role. But 'influences' in political theory may be double edged; what one thinker takes over from another may be less significant than what he consciously rejects. Burke rejected Locke's idea of contract.[10] He could not derive rights from the contract so he had recourse to a variety of other explanations which, taken together, led Burke to equate rights with obligations, and thus to render his philosophy much less individualistic than that of Locke. Furthermore, although Locke believed that the people had the right to reclaim their sovereignty in certain situations, Burke believed that the location of sovereignty was unalterably settled. In the case of Britain, for example, it was vested in the king and in parliament, an arrangement which no earthly power could alter or amend. From Bolingbroke, on the other hand, Burke derived both the ideal of propertied independence and his horror of corruption. He held that the safety of the constitution was bound up with independence but, unlike Bolingbroke, who had idealized the independence of the gentry, Burke championed the independence of the aristocracy. It was the task of government moreover, to protect property, especially the property of the aristocracy, as a means of minimizing the possibilities of corruption in the state. But whereas Bolingbroke saw the saving of the state in his 'Patriot King' Burke had recourse to an aristocratic party. In this manner, the prevailing concerns of political philosophy guided Burke's thought. He pioneered no novel philosophical method, preferring to remain within the bounds of traditional philosophical discussion, maintaining, yet at the same time, beginning to transform, the old Whiggism.

Edmund Burke was born in Ireland in 1729. He arrived in England in 1750 to continue the legal education he had begun at Trinity College, Dublin. This he soon abandoned in favour of a literary career. His name first came before the public in 1756 when his *Vindication of Natural Society* and the *Sublime and Beautiful* were both published. These were minor, yet distinct, successes and introduced the young Burke into London literary circles. In 1757 he wrote his *Abridgement of English History* (although it was not published until 1812) and, in the same year, co-operated with his kinsman, William Burke, in the composition of the *Account of the European Settlements in America*. In 1758 he began to edit the *Annual Register*, for which he received £100 per annum. But the income from his writings was inadequate

---

[10] For the reaction against Locke see H. V. S. Ogden, 'The Decline of Lockian Political Theory in England, 1760–1800', *American Historical Review* (1940), 21–44.

to sustain him. He began to seek employment in the more lucrative sphere of politics. After some rebuffs, he obtained the post of private secretary to the Irish Lord Lieutenant's Secretary and he returned to his native land between 1761–4 when he composed his *Tracts on the Popery Laws*. In 1765 he separated from his patron after a bitter dispute concerning his conditions of employment.

Burke had been a writer for about ten years before he became irrevocably committed to politics in 1765. It is tempting to search his early writings for the kernel of what was to come later, but one searches in vain. In fact, no coherent view of politics informs them and most of them are not political works at all. The *Sublime and Beautiful* was a treatise on aesthetics, the *Vindication* a satirical and polemical attack upon the principles of natural philosophy, the *Abridgement* and the *Account* were works of history. Already the extraordinary variety of Burke's interests was apparent but before 1765 he had not committed himself either on politics or political philosophy.

Nobody would seriously deny, however, that the early writings are in some ways a significant anticipation of Burke's political philosophy. Many commentators have noticed, rightly, that the *Vindication* was an attack upon the *a priori* methods of the rationalist philosophers. It was also an attack upon Rousseau's theory of the superiority of natural to civil society. Burke was reluctant to investigate closely the foundations of society for 'the same engines which were employed for the destruction of religion, might be employed with equal success for the subversion of government'.[11] It is important to notice that Burke merely announced his characteristic suspicion of abstract reasoning: he did not as yet choose to apply it to any particular political problem. In much the same way, Burke tentatively approached the large question of the relation of man to religion and Divine Providence. From his student days onwards, Burke had constantly intimated his awareness of a providential order and his understanding of the social functions of religious observances. 'Civil government borrows a strength from ecclesiastical, and artificial laws receive a sanction from artificial revelation.'[12] And although he understood that 'there is nothing of more consequence in a state than the ecclesiastical establishment'[13] he had not yet even begun to consider in any depth either the nature or the extent of religious toleration which a church establishment could safely permit. The reason why he refused to enter into controversy about rights and refrained from discussing the limits of toleration probably arose from the fact that for Burke at this stage of his develop-

[11] *Works*, I, 5 (*Vindication*).   [12] Ibid., 14.
[13] Ibid., X, 380 (*Abridgement*).

ment, these were not human problems at all. Morality was given directly by God.

> Yet we have implanted in us by Providence, ideas, axioms, rules, of what is pious, just, fair, honest, which no political craft, nor learned sophistry, can entirely expel from our breasts.[14]

How far passages such as this provide an early anticipation of Burke's later 'Natural Law' position must briefly be discussed. His *Tracts on the Popery Laws* are usually taken by commentators to support the view that from an early stage of his career Burke appealed to the Natural Law. There is no doubt that Burke referred to it on a number of occasions but a close analysis of his argument diminishes the significance of these references. His attack on the laws discriminating against Catholics in Ireland was directed against the fact that they struck at the foundation of society itself, at the coherence and existence of the family. Nevertheless, such laws did not offend against the 'Natural Law'. They were merely 'unjust, impolitic, and inefficacious against common right and the ends of just government'.[15] Burke took for his standard the view that 'in all forms of government, the people is the true legislature'. A law directed against the majority of the people was thus against the spirit of the law itself. Such a law loses the force of law and becomes void. The law, therefore, provides its own criterion for judging of executive and legislative action; but this criterion does not exist in a vacuum. It arises from a power 'which it is not in the power of any community, or of the whole race of men, to alter'.[16] Because the *will* of God is superior and anterior to the laws of men, human laws are only declaratory because they 'have no power over the substance or original justice'.[17] How far Burke continued to maintain this view during the rest of his career is an interesting question to which we will return later. For the moment, it is enough to suggest that a remark such as this was an acknowledgement of the existence of God and His Law – rather than a recognition of the *relevance* of that law to practical political problems. In fact, Burke's attribution of a principle to the Natural Law is usually a polemical technique which is designed to reinforce the status of the principle itself rather than to illustrate the workings of the Natural Law. In any case, allusions to the Natural Law were not among the most significant characteristics of his writings in this period.

Of considerably greater importance is Burke's recognition of the

[14] *Works*, I, 35–6 (*Vindication*).
[16] Ibid., 349.

[15] Ibid., IX, 345 (*Tracts*).
[17] Ibid., 351.

importance of history. His early writings had a powerful historical orientation. Indeed, many of them were in some senses historical projects. In addition to the *Abridgement* and the *Account*, he started a history of the laws of England in the mid-1750s which he abandoned. The *Tracts*, indeed are probably all that Burke managed to complete of a projected history of Ireland. Furthermore, his reviews in the *Annual Register* indicated a fairly sophisticated historical sensibility, not least, a healthy scepticism of fashions of historical writing. Such statements as 'Veneration of antiquity is congenial to the human mind,'[18] might appear to be a foretaste of the later Burke whose political philosophy had such strong historical foundations but there is little justification for such a view. Although Burke's historical debt to Montesquieu was obvious in his ascription of events to environmental causes (in the *Abridgement* and the *Account*) he showed little interest in providing any sort of detailed, empirical analysis. There was scarcely a hint in his early historical works of his concept of prescription and barely an intimation that there might exist a relationship between political theory and history. At the same time, there is nothing to anticipate one of the most important and characteristic aspects of Burke's political philosophy, his idea of the fragility of human societies. Furthermore, his conception of the complexity of social and political units is similarly absent from these works. This is said not to belittle the early works. Taken on their own merits there is much of value in them. But it would be fanciful to imagine that they contained the germ of a 'systematic' or 'developing' philosophy. They contain no such things. They contain, as would have been expected, some few broad hints of the Burke to come but most of the characteristics of his later works are absent from all of these earlier writings, except possibly the *Tracts*.

In much the same way, it is difficult to make out any sort of case for the view that Burke's later political exploits have more than coincidental origins in these early years. His main, perhaps his only profound, political concern was for the unfashionable country of Ireland. His comments, moreover, on British domestic politics did not display unusual perspicacity. Although his sympathies were at times with the opposition to the court in the early 1760s (in spite of his post in Ireland) his assessments of the political situation in Britain were sometimes amusingly incorrect.[19] There is no trace here

---

[18] *Works*, IX, 370.
[19] Burke to John Ridge, 23 April 1762, *Correspondence*, I, 168–9. These references are to the excellent, modern edition of Burke's *Correspondence*, general editor, T. W. Copeland. The edition is now complete, thus:

of the great career to come, most of which was spent in opposition. On his return to England in 1765 Burke might have been forgiven for bewailing his plight. His literary promise had seemingly not been fulfilled and he had failed in his second career, that of politician. Although he was accepted into London society (he was friendly with the circle of Mrs Montagu) and although he was penetrating the intellectual establishment of the time (he was friendly with David Hume and corresponded with Adam Smith) Burke was no longer a young man. His early career was littered with fragments of works which he had not been able to complete.[20] It was, therefore, only through a series of incredibly lucky chances that Burke's fortunes were saved and the later flowering of philosophical and political talent made possible. In 1765, partly through his connexion with a friendly politician, Charles Townshend, he was offered the post of private secretary to the Marquis of Rockingham. Burke eagerly seized the opportunity, for Rockingham was a rapidly rising politician and became Prime Minister in July 1765. Burke was at once drawn into the centre of the political world. In the December of Burke's *annus mirabilis*, a friend of Rockingham, Lord Verney, brought him into parliament for the rotten borough of Wendover. It was not long before Burke made an impact on the Commons through his command of fact and the power of his oratory. When the Rockingham ministry fell in July 1766 Burke went into opposition with his master, in spite of offers from the new ministers.

It was not, however, until November 1766 that Burke can be said *finally* to have decided to remain with Rockingham in opposition. (There is some evidence to suggest that he may have been willing to serve with the new ministry.)[21] His rejection of the ministerial overtures

Vol. I to 1768, T. W. Copeland, ed. (1958).
Vol. II, 1768–74, L. S. Sutherland, ed. (1960).
Vol. III, 1774–8, G. H. Guttridge, ed. (1961).
Vol. IV, 1778–82, J. A. Woods, ed. (1963).
Vol. V, 1782–9, H. Furber, ed. (1965).
Vol. VI, 1789–91, A. Cobban and R. A. Smith, eds. (1967).
Vol. VII, 1792–4, P. J. Marshall and J. A. Woods, eds. (1968).
Vol. VIII, 1794–6, R. B. McDowell, ed. (1969).
Vol. IX, 1796–7, R. B. McDowell and J. A. Woods, eds. (1970).

[20] In addition to the works already mentioned, there survives a fragment of *Hints for an Essay on the Drama*.

[21] There is strong evidence to support the view that Burke's connection with the Rockinghams was by no means as close or as complete as the Whig historians of the nineteenth century liked to believe. After the fall of the Rockingham Ministry in July 1766 Burke did *not* irrevocably commit himself to the Whig leader (Burke to Charles O'Hara, 10 August 1766, *Correspondence*,

of November 1766 confirmed Burke in his new and unexpected role, that of party politician, and servant of the Marquis of Rockingham.

I, 264). It was Burke himself who began, a few years later, to put a story around that there had never been any question of his deserting the Rockingham Whigs. (Burke to Dr William Markham, *post*-November 1771, ibid., II, 269–70).

Chapter I

The Philosopher of Party

Edmund Burke had decided his political allegiance but his commitment to the Rockingham Whigs did not carry with it the slightest assurance that he would enjoy predominant influence among them. Indeed, for two hundred years his role in the Rockingham Whig party has been greatly exaggerated; in spite of his great talents and his enormous industry, Burke remained the servant – he did not become the master – of the Whig Lords. He was never considered for a cabinet office and did not believe that his pretensions were sufficient to warrant one. He well understood that the highest offices in the state were not for the likes of an Irish adventurer. In the same way, although Burke was the greatest orator of this period his talents never won him the leadership of his party in the House of Commons. Until his death in 1774, William Dowdeswell, a reliable but dull Worcestershire squire, led the Rockingham party in the lower house, to be succeeded for two years by the charming yet hopelessly inefficient Lord John Cavendish.[1] After 1776 Charles James Fox dominated his party in the Commons.[2] Furthermore, Burke was too personally dependent upon Rockingham ever to think of establishing an independent political career for himself. It was not just that Burke believed that the business of building up an electoral interest based upon landed property was not for men like him. Like other members of his family Edmund was something of a failure as a man of business and he remained of necessity dependent

[1] One of the best loved and least competent members of the Rockingham Whig establishment. He represented various constituencies between 1754 and 1790.
[2] The darling of the radicals and a man whose personal attraction was as compelling for contemporaries as it is inexplicable to historians. Charles Fox began his political career as a ministerialist but gave up his office as a Lord of the Admiralty in 1772. Thereafter he drifted into opposition to North's ministry, made a name for himself by his opposition to the war against America and became a national figure during the Petitioning Movement of 1779–80.

upon the Marquis of Rockingham. Burke was a follower not a leader. He never resented his exclusion from the aristocratic centre of the party for it was never his ambition to find a place for himself within it.

In 1765, however, Burke appears to have thrown himself into his new situation with characteristic force and vigour. The Duke of Newcastle, one of the party grandees, complained that 'Burke was so constantly going to and fro that I could scarcely collect his opinion'.[3] And although he was not responsible for any of the major decisions of the first Rockingham ministry (July 1765–July 1766) he defended its policies with great skill in the Commons. He began to revel in the tumultuous world of politics and began to cut something of a figure upon the public stage. His defence of the ministry's American policy – repeal of the Stamp Act but the passing of a Declaratory Act reserving the constitutional right of the British parliament to impose internal taxation upon the colonists – won him immediate recognition albeit of a modest character. Edmund Burke had arrived in politics; he had won his spurs in parliament and he had won a place for himself in his party.

After 1766 there occurred little alteration in Burke's position in the Rockingham Whig party. The limited nature of his influence was evident during the next few years. In the session of 1767, for example, Burke played little part in the formulation of the Rockinghams' policy towards the East India Company, the greatest issue of the session, and he remained indifferent to his party's factious support of a scheme to reduce the land tax from 4s to 3s in the £. In 1768 he played a similarly passive role both in parliament and at the general election of that year. Most significant of all, in the PETITIONING MOVEMENT of 1769, although he played a considerable role in moving Rockingham to activity, he exerted in fact, little real influence over the tactics adopted by his party in its involvement with this first phase of English radicalism. It was Dowdeswell, not Burke, who was the architect of the party's policy of cautious support for the petitions. As for the counties, it required the endeavours of the Whig Lords in mobilizing their tenants to make a reality of the radical movement. Burke's importance in his party can easily be exaggerated. He never desired a position of over-whelming influence. Even if he had, his Whig masters would never have allowed him to attain it. As Burke himself put it: 'I am no leader my Lord, not do I ever answer for the Conduct of anyone but myself'.[4]

---

[3] M. Bateson (ed.), *The Duke of Newcastle's Narrative of Changes in the Ministry, 1765–7* (1898), 121.

[4] Burke to Dr William Markham, *post*-9 November 1771, *Correspondence*, II, 269–70.

Nevertheless, from the earliest days of his attachment to the Rockingham Whig party Burke, as a writer, had been entrusted by Rockingham
with the task of justifying the activities of his party. As early as 1766
he had written *A Short Account of a Late Short Administration*, a
defence of the record of the first Rockingham ministry. The pamphlet
was unremarkable and succeeded in anticipating nothing of Burke's
later party theory. (The pamphlet did not even mention the word
'party'.) He was defending the record of a particular ministry not a
general concept of government. Thus he recounted the achievements
of the ministry in glowing terms but he failed to explain how such a
successful ministry, enjoying the support of public opinion, failed to
maintain itself in office. As a partisan of the Rockinghams, Burke
discreetly drew a veil over the chronic interval divisions which wracked
the ministry. Although he ascribed all the difficulties faced by the
ministers to the opposition of certain placemen[5] he completely failed
to invest this phenomenon with the significance which he was later
to assign to other manifestations of court intrigue. The absence of
even the glimmerings of a party ideology not only in this early tract
but also in the other writings and speeches of this period strongly
suggests not only that Burke did *not* come to the Rockingham party
with a theory of party to impose upon it but also that he did not embrace
such a theory of party at all at this stage. Yet in 1769 and again in 1770
Burke proceeded to enunciate his theory of party in some detail. The
question naturally arises, therefore, of where Burke derived his idea
of party.

The answer is quite simple; Burke derived it from the experiences
of the Rockingham Whigs themselves. He had not long been among
them when he began to imbibe the myths and the prejudices of the
party, the strongest of which was the myth of the influence of Lord
Bute.[6] It was to the king's *quondam* favourite that the Rockinghams
ascribed the cause of all their difficulties and, in particular, the responsibility for the apparent anti-aristocratic policy of the reign of
George III, a policy which was manifested in the Massacre of the

---

[5] Several of whom had held office under George Grenville (1763–5) and
thus acquired responsibility for his American policy. When the Rockingham
ministry (1765–6) proceeded to reverse his policies, they naturally voted against
it. Burke and others incorrectly ascribed their behaviour to the insidious
plotting of the court.

[6] The king's tutor whom George III brought into politics in March 1761.
He remained by his side until his retirement in April 1763. His close and
affectionate relationship with the young king and the inability of the older
Whigs to displace him in the king's estimation aroused considerable envy
among them.

Pelhamite Innocents[7] and in the fall of the first Rockingham ministry. Of course, they exaggerated Bute's importance – which rapidly declined after April 1763 – but the 'Bute Myth' raised important constitutional questions, such as the extent of the royal prerogative of appointing ministers, the relation between the crown and its ministers, the relation between the ministers and the legislature. It opened a chasm of mistrust between the Rockinghams and George III and contributed largely to their reluctance to take office after 1766. Burke's doctrine of party was a Rockinghamite riposte to Lord Bute: government by party would render government by favourite impossible. In this, as in so much else, Burke was echoing Rockingham's sentiments, not prompting them. In a very real sense, Edmund Burke was his master's voice.

The 'Bute Myth' was not the only Rockinghamite justification for the party's exclusion from power after 1766. The finger of blame also pointed at Lord Chatham, upon whose lack of co-operation Rockingham had partly blamed the downfall of the Rockingham ministry in the summer of 1766. It was towards the end of that year that Burke began to echo the party's catch-phrases about the Great Commoner who had come to power amidst the ruins of the Rockingham ministry. 'Lord Bute, to be sure, is uncertain and unquiet in his Nature; but who *will* do more, who *can* do more, to satisfy him, than the present Minister.'[8] Burke had entered upon the political scene somewhat too late to share to the full his party's hatred of Bute but he was just in time to experience the bitterness which they felt towards Chatham, a man who had suffered the same proscription as themselves at the hands of Bute but who had evidently proceeded to throw in his lot with the court.

In seeking to defend his party against Bute and Chatham, Burke sought to relate the principles of his party to those of traditional Whiggism. As he wrote in 1791 in the *Appeal from the New to the Old Whigs*, 'When he entered into the Whig party, he did not conceive that they pretended to any discoveries.' For Burke it was the duty of good Whigs in the 1760s to preserve the constitution, to maintain the Hanoverian succession and, in their natural function as leaders of society, to govern the country by counselling the king. The king and Bute were guilty of

[7] The dismissal from offices (both in local and central government) of those who voted against the Bute ministry in December 1762 on the issue of peace with France and Spain. On an issue of confidence such as this, it was only reasonable that the court would discipline those office-holders who refused to support the king's administration. The victims of the Massacre, however, were, not unnaturally, disposed to ascribe their martyrdom to the sinister plans of Lord Bute, the king's favourite.

[8] Burke to Charles O'Hara, 23 December 1766, *Correspondence*, I, 284–5.

dangerous innovation in ridding the public service of those who were the traditional rulers of the country. Such sentiments chimed in well with the unspoken assumptions of the aristocratic Rockingham Whig leaders. Burke's application of the Whig tradition to the Rockingham Whigs was beautifully tailored to suit the instinctive cliquishness and the co-operative spirit of the lords of the Rockingham party.

In 1769 and in 1770 Burke published pamphlets which set out his general theory of party. In the former year, his *Observations on a Late Pamphlet Intituled a State of the Nation* was published anonymously followed in April 1770 by his more famous *Thoughts on the Cause of the Present Discontents*. There can be little doubt that suspicion of Chatham was the most powerful single motivation in Burke's mind during his composition of the *Thoughts*. While he was busy putting his party thoughts down on paper, the PETITIONING MOVEMENT of 1769 was proceeding apace, to culminate, the Rockinghams hoped and expected, in the fall of the Grafton ministry[9] and its replacement by a ministry which included both Chatham and Rockingham. Yet who was to lead it? It was to the debate provoked by this question that Burke contributed his party writings. He tried to demonstrate that the Rockinghams had claims to leadership which were superior to those of Chatham. This he strove to do in a subtle and delicate manner, lest Chatham be so offended that he damage the fragile unity of the opposition. This is why Burke attacked the principles rather than the personality of Chatham. In attempting to establish the claims of the Rockinghams to lead the opposition in the peculiar conditions of 1769, therefore, Burke went so far as to *justify* the constitutional principles of the Rockinghams (not to invent them) over and against those of Chatham.[10] To inform himself on party affairs he looked over the party's papers and letters of the last few years to show, as he confided to Rockingham, how 'past experience had informed us of nothing but

[9] The Grafton ministry replaced that of Chatham in 1768. Its unhappy history was marred by the Middlesex election affair of 1768 when the ministry, through its parliamentary majority, attempted to exclude John Wilkes from the parliamentary seat to which he was thrice elected. The Rockingham Whigs, in uneasy alliance with Chatham, Grenville and the metropolitan radicals took the issue to the country. Petitions demanding the dissolution of parliament were raised in a score of towns and counties.

[10] Burke was striving to present to the public the Rockinghams' solution to the 'Discontents' of the age as well as claiming the leadership of the opposition for his master. For an interpretation which concentrates upon the latter almost to the exclusion of the former, see J. Brewer, 'Party and the Double Cabinet: Two Facets of Burke's "Thoughts"', *Historical Journal*, vol. XIV (1971), 484–6.

his Enmity to your whole system of men and Opinions'.[11] Indeed, Chatham's principles were fundamentally different from those of the Rockinghams. He found planned combination in politics an anathema; he wished to maintain his independence and freedom of action until he was summoned by the king to form a ministry, when he would demand the full exercise of the royal prerogative of appointing ministers. Neither Burke nor Rockingham could find any room for compromise with such opinions. Burke's party theory is an explanation and a justification of their refusal to compromise.

Burke had at least one further motive in publicizing his party ideas: he hoped that their impact upon the Rockingham party would strengthen its cohesion. His theory of party was just as much an *apologia* for the Rockingham Whigs as a defence of any *system* of government. This, at least was what Rockingham hoped it would be. He hoped that Burke's ideas would equally justify the present opinions of his friends as much as their past conduct.[12] It was, indeed, at Rockingham's instigation that the *Thoughts* were written at all. 'I think it would take universally, and tend to form and to unite a party upon real and well founded principles', he wrote.[13] Burke thought that he was successful in this. 'It is the political creed of our party', he proclaimed.[14] Yet the party would be nothing without the support of public opinion. 'The public in general have never as yet had a fair State of our Principles laid before them – In my opinion they will like them.'[15] He persuaded himself that they did. In May 1770 he affirmed that the *Thoughts* had won 'the approbation of the most thinking part of the people'.[16] The theory of party, for Burke, had fulfilled its immediate political objectives.

The starting point for Burke's party thought was his conviction that the country was afflicted with the evil consequence of the court's attack upon the aristocracy and the traditional constitution. These 'Present Discontents' could be cured only through the agency of party. Burke began to describe them in the *Observations* when he referred to the plans of the court 'long pursued, with but too fatal a success . . . to break the strength of this kingdom by frittering down the bodies which compose it, by fomenting bitter and sanguinary animosities, and by dissolving every tie of social affection and public trust'.[17] The

[11] Burke to Rockingham, October 1769, *Correspondence*, II, 88.
[12] Rockingham to Burke, 4 November 1769, ibid., 104.
[13] Rockingham to Burke, 15 October 1769, ibid., 92.
[14] Burke to Richard Shackleton, 6 May 1770, ibid., 150.
[15] Burke to Rockingham, *post*-6 November 1769, ibid., 108–9.
[16] Burke to Richard Shackleton, 6 May 1770, loc. cit.
[17] *Works*, II, 11.

malaise of social and political dissensions had in Britain traditionally been associated in the public mind with party conflict but, as Burke wrote in an important passage in the *Thoughts*: 'the great parties which formerly divided and agitated the kingdom are known to be in a manner entirely dissolved'.[18] It was all the more curious then,

> That Government is at once dreaded and contemned; that the laws are despoiled of all their respected and salutory terrors; that their inaction is a subject of ridicule, and their exertion of abhorrence; that rank, and office, and title, and all the solemn plausibilities of the world have lost their reverence and effect . . . that hardly anything above or below, abroad or at home, is sound and entire; but that disconnexion and confusion, in offices, in parties, in families, in Parliament, in the nation, prevail beyond the disorders of any former time.[19]

Burke did not ascribe the political and social instability of the time to the court itself but to the cant of blind and indiscriminate support of government, 'He that supports every Administration, subverts all Government.' Such a man does nothing to strengthen government because he is 'open to continual shocks and changes, upon the principles of the meanest cabal, and the most contemptible intrigue'.[20] Burke denied the court maxim, 'That all political connexions are in their nature factious, and as such ought to be dissipated and destroyed.'[21] He was confident that there existed a large number of honest men who could resist the blandishments of the court and who, through the agency of party, would be willing to play their part in contesting the establishment in Britain of a sinister royal absolutism.

Burke feared not only the principles of the court but also the means by which it sought to translate its loyalist ideals into practical politics. The great object of the court cabal was 'to secure to the Court the un-limited and uncontrouled use of its own vast influence, under the sole direction of its own private favour'.[22] To this end, the court wished to establish a 'double cabinet', a second administration, which would be both separate from, and more powerful than, the responsible ministry, enjoying, as it would, the extensive range of royal influence as a source of bribery and corruption. Through these means, the court cabal would build up for itself a party of 'King's Friends' who would render parliament acquiescent in the whole scheme. Burke believed that the destruction of the constitution presaged the breakdown of government and a military coup. The victory of the court would not

[18] *Works*, II, 220 (*Thoughts*).   [19] Ibid., 220.   [20] Ibid., 326.
[21] Ibid., 329.   [22] Ibid., 231.

result in firm government for the court system, according to Burke, 'not only strikes a palsy into every nerve of our free constitution, but in the same degree benumbs and stupifies the whole executive power: rendering Government in all its grand operations languid, uncertain, ineffective'.[23] The acquiescence of the governed might ultimately have to be effected through force of arms. The court system, for Burke, was thus symptomatic of a new and sinister threat to the liberties and constitution of Great Britain.

How much credence can be given to Burke's analysis of the 'Present Discontents'? He was, of course, perfectly justified in calling attention to the unusual nature of the politics of the 1760s, the instability of ministries, the weakness and unpopularity of government, the fragmentation of connections and, most important of all, the demise of the great parties. None of these, however, had their origin in court plots. Indeed, historians no longer believe in the myth of the 'King's Friends' nor take seriously the idea of a court cabal. There never was a conscious attempt by the court, even in the days of Lord Bute, to undermine the role of parliament in the constitution or to make ministries dependent upon the court. Furthermore, although there can be little doubt that the king and the court disliked party combinations and that they were reluctant to have them in office upon a party basis, there is nothing to substantiate Burke's claim that the court had embarked upon a deliberate policy of taking the powers of government out of the hands of ministers and placing them into those of creatures of its own selection. Even if they had intended to do so, it is very doubtful indeed if George III and Lord Bute had the ability to envisage, let alone to execute, the kind of far-reaching scheme which Burke imputed to them. In long-term political planning they were woefully deficient. They had neither the political skill nor the personal nerve seriously to undertake a constitutional revolution.

Why did Burke indulge in this kind of misrepresentation? To a considerable extent he was merely echoing some of the traditional 'country' prejudices of the century. A generation earlier Bolingbroke had raised his standard in opposition to the luxury and the wealth which gave rise to the corruption which, he alleged, maintained his arch-enemy, Walpole, in office. It is important to recognize that such conceptions were an integral and essential part of the political language of the age. The influence of Machiavelli, or, at least, the eighteenth-century version of Machiavelli, was such as to rivet public attention to the morality of the leading men of the age, whose corruption led to national degeneracy and whose virtue led to national well-being. The

[23] *Works*, II, 271 (*Thoughts*).

eighteenth-century mind was concerned less with the morality of individuals than with the corruption of individuals as a symptom of a deeper malaise: the corruption of the state through the unbalancing of the delicate system of checks and balances which maintained the mixed constitution. Burke was saturated in this kind of thinking. He believed that the sinister operations of the court cabal and the engine of royal influence were spreading corruption like an infectious disease through the state. Bolingbroke had looked to his 'Patriot King' to effect the restoration of virtue. Edmund Burke called upon the principles of party to do the same. In so doing he was following a popular contemporary belief that a state which had 'fallen' could only be reformed or restored if it returned to the principles upon which it had been founded. Almost inevitably, therefore, Burke's solution of the problem of the 'Present Discontents' involved a reassertion of traditional principles, in this case those of the Whigs of the period of the Glorious Revolution.

Burke was, therefore, perhaps more inclined to define what a party ought to *be* rather than to explain what a party ought to *do*. It is no accident that the best known aspect of his party theory is his *definition* of party: 'a body of man united for prompting by their joint endeavours the national interest, upon some particular principle in which they are all agreed'.[24] In defending the principledness of party Burke was careful to protect himself from the charge that a strict adherence to party dogma violated that independence of judgement which the eighteenth century valued so highly:

> as the greater part of the measures which arise in the course of public business are related to or dependent on some great *leading general principles in Government*, a man must be peculiarly unfortunate in the choice of his political company if he does not agree with them at least nine times in ten.[25]

The function of party men was not to nurse their untainted virtue in opposition but, by every constitutional and legal means, to seek power. A party ministry need not absolutely exclude non-party men but the large majority of places would go to party men. But, the most important offices must not go to men 'who contradict the very fundamental principles upon which every fair connexion must stand'.[26] Party enabled honest men to achieve a reassertion of the fundamental principles of the constitution. The 'Present Discontents' would disappear once there came into office a ministry dependent for its existence not upon the whim of a favourite but upon the support of a majority in the

[24] *Works*, II, 335.   [25] Ibid., 339.   [26] Ibid., 336.

House of Commons, for not only the strength and energy but also the representative nature of the British constitution would be re-established.

Two aspects of Burke's doctrine of party have been much mis-understood by commentators, the question of the ubiquity of party and the question of the permanence of party. On one level, Burke argued that in any state parties were essential to the preservation of freedom. He refuted the view that they were vicious aberrations from normal political life. 'Party divisions, whether on the whole operating for good or evil, are things inseparable from free government.'[27] They 'have always existed and they always will'.[28] The ubiquity of parties in free states did not logically entail, however, that parties should be a *permanent* part of every free constitution. As he wrote in the *Thoughts*: 'It is not every conjuncture which calls with equal force upon the activity of honest men; but critical exigencies now and then arise, and I am mistaken if this be not one of them.'[29] Party was, therefore, an ever-present political practice to which recourse might be had in exceptional circumstances.[30] There is no need to assume that Burke believed that party should be permanent.

Indeed, we should avoid the temptation to jump to the conclusion that Burke thought in terms of a party *system*. He conceived of party as a temporary expedient, a means of resolving problems within a static political system. He did not think of party in the context of a developing constitution. He did not think of party as a dynamic force, affecting the development of the British constitution. If the British political system were in need of reform, then reforming endeavours must be directed towards restoring the constitution to its original principles not towards changing the nature of the constitution itself. Party was, therefore, a profoundly conservative force. The idea that the British political system might move towards a two party system of government was entirely absent from Burke's mind. The *restoration* of the constitution which Burke envisaged was to be achieved not through the institutionalization of party conflict but by bringing

[27] *Works*, II, 9 (*Observations*).
[28] Burke to Richard Shackleton, 25 May 1779, *Correspondence*, IV, 79.
[29] *Works*, II, 341 (*Thoughts*).
[30] This interpretation of Burke's idea of party differs slightly from that of Dr Brewer (*supra n.* 10) who comments that because none of Burke's colleagues in the Rockingham party expressed surprise at Burke's references to party in the *Thoughts* then Burke was less interested in pioneering a novel concept of party than in claiming the leadership of the opposition for the Rockinghams. Burke's idea of party, of course, was *not* a novel concept and there was, therefore, no reason for his colleagues to express surprise at it.

virtuous men into government through the agency of party, and thus by ending, not prolonging, the political partisanship of the reign of George III. Party was Burke's vehicle for annihilating conflict and, as such, was not capable of political change or constitutional development, in his political theory.

These considerations help to explain what is otherwise inexplicable – Burke's neglect of the organizational side of party. He never seriously entertained the prospect that a party ought to seek to augment its numbers in the lower house, preferring to rely, with astonishing sanguinity, upon the good-will of other groups. In an intellectual and political climate which accepted the assumption that political power stemmed from property and not from people – an assumption which Burke keenly defended – it was impossible for him to conceive of a ministerial party, independent of the king, resting upon a parliamentary majority, representing the body of the nation. Burke thus appears to reject the concepts and developments which later generations have come to associate with party government. In fact, he became unhappy when, in the 1790s, politics acquired a superficial polarity during the contest between Pitt and Fox 'and that there appears a sort of necessity of adopting the one or the other of them, without regard to any public principle whatsoever. This extinguishes party as party'.[31] It is, therefore, extremely doubtful if Professor Cone's assessment can be accepted: that Burke in 1770 'already perceived the lines which England's political and constitutional development would follow'.[32] It does Burke's reputation no good both to claim too much for his perspicacity and also to attribute to him ideas which he explicitly rejected.

Edmund Burke's traditional title to the role of prophet of the two party system is thus unacceptable – and not only because he did not believe in a party system. He may have been the greatest but he was certainly not the first propagandist of party. Since the later seventeenth century the isolated individuals who defended the principle of party had become a steady trickle. The early stalwarts of party thought in terms of a state divided by *religious* parties, a state in which toleration could only be established by one church 'balancing' another. Gradually, however, as parties developed in England, especially after 1688-9, so an initial reluctance to admit their legitimacy gradually lapsed into a critical acceptance of their constitutional functions. The ambivalent attitude of the eighteenth century towards political parties was reflected in the fact that the Walpolean Whigs who condemned opposition

[31] Burke to Lord Fitzwilliam, 2 September 1796, *Correspondence*, IX, 77-80.
[32] Carl B. Cone, *Burke and the Nature of Politics: The Age of the American Revolution* (University of Kentucky Press, 1957), 203.

parties regarded party organizations among their own number in a favourable light[33] and even that great scourge of party, Bolingbroke, not only admitted the legitimacy of opposition but also acknowledged the permissibility of a 'national' party.[34] Already, in Bolingbroke, exists the distinction between opposition to the throne and opposition to the crown's ministers.[35] The only possible conclusion, therefore, is that not only the principles of the Rockingham Whigs but also the conception of party itself had become political commonplaces even before Burke.

The novelty of Burke's idea of party consists less in its content than in the circumstances of its exposition. The fact that Burke was applying to the political problems of his day a traditional nostrum does not render his theory of party spurious. There can be no doubt that Burke was completely sincere in what he wrote although his work represented an accurate, if highly elaborate synthesis of Rockinghamite principles, myths, grudges and prejudices. Similarly, there can be no doubt that the political philosophy which he fashioned from these unpromising materials was advanced in no self-interested manner. For Burke's enunciation of the theory of party damaged the relations of his party with Chatham and with the radicals.

As we have seen, the *Thoughts* was nothing less than a public rejection of Chathamite political principles. He attacked the Chathamite maxim, 'Not Men but Measures' as 'a sort of charm, by which many people get loose from every honourable engagement'.[36] He admitted that 'power arising from popularity', the Chathamite principle, was just as much a security for the rights of the people as the Rockinghamite maxim of 'power arising from connexion'. The weakness of Chathamite principles was that they depended entirely upon the personal, and therefore, transient, power and reputation of one man. Those of the Rockinghams were rooted in the country.[37] This did not mean that Burke neglected the importance of personality in politics. On the contrary, his conception of party embraced a profound appreciation of its significance: 'Constitute Government how you please, infinitely the greater part of it must depend upon the exercise of the powers which are left at large to the prudence and uprightness of Ministers of State. Even all the use and potency of the laws depends upon them'.[38] And he went on to insist:

Before men are put forward into the great trusts of the State, they

---

[33] I. Kramnick, *The Politics of Nostalgia: Bolingbroke and his Circle* (Harvard, 1968), 121–4.

[34] Ibid., 59.

[35] Ibid., 153–63, *passim.*

[36] *Works*, II, 337 (*Thoughts*).

[37] Ibid., 239.

[38] Ibid., 260.

ought by their conduct to have obtained such a degree of estimation in their country, as may be some sort of pledge and security to the public, that they will not abuse those trusts. It is no mean security for proper use of power, that a man has shown by the general tenor of his actions, that the affection, the good opinion, the confidence, of his fellow citizens have been among the principle objects of his life; and that he has owed none of the gradations of power or fortune to a settled contempt, or occasional forfeiture of their esteem.[39]

Burke, of course, argued that this security is best obtained in party combination. How, he asked, could a man sit for years in parliament 'without seeing any one sort of men, whose character, conduct, or disposition, would lead him to associate himself with them, to aid and be aided, in any one system of public utility' ?[40] The function of party, therefore was, 'To bring the dispositions that are lovely in private life into the service and conduct of the commonwealth; so to be patriots, as not to forget we are gentlemen.'[41]

It was therefore, not merely political institutions that needed changing. Indeed, the institutions ought not to be tampered with. It was the *men* who needed to be changed. Party was the vehicle by which this change would be effected:

> Whilst men are linked together, they easily and speedily communicate the alarm of an evil design. They are enabled to fathom it with common counsel, and to oppose it with united strength. Whereas, when they lie dispersed, without concert, order, or discipline, communication is undertaken counsel difficult, and resistance impracticable. . . .
>
> In a connexion, the most inconsiderable man, by adding to the weight of the whole, has his value, and his use; out of it, the greatest talents are wholly unserviceable to the public.[42]

The virtuous men of the Rockingham party, then, were Burke's answer to the political corruption and moral degeneracy of the age.

Burke never wearied of underlining how acting in corps strengthened a man's principles and stiffened him sufficiently to resist the temptations of court emoluments. Party was made for man's weakness for without it he was too weak and vulnerable to maintain correct political principles in the world. Party enabled him to develop his political and moral capacities to the full.[43] Burke's idea of party, therefore, conformed to his view of human nature. Of parties, he noted in 1779,

[39] *Works*, II, 264–5 (*Thoughts*).   [40] Ibid., 340.   [41] Ibid., 340–1.
[42] Ibid., 329–30.   [43] Ibid., 328–32.

I have observed but three sorts of men that have kept out of them. Those who profess nothing but a pursuit of their own interests, and who avow their resolution of attaching themselves to the present possession of power, in whose ever hands it is, or however it may be used. The other sort are ambitious men, of light or no principles, who in their turns make use of all parties, and therefore avoid entering into what may be construed an engagement with any. The other sort is hardly worth mentioning, being composed only of four or five Country Gentlemen of little efficiency in public business.[44]

Burke derived his theory from no abstract source and he sought for no external criterion of behaviour outside the nature of man himself. This is hardly surprising since the 'Present Discontents' were at bottom, a breakdown in man's public responsibility and a lapse of his moral control. Party will remedy these failings because it is rooted in man and designed to further the standards of his public activities.

Burke's reluctance to embrace the increasingly popular radical ideas for curing the 'Present Discontents' may now become clear. We should remember that the temptation for Burke to have included in his political manifesto some of the radical demands must have been very strong. During the Petitioning Movement of 1769 the Rockinghams had attempted to work with the radicals in the country. If they had embraced some part of the radical programme then they would have received that enthusiastic, popular following of which the aristocratic Rockingham Whigs always stood badly in need. Yet there was far more to Burke's rejection of radicalism than his reflection of the aristocratic prejudices of the Rockingham party. Fundamentally, he did not believe that the various planks in the radical programme would do anything to reduce the 'Present Discontents'. More frequent elections, for example, would simply allow the court a more frequent opportunity of corrupting electors. This prospect deeply alarmed Burke for he believed that any extension of court influence would only serve to undermine the power of the landed interest.[45] He was prepared to take place bills much more seriously. Nevertheless, the desire to enhance the right of free election clashed with another constitutional maxim, the principle of the mixture of powers in the constitution. Burke was not opposed in principle to a ministry having some influence with the lower house so long as the influence in question was open and visible. He would have retained the system by which

[44] Burke to Richard Shackleton, 25 May 1779, loc. cit.

[45] For Burke believed that the country gentlemen would be no match for the court interest in prolonged and violent electoral struggles. *Works*, II, 319–20 (*Thoughts*).

ministers and office-holders retained their relationship with the legis-lature.[46] Burke was haunted by the curious fear that the mixed con-stitution revered by the Whig theorists, would give way to a legislature completely independent of (and in danger of confrontation with) the executive. As for the radical demand for the widening of the franchise, Burke could not see how increasing the numbers could lead to a freer parliament. Burke, in fact, would have *reduced* rather than increased the size of the electorate.[47] No wonder that the radicals of the metro-polis, having recently rediscovered their intellectual heritage of the seventeenth century, reacted strongly when Burke's mordant logic threatened to make nonsense of their principles. No wonder that one of the most immediate, yet longest lasting, consequences of Burke's publication of his party ideas was the weakening of the relationship between the Rockinghams and the radicals. Burke's redefinition of Whiggism, therefore, patently left no room within it for radical ideology.

So far we have considered only those aspects of Burke's theory of party which were rooted in the political circumstance of the Rocking-ham Whigs in the decade of the 1760s. There remain to be discussed certain general themes within it which cannot immediately be related to political matters. Among these must be included Burke's peculiar conception of history. This appears to have operated at more than one level. For example, he acknowledged his indebtedness to the common law school of the seventeenth century. Its adherents believed in the ancient constitution of Anglo-Saxon times, whose freedom from corruption and whose popular basis contrasted strongly with the sterile and corrupt political system of Hanoverian England.[48] It is by no means clear that the reader ought to accept naively Burke's belief in the Anglo-Saxon constitution. It is not clear how seriously Burke took it himself.

Many a stern republican, after gorging himself with a full feast of admiration of the Grecian commonwealths and of our true Saxon constitution, and disgorging all the splendid bile of his virtuous indignation on King John and King James, sits down perfectly satisfied to the coarsest and homeliest job of the day he lives in.[49]

[46] *Works*, II, 321-3 (*Thoughts*).
[47] Ibid., VIII, 140-1 (*First Letter on a Regicide Peace*).
[48] These ideas had been perpetuated and popularized in eighteenth-century England by none other than Bolingbroke. See I. Kramnick, op. cit., 177-81. For the seventeenth-century origins of the common law school see the classic statement by J. G. A. Pocock, *The Ancient Constitution and the Feudal Law* (Cambridge University Press, 1957), especially chapters two, three and four.
[49] *Works*, II, 226-7 (*Thoughts*).

More seriously, Burke ransacked history for examples which would support his arguments. He affirmed that in ancient times parties were well known and much respected.[50] More recently, during the reign of Anne, parties had been an integral part of the British political system.[51] The reason for this lay deep in the fabric of the constitution after the Glorious Revolution. In a crucial passage in the *Thoughts* Burke describes how after the Glorious Revolution, the monarchy was too weak to manage a distracted kingdom:

> The Court was obliged therefore to delegate a part of its powers to men of such interest as could support, and of such fidelity as would adhere to, its establishment. Such men were to draw in a greater number to a concurrence in the common defence. This connexion, necessary at first, continued long after convenient; and properly conducted might indeed in all situations, be a useful instrument of Government. At the same time, through the intervention of men of popular weight and character, the people possessed a security for their just proportion of importance in the State. But as the title to the Crown grew stronger by long possession, and by the constant increase of its influence, these helps have of late seemed to certain persons no better than incumbrances.[52]

Historic precedent, constitutional necessity and political practice, therefore, vindicated party government. Although Burke could not claim that the court system violated 'the letters of any law', he was confident that it offended against the *spirit* of the constitution established at the Glorious Revolution.

It also offended against Burke's elitist concept of aristocratic government.[53] He was naturally concerned to defend the Whig aristocracy, especially after the misfortunes they had suffered at the hands of George III, but his justification of Whig aristocratic power was far more complex and far more subtle than political convenience alone required. For Burke it was both natural and desirable that government would reside in the hands of the aristocracy. 'While they are men of property, it is impossible to prevent it.'[54] Burke accepted the assumption of his age that political power should correspond to property and not to opinion. Yet for him the political power of the aristocracy was not merely a crude manifestation of its propertied power. Its influence should rest upon the favour of the people, who should 'never be duped into an opinion, that such greatness in a Peer is the despotism of an

---

[50] *Works*, II, 332–3.   [51] Ibid., 334.   [52] Ibid., 230.
[53] Burke to William Weddell, 31 January 1792, *Correspondence*, VII, 50–63.
[54] *Works*, II, 245 (*Thoughts*).

aristocracy, when they know and feel it to be the effect and pledge of their own importance'.[55] Nevertheless, Burke was aware of a host of good reasons why the aristocracy enjoyed a natural right to govern.

> Long possession of Government; vast property; obligations of favours given and received; connexion of office; ties of blood, of alliance, of friendship . . . the name of Whig, dear to the majority of the people; the zeal early begun and steadily continued to the Royal Family.[56]

Party for Burke was a means of placing at the disposal of the state these attributes of the aristocracy. Late in his life he reflected upon his party career:

> The party with which I acted had, by the malevolent and unthinking, been reproached, and by the wise and good always esteemed and confided in – as an aristocratic Party. Such I always understood it to be in the true sense of the word. I understood it to be a Party, in its composition and in its principles connected with the solid permanent long possessed property of the Country . . . attached to the ancient usages of the Kingdom, a party, therefore essentially constructed upon a ground plot of stability and independence.[57]

In relating his theory of party so closely to the Whig aristocracy Burke has laid himself open to the charge not only that he was behaving obsequiously towards the Lords of the Rockingham party but that he was attempting to reduce the influence of the crown in order to strengthen that of the aristocracy. Had Burke ever troubled to reply to this charge he would have pointed out that such a transfer of power would not have damaged the constitution, that it would only have served more strongly to safeguard the rights of the people, and that it would have corrected the balance of the constitution which had been upset by the activities of the court cabal in recent years. Burke is, perhaps, more open to criticism for his unquestioning acceptance of the divine right of the owners of hereditary property to govern the country. He did not defend the principle; he regarded it as self-evident, not troubling to inquire into the status of inherited privilege, still less to question the humanity, justice and efficiency of aristocratic government. His failure to do so is striking. For Burke knew the aristocracy well. Indeed, in his private correspondence he frequently criticized the leaders of his own party for their irresponsibility, their laziness, their inattention to business, their short-sightedness and their

---

[55] *Works*, II, 246. [56] Ibid., 238.
[57] Burke to William Weddell, 31 January 1792, loc. cit.

selfishness. Why, then, should he so readily have allowed them the enormous responsibility of governing the country?

The answer is that there appeared to be no dispute about the matter. The Whigs had been the party and Whiggism had been the creed of government for half a century when Burke wrote. Yet to justify the political activities and to defend the principles of the Rockingham Whigs it was necessary for Burke to convert an ideology of government into an ideology of opposition. This he did by reviving the pre-Walpolean 'country' aspects of Whiggism which had placed considerable emphasis upon limiting the royal authority and stressing the popular responsibilities of political power. Both of these objectives could safely be achieved by the aristocracy acting through the agency of party. Party, for Burke, therefore, was not an end in itself. His primary intention was to restore the balance of the constitution. Party was only a means towards that end. In the same way, he did not defend aristocracy *per se*. Indeed, he once said of the aristocracy: 'I hold their order in cold and decent respect. I hold them to be of an absolute necessity in the Constitution; but I think they are only good when kept within their proper bounds.'[58]

We should not be misled by the fact that Burke leapt to the defence of popular liberties 'threatened' by the court for political reasons. He lived contentedly with the assumption that the opinions of the country, together with the affections and the confidence of the people, were represented by the landlords, who were the patrons, protectors and paternal guardians of the countless communities which together made up the kingdom. These men should lead the country and guide its opinions; they should not slavishly follow the transient whims of popular prejudice. Politics, and thus party, started and stopped with the aristocracy. Because he wished to maintain the unity of their order Burke did not believe it to be the business of politicians to legislate on contentious issues. Their business was to preserve the constitution by safeguarding its principles. Political action, for Burke, meant the removal of abuse not the implementation of a programme, the restoration of a theoretically ideal constitution, not a series of humanitarian reforms. For Burke, as we have been reminded, 'the programme of a party is to be found in its history . . . not in its plans for the future'.[59] Because of his preoccupation with precedent, therefore, Burke was uninterested in considering certain critically important constitutional

[58] Speech on the Repeal of the Marriage Act, 1781, *Speeches* (4 vols 1816), II, 279.

[59] Harvey Mansfield Junior, *Statesmanship and Party Government* (Chicago, 1965), 188.

issues with which party men might have to deal. He had, for example, little to say about the whole question of the relationship between the king, the ministers and parliament. He did not face up to the fact that there was an inherent contradiction between the conception of a party ministry and the royal prerogative of appointing ministers because he failed to conceive of the possibility that party might become a permanent part of the constitution.

We should not, however, allow critical observations to conceal the more positive aspects of Burke's theory of party. The notions of party and opposition once more obtained currency in the political language of the period. In establishing a measure of ideological unity for his party, Burke fashioned a theory out of the disparate experiences and prejudices of the Rockingham Whigs which, in its very ambiguity, permitted of flexible development at the hands of future generations. It is immaterial that his diagnosis of secret influence was hopelessly exaggerated. Historically, what matters is that his ideas took root in the minds of the Rockingham Whigs. That later generations credited Burke with the intellectual paternity of the two party system, however, is merely one of the paradoxes of modern British history, for Burke would have denied not only the paternity but perhaps also the legitimacy of the offspring.

After 1770 Burke slowly began to change his mind about party. Although on public occasions he continued to assert the indispensability of party, his private opinions began to diverge from his public utterances. In 1777, for example, he wrote to one of his closest friends in an unusually frank and delightfully sincere vein:

Also my dear friend those whom you and I trust, and whom the public ought to love and trust, have not that trust and confidence in themselves which their merits authorise, and which the necessities of the Country absolutely demand. . . . But still, as you say, they are our only hope; on my conscience, I think the best men, that ever were. We must therefore bear their infirmities for their virtues, and wait their time patiently. I believe you know that my chief employment for many years has been that woeful one, of a flapper. I begin to think it time to leave off. It (advice) only defeats its own purpose when given too long and too liberally; and I am persuaded that the men who will not move, when you want to teize them out of their inactivity, will begin to reproach yours, when you let them alone. Perhaps, they would not, after all, be so right; if one had in his own mind a distinct plan, when he could propose to others, and make it a point with them to pursue. I do not remember to have found myself at a loss in my own Mind about our Conduct, until now. I confess it; I do not know how to push others to resolution, whilst I am unresolved myself.[60]

It was not until 1780, however, that events first began seriously to weaken Burke's party attachment. In that year parliamentary reform first emerged as an issue which threatened to destroy the unity of the Rockingham party. Its acceptance by some of the party leaders horrified Burke. In 1780, too, he lost his prestigious seat at Bristol. He became even more dependent upon Rockingham, whose pocket borough of Malton he represented for the next fourteen years. Even when the Rockinghams returned triumphantly to power in 1782 Burke felt little jubilation. 'The Arrangement', he remarked, 'has not been wholly in Lord Rockingham's hands. But on the whole, things have turned out much better than could be expected.'[61] But not for him. 'I am a placeman of some rank; but have no share whatsoever, except what belongs to me a member of Parliament, in the conduct of public affairs.'[62] When Rockingham died in the summer of 1782 Burke was stunned. To the Marquis he had owed his career. Although he continued to support the party loyally his authority within it diminished and his ardour for the party battle declined. Although the infamous Fox–North coalition owed nothing to Burke it was he who retained most of the odium for the ill-fated India bill of 1783. After the disastrous general election of 1784, which resulted in about one hundred losses for the party of Fox and North, Burke had had enough of the fruitless party battle of which he had been the first casualty.

I consider the House of Commons as something worse than extinguished. We have been labouring for near twenty years to make it independent; and as soon as we had accomplished what we had in View, we found that its independence led to its destruction. The people did not like our work, and they joined the Court to pull it down. The demolition is very complete. Others may be more sanguine; but for me to look forward to the Event of another twenty years toil – it is quite ridiculous. I am sure the Task was more easy at first than it is now. The examples which have been made must operate. I can conceive that men of spirit might be persuaded to persevere in a great and worthy undertaking for many years, at the hazard, and even with the certainty of the utmost indignation of a Court; but to become Objects of that indignation only to expose

[60] Burke to William Baker, 12 October 1777, *Correspondence*, III, 388–9.
[61] Burke to John Lee, 25 March 1782, ibid., IV, 427.
[62] Burke to John Hely Hutchinson, *post*-9 April 1782, ibid., 440–1.

themselves to popular indignation, and to be rejected by both Court and Country, is more perhaps than any one could expect, certainly a great deal more than one will meet, except perhaps in three or four men, who will be more marked for their singularity and obstinacy, than pitied for their feeble good intentions.[63]

This was the end of Burke's consistent and continuous party campaigning. He continued to support the party of Fox but his energies were involved in issues which transcended party, such as the impeachment of Warren Hastings, the question of Ireland and, of course, the French revolution. Nevertheless he continued to believe in the doctrine of party although he left others to undertake the detailed work which he had outlined in the later 1760s. After the outbreak of war between Britain and revolutionary France, however, Burke became increasingly indifferent to party politics, feeling, as he did that European civilization was endangered by the contagion of atheistic Jacobinism. Shortly before his death, he was convinced that a new and dangerous polarity existed in politics. The old parties had become defunct:

... these parties, which by their dissensions have so often distracted the kingdom, which by their union have once saved it, and which by their collusion and mutual resistance have preserved the variety of this constitution in its utility, be (as I believe they are) nearly extinct by the growth of new ones, which have their roots in the present circumstances.[64]

In this crisis, the old party conflicts must be forgotten. Whigs and Tories should unite against the common enemy, the Jacobins. Much to Burke's satisfaction, the larger part of Fox's party formed a coalition with the Younger Pitt in 1794. Only a rump of the Whigs remaining loyal to him, Fox endured over a decade of fruitless opposition. In effect, party was dead.[65] Although in a subtle way, the old Whig party continued to exist as a refuge of moral and political principle,[66] in practice, the party no longer mattered.

To what extent the party of Rockingham and of Fox had been able to achieve what Burke had intended for it is not easy to decide. His own personal and political disappointments, the death of Rockingham

[63] Burke to William Baker, 22 June 1784, *Correspondence*, V, 154.
[64] Speech on the Quebec Act, 11 May 1791, *The Parliamentary History*, XXIX, 421.
[65] The Foxite Whigs numbered only about 50–60 members of parliament in the period 1794–1804, the only group in systematic opposition to the conservative coalition which governed Britain during the revolutionary period.
[66] Burke to Lord Fitzwilliam, 2 September 1796, loc. cit.

in 1782 and the military crisis of the 1790s had obscured the natural operations of party. What Burke had described in 1769–70 as the only means of saving the country had become a political luxury which the safety of the constitution could not afford. The significance of Burke's idea of party, however, does not end with the apparent disappointment of Burke's party expectations. It provided the starting point for Burke's analysis of the British constitution; it elicited from him a wide ranging discussion of the nature of the British polity. The party situation of the Rockingham Whigs, in fact, forced Burke to reinforce his party notions with a new Whig theory of the British constitution.

Chapter II

The British Constitution

The supreme practicality of Burke's thought is nowhere better illustrated than in his solicitousness to explain – and in explaining, to defend – the British constitution. At all times he was moved by political considerations in his theoretical activities. Early in his political career he placed his party philosophy within a framework of constitutional ideas. This he proceeded to define under the pressure of circumstances, especially the campaigns for economical and parliamentary reform. Later, Burke defended the British constitution from the Jacobins at home and abroad in such works as *Reflections on the Revolution in France* (1790) and the *Appeal from the New to the Old Whigs* (1791). Not only were Burke's inquiries always undertaken for pressing political reasons; they were directed towards the solution of practical questions, such as the degree of representation or the extent of toleration permissible within the British state. Burke was uninterested for the most part, in such theoretical questions as the location and distribution of sovereignty in the state.

His lack of interest does not only arise from his personal dislike of abstract inquiries; for him, such questions were already and unalterably settled. Sovereignty, for example, was vested in king and parliament. Burke did not regard the British constitution as perfect; he nevertheless looked upon it as perfect for Englishmen. He viewed it as the product of the ages, as a fully developed and fully matured entity rather than as a continually changing political structure. To understand fully this idiosyncratic conception of the British state it will be useful to examine the sub-structure of socio-economic considerations from which his political theory arose.

Burke had been interested in economics since his student days and had acquired both first-hand experience and specialist knowledge of the subject during his years in his native country in the sixties. His reviews in the *Annual Register* showed a keen appreciation of economics. (He reviewed Adam Smith's *Theory of Moral Sentiments*

45

favourably in 1759.) In these early days Burke adopted some fundamental axioms from which he never subsequently moved. He accepted
the socio-economic framework without question. His deep conviction
of the value of class harmony and social cohesion overrode any considerations of popular rights which he may have entertained. For
Burke, the poor were both too ignorant and too numerous to aspire
to economic or political power. Social inequality held no terrors for
Burke. In fact, it was part of the natural order of things. There was no
difference of *interest* between the rich and the poor because the rich
act as the trustees of the poor, as their protectors and as their providers,
taking, in their profits, a just commission for these responsibilities.
Inequality also had an historical vindication. Burke wrote of 'the
inequality, which grows out of the *nature of things* by time, custom,
succession, accumulation, permutation and improvement of property'.
Such inequality was, for Burke, 'much nearer that true equality,
which is the foundation of equity and just policy, than any thing
which can be contrived by the Tricks and devices of human skill'.[1]
Burke would not therefore seriously entertain the possibility that a
conflict of interest could arise between the producer and the consumer,
the employer and the labourer, the rich and the poor, that could not
be settled by some mutually acceptable and equitable compromise. As
he put it towards the end of his life:

> There is an implied contract, much stronger than any instrument,
> or article of agreement between the labourer in any occupation and
> his employer, that the labourer, so far as that labour is concerned,
> shall be sufficient to pay to the employer a profit on his capital and a
> compensation for his risk.[2]

Burke therefore, regarded society as a self-regulating mechanism, a
totality in which harmony could be found even in the most unequal
of relationships.

Social harmony was not thus the product of government intervention.
It was a function of the market. Governments ought not to interfere
with its operations for the market was governed by mysterious,
beneficent laws which steadied prices, allowed just profits and, indirectly, protected property. Government regulation which depressed
prices artificially would both impoverish the manufacturer and lead
to unemployment. Government regulation to raise wages would have
the same effect. On the other hand, regulation either to raise prices or

[1] Edmund Burke to John Bourke, November 1777, *Correspondence*, III,
402–4.
[2] *Works*, VII, 380 (*Thoughts and Details on Scarcity*).

reduce wages would have equally unfortunate results: the reduction of demand and the creation of unemployment. From these rough and ready and perfectly commonplace notions Burke was to construct a non-interventionist philosophy of government in which the role of the executive was limited and in which far-reaching and theoretical schemes of political and social reform thus became quite irrelevant. From these basic notions, too, Burke was to devise an imperial outlook which limited the role of the British parliament, permitting colonial commerce, left to itself, to flourish. There was thus nothing idealistic or utopian about Burke's view of government and society. Much of it, indeed, was little more than a reflection and a refinement of contemporary attitudes. For Burke gave an enormous presumptive advantage to existing institutions. He was not prepared to be over-critical of them if, in general, they were able to achieve the limited aims which he set for them.

Burke was thus much more concerned with the presumptive rights of government than with theoretical discussions of the origins or the nature of government. The origins of government, indeed, were not to him a matter of practical concern. He wrote little about them before the 1790s and, even then, refused to say anything very significant on the subject:

> The foundations on which obedience to government is founded are not to be constantly discussed. That we are here, supposes the discussion already made and the dispute settled. We must assume the rights of what represents the public to controul the individual, to make his acts and his will to submit to their will, until some intolerable grievance shall make us know that it does not answer its end, and will submit neither to reformation or restraint. Otherwise we should dispute all the points of morality, before we can punish a murderer, robber and adulterer.[3]

That there attaches a clear, presumptive right in favour of established institutions is a proposition which Burke does not find it necessary to demonstrate further. The functions of government itself are determined by the practical needs of the state and, for Burke, they should be confined

> to what regards the state, or the creatures of the state, namely, the exterior establishment of its religion; its magistracy; its revenue; its military force by sea and land; the corporations that owe their existence to its fiat; in a word, to everything that is truly and *properly*

[3] *Works*, X, 51-2 (Speech on the Unitarians Petition, 11 May 1792).

public, to the public peace, to the public safety, to the public order, to the public prosperity.[4]

This amounted to little more than the state's right to perpetuate itself and its institutions. There was no hint here of social reform, no intimation of consulting the wishes of the people, no conception of a changing or developing polity. The function of government was to preserve the state and its institutions. Necessary adjustments, adaptations and changes might occur but, ultimately, existing institutions must survive.

This first duty of government, however, was not a matter of legislation:

> Nations are not primarily ruled by laws; less by violence. Whatever original energy may be supposed either in force or regulation; the operation of both is, in truth, merely instrumental. Nations are governed by the same methods, and on the same principles, by which an individual without authority is often able to govern those who are his equals or his superiors; by a knowledge of their temper, and by a judicious management of it; I mean, – when public affairs are steadily and quietly conducted; not when Government is nothing but a continued scuffle between the magistrates and the multitude; in which sometimes the one and sometimes the other is uppermost; in which they alternatively yield and prevail, in a series of contemptible victories, and scandalous submissions.[5]

Indeed, Burke did not think about *government* as some of his contemporaries did, as the application of the maxims of jurisprudence and statecraft to particular situations. Burke did not regard government as a science. He had an elevated conception of the art of politics and saw it as a process which required the exercise of all the great qualities of the human mind[6] whose aim was to secure the confidence of the governed as a step towards pursuing 'the interest and desire of common prosperity'. How this in all circumstances was to be achieved was a problem of statesmanship. Until the period of the French Revolution Burke had little to say about the theoretical aspects of politics. His silence on the subject can be accounted for in part because for many years his concerns were largely those of the practical politician whose interest focused upon the problems of Britain and the British Empire. In so far as Burke may be deemed to have professed a political theory

---

[4] *Works*, VII, 416 (*Thoughts and Details on Scarcity*).
[5] Ibid., II, 218–19 (*Thoughts on the Cause of the Present Discontents*).
[6] Speech on the Regulation of the Civil List, 15 February 1781, *Speeches*, I, 213.

of the state before the French revolution, therefore, it was a political theory of the British constitution.

One of the most fundamental assumptions of Burke's political theory derived from Bolingbroke. This was the assumption that the 'great parties' of the reign of Queen Anne were dead and with them the shibboleths of the time. The Glorious Revolution and the Revolution Settlement had together established a new consensual framework for British politics in which the party passions and party principles of the late seventeenth and early eighteenth centuries were no longer relevant to politics. The principles of traditional Whiggism ('The power and majesty of the people, an original contract, the authority and independency of Parliament, liberty, resistance, exclusion, abdication, depositions') and Toryism ('Divine, hereditary, indefeasible right, lineal succession, passive obedience, prerogative, non-resistance') no longer mattered.[7] Burke did not, therefore, adopt a two party distinction in his discussion of eighteenth-century politics, preferring to speak the customary language of the 'balance of the constitution'. Bolingbroke, indeed, had already attacked Walpole for using 'influence' to upset the balance of the constitution established at the Revolution. Walpole's scribblers had responded to such charges by pointing out that 'balance' did not mean the *separation* of the parts of the constitution. Influence, they argued, was necessary to make the parts of the constitution work together. Government could not be carried on unless ministers were permitted some influence over the deliberations of the lower house. Although Burke used such language and adopted such concepts he did not think in mechanistic terms of the balanced constitution. Early in his career he thought in terms of a confrontation between the crown and the aristocracy, and, later in his career, in terms of a confrontation between the people and the aristocracy.

In the absence of organized parties, Burke's discussion of the balanced constitution inevitably considered the role of the monarch within it, and, in particular, as the repository of emergency and discretionary powers. Burke regarded this as a regrettable necessity, an outcome of the need to repose these powers *somewhere* out of the way of everyday political conflict. Furthermore, he insisted that these powers should be exercised upon public principles and national grounds. This could best be done by placing the exercise of these powers in the hands of the ministers. The just and proper influence of the crown – sufficient to maintain its dignity, to pay its household and to maintain itself in a manner appropriate to the national dignity –

[7] H. N. Fieldhouse, 'Bolingbroke and the Idea of Non-Party Government', *History*, XXIII (1938), 46.

this was acceptable to Burke. What he objected to was the influence of the crown being held out 'as the main and chief and only support of Government'.[8] Furthermore, he protested not merely against the increasing influence of the crown but also against the fact that this influence was falling into the wrong hands. Burke believed that the influence of the crown should be bestowed only upon the highest orders of men in the state but 'It has now insinuated itself into every creek and cranny in the kingdom'.[9] He feared that the purpose of 'influence' was being lost sight of – that of facilitating a political connection between the ministers and the Commons – as its volume increased.

Nevertheless, Burke spent the second half of his career fighting not the influence of the crown but the influence of the people. He fought the second rather more vigorously than he fought the first for the aristocratic power which he championed had more in common with royal power than with popular politics. Both rested upon traditional practices, established institutions, landed wealth and the distribution of offices and sinecures. Essentially, Burke believed that government ought to be in the hands of the aristocracy rather than in the hands of the people. The sober conduct of business, to say nothing of the independence of parliament, might be severely compromised if government had constantly to attend to the popular voice. In adopting this view, Burke was, consciously or not, echoing the elitist sentiments of Walpolean writers, echoes which reverberated in other, related, areas of Burke's thought, most particularly in his attitude towards parliament.

From a different and more philosophical, point of view, however, Burke argued that not only the Commons but all the political and legal institutions of the country had a popular origin. How does this relate to the anti-popular drift of so much of his thinking? Burke explained:

> The king is the representative of the people; so are the lords; so are the Judges. They are all trustees for the people, as well as the Commons; because no power is given for the sole sake of the holders.[10]

Furthermore, the popular aspects of government were not centred exclusively upon the lower house: 'although Government certainly is an institution of Divine authority, yet its forms and the persons who administer it, all originate from the people'.[11] The popular nature of

---

[8] Burke to Rockingham, 14 February 1771, *Correspondence*, II, 194.
[9] Speech on a Plan of Economical Reform, 15 December 1779, *Speeches*, II, 5.
[10] *Works*, II, 288 (*Thoughts on the Cause of the Present Discontents*).
[11] Ibid.

the House of Commons could not, therefore be gainsaid. The House could only fulfil its proper political objectives of exercising vigilance over the executive and giving expression to the grievances of the people if it reflected 'the express image of the feelings of the nation'.[12] The Commons, therefore, was the most important part of the constitution. This was one more reason why Burke, although he accepted the rights of the crown, the Lords, and the Commons, could not accept the idea of a precise balance of their respective powers, for balance implied equality.

These principles Burke regarded as fixed and unchanging, beyond the power of man to alter or amend. It was for this reason, among others, that he criticized the ministerial attack upon the rights of electors in 1768-9.[13] He did not accuse the ministers of acting illegally. Indeed, what they had done was not self-evidently illegal but, equally self-evidently, what they had done operated against the spirit of the constitution itself, a factor which transcended questions of legality.

> We do not *make* laws. No; we do not contend for this power. We only *declare* law; and, as we are a tribunal both competent and supreme, what we declare to be law becomes law, although it should not have been so before.[14]

There exist powers beyond and outside the laws with which the law and with which parliament may not tamper. The rights of electors were among these rights, whose exercise was essential to the proper identity of the lower house. It was beyond the competence of that house to change its own nature, although this was what the ministers were effectively seeking to achieve. In exactly the same way, Burke retrospectively criticized George III's elevation of Bute, a minister who had no connection with the people and who owed his office to court favour alone. Burke did not consider the possibility that such a minister might have just as wise a conception of the public good as a minister given by the people to the king. For Burke, what was important was that a minister must come to power on public and national rather than on private grounds.

Burke frequently adverted, therefore, to a standard of judgement whose criterion is how far parliament is able to maintain its historic character. For example, Burke condemned the court system and its 'rule of indiscriminate support to all Ministers'[15] because it weakened the function of the Commons as a check upon the executive. It prevented parliament from exercising its right to withhold support from govern-

---

[12] *Works*, II, 228.   [13] See above, p. 24.
[14] *Works*, II, 303 (*Thoughts on the Cause of the Present Discontents*). [15] Ibid., 290.

ment 'until power was in the hands of persons who were acceptable to the people'.[16] Burke's thinking operated permanently, therefore, within the classical eighteenth-century framework of king, parliament and people. He did not envisage a dynamic and changing political system. He was content to allow the various parts of the constitution to perpetuate themselves. His constitutional crusades sought to *restore* to parliament its original characteristics. Burke protested against the innovation of 'the rule of indiscriminate support to all ministers' because it threatened to change the nature of parliament and although it was not illegal through precedent it *must* be illegal of its nature. Anything which weakened the essential characteristics of parliament, such as its control over its own membership, its necessary connection with the opinions of the people, *must* be illegal. This is clear enough and explains why Burke regarded certain actions as illegal. But what gave to the constitution the enormous authority and prestige with which Burke credited it? The answer can be found in Burke's idea of prescription.

His conception of prescription validated the titles to authority of existing institutions by their use and longevity. Unlike the Natural Law philosophers, Burke was uninterested in the original titles to authority or even property. For Burke, usage alone validated a title. (For earlier thinkers the *manner* in which property and power had been acquired had been an important element in establishing title.) Prescription slots neatly into Burke's philosophy for it legitimized the property and the powers of the heirs of the Glorious Revolution; it protected their property from seizure either by the crown or by the people. Prescription became a bulwark of aristocratic privilege at the hands of Burke. Property became sacrosanct. The propertied basis of aristocracy, indeed, of British society, rested upon a prescriptive foundation.[17] He specifically denied that the British constitution rested upon a Natural Law foundation because 'it is a prescriptive constitution, whose sole authority is, that it has existed time out of mind'.[18] And it is not only the authority of the constitution but the distribution of power within it which can claim such a prescriptive authority. 'Your king, your lords, your judges, your juries, grand and little, all, are prescriptive.'[19] How did Burke try to prove this assertion? He proceeded from the observation that because it was not then known how parliament had come into existence, it was the *fact* of its coming into existence together with the fact of its survival which demonstrated the plausibility

[16] *Works*, II, 261 (*Thoughts on the Cause of the Present Discontents*).
[17] Ibid., X, 96 (Speech on Parliamentary Reform, 7 May 1782).
[18] Ibid.   [19] Ibid.

52

of the idea of a prescriptive constitution. Prescription had its peculiar attractions for Burke because it was,

> ... an idea of continuity which extends in time as well as in numbers and in space ... a deliberate election of ages and of generations; it is a constitution made by what is ten thousand times better than choice, it is made by the peculiar circumstances, occasions, tempers, dispositions, and moral, civil, and social habitudes of the people, which disclose themselves only in a long space of time.[20]

It was not difficult for Burke to relate the social function and the hereditary property of the aristocracy to the principle of prescription. He once wrote of the aristocracy that, 'their houses become the public repositories and offices of Record for the constitution' which had been safeguarded as much by the 'traditionary politics of certain families as by anything in the Laws and order of the State'.[21] This did not dispense with the law because the accumulation of property itself provoked envy: 'But still we must have laws to secure property; and still we must have ranks and distinctions and magistracy in the state, notwithstanding their manifest tendency to encourage avarice and ambition.'[22] Prescription, therefore, brought stability and order both to society and to politics. In particular, prescription underpinned the framework of the social order which made both rights and duties possible in a civilized society. Liberty might be an integral element in the political and constitutional structure of Great Britain. Prescription was its very foundation.

Burke's doctrine of prescription was translated into the circumstances of the British constitution and applied to the ideology of Whiggism. Not that Burke concerned himself with the speculative niceties of Whig doctrine. It was not his manner to involve himself in sterile controversies. His definition of Whiggism was almost platitudinous: the promotion of 'the common happiness of all those, who are in any degree subjected to our legislative Authority; and of binding together in one common tie of Civil Interest, and constitutional Freedom, every denomination of Men amongst us'.[23] Ambiguous his formulation of Whiggism may have been but it played a vital role in his thought. The most important aspect of Whiggism, for Burke, was its prescriptive aspect: the idea of hereditary trusteeship. Burke had written in the *Thoughts* that

---

[20] *Works*, X, 97.
[21] Burke to the Duke of Richmond, 15 November 1772, *Correspondence*, II, 372–8.
[22] *Works*, X, 140 (Speech on the Repeal of the Marriage Act, 1781).
[23] Burke to John Noble 24 April 1778, *Correspondence*, III, 437–78.

government originates with the people and that it should be conducted on public rather than on private grounds; nevertheless he refused to admit the people to any share in government. This did not mean that the wishes, still less, the interests of the people should not be consulted. Political power should be held in trust for them: 'The king is the representative of the people; so are the lords, so are the judges. They are all trustees for the people, as well as the Commons, because no power is given for the sole sake of the holder.'[24] One aspect of Burke's conception of prescription, therefore, is that of hereditary responsibility. Burke's veneration of the historic process constantly underpinned his unswerving concern for the preservation of the prescriptive constitution. For Burke, the hereditary aristocracy acted as the repository of the accumulated experience of time, as trustees for the values and the wisdom of the community.

The notion of trusteeship, however, did not remain an exclusive and narrow conception. Burke gave it new vigour and a new relevance by investing it with some of the newer humanitarian elements which were beginning to dissolve the old political certainties. Burke revived Whiggism. To men of his generation, he must have appeared to be a man of advanced opinions, believing as he did not only in limited monarchy and government by consent, but in social justice, social harmony, liberty, religious toleration and the reform of government. The framework of Whig trusteeship was traditional. Its content was modern. The great message of Edmund Burke – that power was to be exercised on behalf of the people – needed reasserting after two generations of aristocratic rule. To grasp the significance of Burke's notion of trusteeship allows one to escape from the sterile discussions concerning Burke's 'consistency'. To understand that notion throws light on the simple fact that both Burke's early defence of parliament and people and his later defence of authority were simply different methods of resisting attacks upon aristocratic trusteeship.[25] The enormous responsibilities which rested upon politicians arose directly from the heavy powers and obligations with which they had been invested. The politician was the servant, in some ways, the agent, of society and property. He did not exist to serve his own purposes.

One of the most famous and influential aspects of Burke's political philosophy flows logically from his concept of trusteeship, his idea of representation. For Burke, representation, did not involve, quite

[24] See above, p. 50.
[25] Perhaps Burke's deep religious feelings and passionate humanitarian instincts were the crucial characteristics of his philosophy which rescued it from the dull sterility of so much contemporary thought.

literally, the representing of all people, places and interests in the kingdom. Rather it involved doing justice to all on the grounds of the general good and the public welfare.

> Virtual representation is that in which there is a communion of interests, and a sympathy in feelings and desires between those who act in the name of any description of people, and the people in whose name they act, though the trustees are not chosen by them.[26]

The representative system was not, therefore, primarily a mechanism for registering the opinions of the country. It was first and foremost the arena for reconciling different interests in the state. Although political power must be exercised for the good of the people, it ought to be exercised neither by them nor under their surveillance. 'I shall always follow the popular humour, and endeavour to lead it to right points, at any expence of private Interest, or party Interest, which I consider as nothing in comparison.'[27] But Edmund Burke would never allow the crowd to choose his principles for him.

The best known part of Burke's attitude towards representation is his conception of the duty of a member of parliament. It would be well, however, to make two cautionary statements. One is that his conception did not achieve the fame and prominence for contemporaries that it did for subsequent generations. The other is that Burke was arguing for the independence of an MP not only from his constituents but also from his patron or patrons. Burke faced the practical problem of relations between himself and his constituents while he represented Bristol from 1774 to 1780. For the rest of his career Burke's relations with his patrons, Verney, Rockingham and Fitzwilliam were more important than those with his constituents. Yet Burke believed that an MP ought 'to live in the strictest union, the closest correspondence and the most unreserved communication with his constituents'.[28] Furthermore, the wishes of his constituents 'ought to have great weight with him; their opinions high respect; their business unremitted attention', but he should not sacrifice to them 'his unbiased opinion, his mature judgement, his enlightened conscience'. In the last analysis, these faculties should be exercised at the discretion of the member. Burke asserted that 'They are a trust from providence, for the abuse

[26] *Works*, VI, 360 (Letter to Sir Hercules Langrishe, 1792).
[27] Burke to the Duke of Portland, 3 September 1780, *Correspondence*, IV, 274.
[28] *Works*, III, 18 (Speech at the conclusion of the Poll, Bristol, 1774). For Burke's activities as MP for Bristol see P. Underdown, 'Edmund Burke, the Commissary of his Bristol Constituents, 1774–80', *English Historical Review* (1954) where the author demonstrates the very great industry which he expended on behalf of his constituents.

of which he is deeply answerable' because government was not a matter of will but 'of reason and judgement, not of inclination'. And he stated in famous words that parliament was 'not a *congress* of ambassadors from hostile and different interests' but 'a deliberative assembly of *one* nation, with *one* interest, that of the whole' in which 'the general good, resulting from the general reason of the people' should prevail.[29] Burke, therefore, believed that members must not act purely from local or from sectional considerations but 'upon a *very* enlarged view of things'. Burke, as will have become apparent by now, was more concerned to represent the best interests of the people rather than their opinions. The two need not, of course, be the same. 'I maintained your interest, against your opinions', he proudly told his Bristol constituents.

It was, to say the least, slightly perverse for Burke to declare his indifference to the opinions of his constituents at just that moment in history when, after half a century of apathy, the constituencies were once again beginning to stir. In the same way, it was perhaps unwise for Burke to begin to idealize the representative system of the age and to ignore the glaring abuses within it at just that moment when voices were being raised demanding its extensive reform. Burke's theory of representation had much to do with the fact that the Rockingham Whigs were unable effectively to co-operate with the radicals who demanded the reform of parliament as doggedly as Burke and the Rockinghams constantly rejected it. Burke, with all his talk of trusteeship, ignored the wishes of the people whenever it suited him to do so. Public opinion, for example, clearly supported a coercive policy towards America but the Rockingham Whigs opposed coercion. Here was a gulf of sentiment between the Rockingham Whigs and the people. Here was a breakdown in Burke's 'logic'. For it was possible to explain away the huge majorities which Lord North continued to enjoy as the operation of royal influence corrupting members of parliament but it was scarcely possible to indict a whole people as corruptible. Burke was painfully aware of the fact that it was impossible to change the public mood. Only a military disaster in America could effect such a transformation.

By the mid seventies it was clear that his suggested panacea for the 'Present Discontents', party, had not succeeded in attaining the objectives which Burke had laid down for it. This realization however, did not lead Burke to embrace ideas of radical reform.

You know how many are startled with the idea of innovation.

[29] *Works*, III, 360-1 (Speech previous to the Election, Bristol, 1780).

Would to God it were in our power to keep things *where they are*, in point of form; provided we are able to improve them in point of Substance. The Machine itself is well enough to answer any good purpose provided the Materials were sound.[30]

Long before the French Revolution revealed starkly to Burke the excesses to which innocently motivated reform could run, he had already pronounced his stern refusal to tamper with the framework of the constitution or to admit a reform which effected even the slightest change in the hierarchical structure of society and politics. He constantly deplored the fact that reformers 'turned their thoughts towards a change in the Constitution, rather than towards a correction of it in the form in which it now stands'.[31] He not only resisted but resented the climate of opinion which fostered attacks upon existing institutions. He was fond of ridiculing the parliamentary reformers for their attacks upon the House of Commons, the freest and most representative part of the constitution, while they neglected the Lords. He poured scorn upon radical fantasies about the 'Anglo-Saxon constitution', preferring to derive his own notions of reform from the known history of the constitution. As he once put it: 'I will not take their *promise* rather than the *performance* of the constitution.'[32] Burke detested radicals. He thought them unreliable, treacherous men who had no stake in the country, whose rantings threatened the principle that political power should be closely related to the ownership of property. He profoundly suspected their motives:

I like a clamour whenever there is an abuse. . . . But a clamour made merely for the purpose of rendering the people discontented with their situation, without an endeavour to give them a practical remedy, is indeed one of the worst acts of sedition.[33]

Fundamentally, as Burke admitted to the Commons in 1779 'I am . . . cautious of experiment, even to timidity, and I have been reproached for it.'[34] Yet by the end of the 1770s the failure of his party schemes to have the effects he had desired persuaded even Burke to take up the cause of reform.

The only type of constitutional reform which Burke thought to be permissible in the context of the English political system was economical

[30] Burke to Joseph Harford, 27 September 1780, *Correspondence*, IV, 294–9.
[31] Burke to Joseph Harford, 4 April 1780, ibid., IV, 218–22.
[32] *Works*, X, 101 (Speech on Parliamentary Reform, 7 May 1782).
[33] Ibid., 127 (Speech on the Juries Bill, 1771).
[34] Ibid., II, 7 (Speech on Economical Reform, 15 December 1779).

reform[35] undertaken by the Rockingham Whig aristocracy. Legislation would curb the opportunities for corruption and thus limit the ever-present threat of increasing royal influence. At the same time, it would safeguard the independence of parliament and enable it to act as a control both upon the crown and the people. Although economical reform had a respectable history in the Rockingham party stretching back to 1768 it was only brought forward as a comprehensive party policy late in 1779. That it should have been so was itself interesting. It indicated that Burke and his party only dared to take a reforming initiative if they were sure of enjoying the support of a public opinion which might otherwise have been seduced by the parliamentary reformers. The disasters of the American war, the growing paralysis of North's ministry and Britain's virtual helplessness against the Bourbon powers in Europe enabled the Rockinghams to bring forward their great plan for economical reform.

Burke entertained the highest expectations of his plan of economical reform, hoping that it would reduce the influence of the crown and strengthen the role of parliament, and especially the Commons, in the constitution. Yet, to be effective, Burke thought, the reform must be moderate; only by being so could it be permanent. It was not for self-educated reformers to tear up by the roots hallowed institutions which had stood the test of time and which were capable of still further development. Burke's position can easily be misrepresented. It was not his intention blindly to preserve *any* institution. He never denied that change was an integral part of the social process. The British constitution, which he so greatly admired, was itself the product of ages of growth, change and development. But what Burke *did* deny was that the essential principles upon which the constitution had been founded should ever be threatened by the hasty experiments of radical reformers. Economical reform contained none of these dangers. It offered one considerable attraction to Burke and his party. It was loudly demanded – and certain to be popular – in the country:

> I cannot indeed take upon me to say I have the honour to *follow* the sense of the people. The truth is, *I met it on the way*, while I was pursuing their interest, according to my own ideas.[36]

Economical reform was an old cry of the country party. It was not the invention of the radicals of the age of the American Revolution. It went back to the reign of Anne. To espouse the cause of economic reform was the natural reaction of an opposition party. But it is

[35] Strictly speaking, to attain cheaper and thus less corrupt government.
[36] Speech on Economical Reform, 11 February 1780, *Speeches*, II, 23–4.

significant that Burke had not been among those members of the Rockingham party who had earlier taken up the cry for economical reform.[37] The demand for economy, retrenchment, the ending of corruption – these were all among the platitudes of contemporary political discussion. It is too frequently forgotten that none other than George III came to the throne in 1760 with a bundle of naive intentions which are not dissimilar to the main planks of the economic reform platform. Given, therefore, the military disasters of the years 1777–9 and the rapidly worsening economic situation in the country it was almost natural for both public opinion and an opposition party which had inherited many of the 'country' slogans of the reign of Queen Anne to revert to the customary cures for the ills of the constitution.

Burke was always careful, however, to keep the popular tumult under the guidance of sober members of the landed class, and, in particular, of course, the more substantial members of his own party. Such leadership of the popular movement would ensure that the constitution was saved:

> Is not every one sensible how much authority is sunk? The reason is perfectly evident. Government ought to have force enough for its functions, but it ought to have no more. It ought not to have force enough to support itself in the neglect, or the abuse of them. If it has, they must be as they are, abused and neglected. . . . The minister may exist but the government is gone.[38]

Economical reform was necessary, therefore, in the interests of good government in the long run, as well as in the interests of healing the divisions and curing the abuses in the state in the short.

Burke proposed in 1779 to abolish superfluous offices and outdated jurisdictions and franchises, proceeding on the principle that 'when the reason of old establishments is gone, it is absurd to preserve nothing but the burthen of them'.[39] Parliamentary scrutiny was to diminish wastefulness and reduce extravagance on the Civil List. This alone, according to Burke's sanguine prediction, would save 'a quantity of influence equal to the places of fifty members of parliament'.[40] What he was prepared to reform, however, was, in some

[37] It had, in fact, been the ex-Tory, William Dowdeswell, who had launched this little known campaign in 1768–70.

[38] Speech on Economical Reform, 15 December 1779, *Speeches*, II, 6.

[39] Speech on Economical Reform, 11 February 1780, *Speeches*, II, 22–8 for Burke's discussion of the principles upon which he based his economical reform bills.

[40] Speech on Economical Reform, 15 December 1779, *Speeches*, II, 8.

ways, less significant than what he was not. He had no intention of reducing the personal influence of the monarch. 'The crown shall be left an ample and liberal provision for personal satisfaction.'[41] Furthermore he did not propose to wield his reforming axe upon the pensions granted by the monarch on grounds of merit. Rewards for political service remained in the gift of the king. Essentially, Burke did not propose to change fundamentally the role of the monarch in the constitution and there remained the possibility that the king might still have the power to influence not only the personnel of the administration but also the proceedings of parliament. It was the abuse and the excesses of royal influence that Burke proposed to remove, not the influence of the crown in politics. Burke did not envisage a political system in which the crown counted for nothing. He did not conceive of novel government forms, still less did he embrace the notion of constitutional monarchy which became current in the nineteenth century. Indeed the conclusion is irresistible that Burke was less concerned to refashion the institutions of the state than he was to effect a timely reform which would quieten the popular tumult for radical reform.[42]

The political crisis of the years 1779–85, particularly the widespread demand in the country for radical change, forced Burke to define his attitude to parliamentary reform even more clearly than he had done in his writings of 1769 and 1770.[43] Burke – and the importance of the fact can hardly be exaggerated – was himself at the centre of a furious political storm in which the parliamentary reformers, especially those in Rockingham's own county of Yorkshire, demonstrated their dissatisfaction with economical reform. The division of opinion in his party between the parliamentary and the economic reformers deeply distressed Burke. For the first time he expressed a wish to retire from politics.[44] On the issue of parliamentary reform he would not compromise at all. He warned the Commons that the effects of extending the representation would be disastrous: 'either that the Crown by its constant stated power, influence, and revenue, would wear out all opposition in elections, or that a violent and furious popular spirit would arise'.[45]

We have already examined briefly the objections which Burke

[41] Ibid., 9. [42] Ibid., 2. [43] See above, pp. 36–7.
[44] For Burke's general political situation at this time, see N. C. Phillips, 'Edmund Burke and the County Movement', *English Historical Review*, LXXVI, 254–78.
[45] 8 May 1780, *The Parliamentary History*, XXI, 605.

raised in 1770 to proposals for the reform of parliament. To what extent had his views been affected by the reform movement of the later years of the American War of Independence? Were his private opinions of reform identical to his public utterances? In fact, his real opinions of reform were considerably more complicated than quotations, such as that given above, imply. For one thing, as is well known, he was fully aware of the obvious abuses in the electoral system of the day. For another, he was prepared, or so he said, to listen to the people for their opinions upon the desirability of reform: 'I most heartily wish that the deliberate sense of the kingdom on this great subject should be known. When it is known, it *must* be prevalent.'[46] Elsewhere, he stated that he was not opposed *in theory* to some change in the representation.[47] Perhaps Burke was trimming his sails to catch the winds of public opinion. Nevertheless, he denied that parliamentary reform *was* the wish of the people. Of shorter parliaments, he wrote, 'I do not know anything more *practically* unpopular.'[48] This was one way of escaping from the logical conclusion of his own admission. There was another. This was to set at naught the wishes of the people. In effect, Burke could say that he would follow the opinions of the people if those opinions were worth following. He had absolutely no intention of 'leaving to the Crowd, to choose for me, what principles I ought to hold, or what Course I ought to pursue for their benefit'.[49] What terrified Burke was the prospect, however remote, of a weak and unpopular government being rushed into ill thought out schemes of radical reform by the cries of the mob: 'They are men; it is saying nothing worse of them; many of them are but ill-informed in their minds, many feeble in their circumstances, easily overreached, easily seduced.'[50] It was thus the *consequences*, rather than the *principle*, of parliamentary reform which Burke abhorred.

Burke believed that government should exist for the good of the people but not that it should be controlled by the people. His firm belief that government should rest upon public principles did not mean that the people should be consulted constantly, 'as to the detail of particular measures, or to any general schemes of policy, they have neither enough of speculation in the closet, nor of experience in business, to decide upon it.[51] Burke's deep-rooted suspicion of the people must

[46] Burke to the chairman of the Buckinghamshire County Committee, 12 April 1780, *Correspondence*, IV, 226-9.
[47] Burke to Joseph Harford, 27 September 1780, loc. cit.   [48] Ibid.
[49] Burke to the Duke of Portland, 3 September 1780, loc. cit.
[50] *The Parliamentary History*, XXI, 607.
[51] *Works*, X, 76 (Speech on Sawbridge's Motion for Parliamentary Reform).

have been confirmed by three occurrences of the year 1780, just when there appeared to be *some* possibility, however remote, that his opinion might be on the point of change. The Gordon riots of June endangered the security of the capital for several days, an event which shocked and terrified large sections of the propertied classes of the nation. The parliamentary reformers whom Burke and his party had done much to conciliate only proceeded to oppose them in several constituencies in the general election of September. Finally, Burke's humiliation in losing his seat at Bristol at the election disillusioned him considerably. He had become the most famous casualty of the new force of public opinion. Burke's hostility to parliamentary reform, then, was neither so fanatical – at least before 1780 – nor so ideological as we tend to assume. Not surprisingly, his own political experiences played a large part in shaping and in confirming his opinions.

Perhaps our suggestion that Burke's hostility to parliamentary reform was neither so deep-rooted nor so 'ideological' as commentators have usually assumed is really not so surprising. After all, triennial parliaments had formed an integral part of the Revolution Settlement, which Burke always claimed to defend. (The Septennial Act could hardly be regarded as one of the fundamental laws of the constitution.) His argument that only the court would benefit from a wider franchise was nonsensical. A wider franchise would be likely to give considerable electoral advantages not to the court but to local patrons. Burke himself knew this very well.[52] But it does not seem to have occurred to him that it was exactly men like the Marquis of Rockingham who would have benefited from parliamentary reform, albeit at the cost of greater exertions and greater expenditure than they were accustomed to making. Burke's curious inconsistency on this subject was reflected yet again in his assertion that the constitution would not survive five triennial elections.[53] In the reigns of William and of Anne, however, the constitution had survived more than five triennial elections. His gloomy prognostications upon the likely effects of triennial parliaments, at least – and perhaps upon other reform proposals, too – should not be taken on their face value. It was ironical that in 1785, when Burke opposed Pitt's proposals to reform parliament, he was in the unaccustomed situation of defending George III against a reforming minister. Burke's hostility to parliamentary reform is enigmatic. But it is more than that. More than anything else it provides a link between the earlier part of his career when he was the liberal, party reformer, struggling to preserve freedom throughout the empire and the later

---

[52] *Works*, X, 78–9.   [53] Ibid., 83–7.

Burke who vigorously defended the established political system of Britain and Europe.

To depict Burke simply as the reactionary scourge of the radicals is, of course, to make a nonsense both of the man and his career. He was concerned not only with the defence of the political establishment but no less strongly with the defence and protection of the individual conscience. He addressed himself to this problem largely through the successive issues of religious toleration which agitated politics during the later eighteenth century. If it is fairly difficult to generalize with confidence about Burke's attitude to parliamentary reform, it is still less easy to pronounce with certainty upon his attitude to religious toleration. The reasons for this are many. First, it is not possible to find in his early writings much of a clue towards his later attitudes. Second, his ideas were set out unsystematically – as one might expect – in response to a series of unconnected issues and enunciated publicly when it may not be unfairly claimed that he may have been striving after rhetorical effect. Third, his ideas on toleration were neither systematic nor original. They derived from a variety of sources, especially from Locke. And although it is impossible to deny the presence in Burke's thought of certain recurring themes – the need to preserve the established church, the necessity of weighing with great caution the likely consequences of the slightest change in the church establishment, the wisdom of preserving a wide degree of freedom of opinion on religious matters – nevertheless, these do not constitute related aspects of a coherent theory of toleration. Indeed, his lack of system in this area of his thought is surprising. Before the 1790s, for example, he did not attempt a reasoned defence of the established church. His attitude towards the Anglican church was typically Burkean: it was an existing, workable institution which enjoyed a prescriptive right to endure. To this he attached a Lockian idea of the right of the individual to his own religious opinions. This kind of attitude was perfectly typical of the latitudinarian outlook of the period. Most contemporaries still accepted the right of the Anglican church to enjoy a privileged position in the state because of its landed wealth, its prestige and its status, its traditions of learning, theology and scholarship. Its privileged status need not, however, preclude a generous treatment of Dissenters, consistent with the security of the church. Burke reflected many of these attitudes. It was only when issues of religious toleration became matters of political controversy that he began to enunciate his own views upon toleration. That his ideas were formulated in this manner meant that they were inevitably rather less than systematic. Even one of the most consistent – and praiseworthy –

of his attitudes, his very real sympathy for the Irish Catholics, led him to adopt a view of toleration which was, in fact, inconsistent with other aspects of his political thought.

In the early 1770s a series of issues concerning toleration aroused Burke to express a somewhat inconsistent view of the rights of the individual measured against the rights of the church establishment. In 1772 certain Anglican clergymen petitioned parliament for relief from subscribing to the thirty-nine articles. He reacted in an extravagant and melodramatic manner. He criticized the petitioners for enjoying the benefits of establishment, accusing them of seeking preferment within an established church to whose basic rules they would not conform. 'Dissent', he bellowed, 'not satisfied with toleration, is not conscience but ambition.'[54] How could the grievances which the petitioners complained of be intolerable if they were not even suffered? For Burke, indeed, the question was not one of toleration. It was a question of safeguarding the church and the state. Once again, Burke invoked the principle of majority which later in his life he was thoroughly to repudiate. As a tactical ploy to reject the petition, Burke asserted that a lawful establishment could only be changed when a majority of the people living under it agrees that abuses have become intolerable.

On another occasion, however, Burke adopted a rather different principle: that the established church might make concessions if the extent of the relief demanded was insignificant. In 1772 certain Protestant Dissenters requested such a slight measure of relief. Burke, feeling that he could afford to be generous, declared that toleration should be an integral part of any establishment, claiming that the observances of the church were an accident of history rather than the creation of the Almighty.[55] To what a considerable extent, then, could Burke's religious thought be affected by the occasion which called it forth. In the same way, when the English Catholics petitioned for relief from the penal laws in 1780 Burke supported 'one of the most sober, measured, steady, and dutiful addresses that was ever presented to the crown'. And he affirmed that, in the emergency of war-time, 'the supreme power of the state should meet the conciliatory disposition of the subject'.[56]

Burke's ideas on toleration, in his earlier career, at least, lack both depth and coherence. His attitude towards the Irish Catholics arose,

---

[54] Speech on behalf of the Protestant Dissenters, 1772, *Speeches*, I, 108.

[55] This question of Burke's religious beliefs and observances entirely awaits detailed investigation. We know surprisingly little of his private, religious opinions and devotions.

[56] *Works*, III, 391 (Speech at Bristol Previous to the Election, 1780).

of course, not from his philosophy but from his background and his nationality. Indeed, he was prepared to concede to the Irish Catholics a far greater measure of toleration than he would have ever dreamed of allowing the English Dissenters. The reason for this almost certainly relates to the fact that his great objective in Irish affairs for many years was to reconcile to the Protestant Ascendancy the mass of Irish Catholics. Burke was thus not merely prepared to extend toleration but, indeed, to create in Ireland the kind of liberal society of which in other circumstances he was terrified. In the special case of Ireland, and in this case only, Burke was prepared to change existing institutions and customary practices. But how could he consistently defend such a proceeding? He could not, and therefore he invoked the Natural Law. It was safer to appeal to the Almighty than it was to assert the principle of majority. For Burke was prepared to concede to the Catholics the right to hold civil offices, to allow them the free and unhindered practice of their religion, to permit them to organize their own episcopate and to educate their own children. But may it not have been the case that the real impetus behind Burke's generosity was less the Natural Law than his profound fear that his fellow-countrymen might emulate the Americans unless their grievances were remedied in time?[57] Furthermore, Burke believed that he was not innovating. He was merely restoring to the Irish the rights which they had lost when they were deprived of their original constitution at the end of the seventeenth century. The *suspension* – for that was what it was – of the rights of the Irish Catholics was of too recent an origin to have acquired a prescriptive authority. With more truth than he perhaps realized Burke stated:

> I am perfectly indifferent concerning the pretexts under which we torment one another; or whether it be for the constitution of the Church of England, or for the constitution of the state of England, that people choose to make their fellow-creatures wretched. . . . The diversified but connected fabric of universal justice is well cramped and bolted together in all its parts.[58]

But Edmund Burke's idea of toleration is not 'well cramped and bolted together in all its parts'. The same reservation may be made about his constitutional ideas in general. Even before the French Revolution wrought a great change in his thought on matters such as toleration, it is impossible to credit him with a coherent approach to

[57] In passing, it is worth remarking that Burke rarely, if ever, mentions the Natural Law during the 1770s either in British or imperial affairs.
[58] *Works*, III, 419 (Speech at Bristol previous to the Election, 1780).

political theory. He would allow one measure of toleration to one sort of Dissenter, a different measure to another, a completely different one to the Irish Catholics and in some cases hardly any relief at all. Such 'flexibility' can be accounted for by the circumstances in which he expounded his ideas – as we have remarked already – and by his commitment to a prescriptive idea of the British constitution. His concern for its preservation provoked him to express ideas in its defence which were not always strictly consistent with each other.

Burke's political philosophy may be described in many ways: as a – or the – Whig theory of the constitution; as the Whig doctrine of trusteeship; or as the theory of the balanced constitution. It lends itself to a variety of descriptions. But what it may not be described as is equally clear and much more important. It is not, and has little in common with, the modern doctrine of responsible government. Burke's thinking operated within the framework of the 'balanced' constitution of the eighteenth century. As we observed earlier, Burke sought to restore the old political order not to invent a new one. He completely failed to read the direction in which history was moving. The modern two-party system with alternating ministries, a prime minister, an impartial civil service and an apolitical monarch was completely unknown to – and unforeseen by – Burke, for he wished to restore the traditional constitution of the past, no less and no more.

Chapter III

The Imperial Problem: America

Edmund Burke's reactions to the imperial problems of his age, of America, of Ireland and of India, were seemingly indistinct and unconnected. The imperial statesman who preached conciliation with America appears to have little in common with the nationalist politician who strove to secure toleration for Irish Catholics or the great humanitarian who tried to reform the government of India. Burke's approach to imperial problems varied in time and according to the issue in hand. It is a large and dangerous assumption that Burke must have had a systematic, imperial 'theory'. It may be more rewarding however to examine Burke's general approach to problems of empire and the methodology he adopted in his imperial inquiries. Not surprisingly, his method was characterized by a fund of common-sense, practicality and a distaste for abstract theorizing. Burke never questioned the purpose of empire. He tacitly accepted Britain's *right* to her empire, her right to maintain it and to extend it. He assumed that the empire should (and did) bring peace, good government and justice to its inhabitants, according to the local conditions. He never entertained the opinion that only one type of administration would suit the diverse provinces of the emprie, 'I was never wild enough to conceive, that one method would serve for the whole; that the natives of Hindostan and those of Virginia could be ordered in the same manner.'[1]

Burke's method of treating the American problem was that of the practical politician rather than that of the speculative philosopher. He avidly consumed materials on the historical and political background of each colony. For Burke, imperial policy ought to derive partly from a statesmanlike awareness of history and experience but also from a prudential assessment of imperial interests throughout the British

[1] *Works*, III, 182 (Letter to the Sheriffs of Bristol, 1777).

dominions. He did not wish to concern himself with abstract rights, divorced from political, social and historical realities. He brought to bear upon imperial questions no set ideas and no preconceived notions. 'I was obliged to take more than common pains to instruct myself in everything which related to our colonies. I was not the less under the necessity of forming some fixed ideas concerning the general policy of the British empire.'[2] Indeed, his practical experience of the American problem included the period from December 1770 to August 1775 when he acted as colonial agent for the colony of New York, 'I think I know America. If I do not, my ignorance is incurable for I have spared no pains to understand it.'[3] Burke's imperial thinking, therefore, was not fixed and rigid; it grew with the problem itself.

In an age when the protection of property was the first duty of the law it was natural for men to think spontaneously in terms of *rights*; at such a time, the pragmatism of Burke was far more novel than we are inclined to assume. Although most of his contemporaries debated the American question in terms of the mother parliament's right to tax the colonists, Burke was prepared to ignore the question of right entirely, 'I am resolved this day to have nothing at all to do with the question of the right of taxation. Some gentlemen startle – but it is true; I put it totally out of the question. It is less than nothing in my consideration.'[4] The reasons for Burke's dislike of abstract discussion are clear: such discussions incited differences of opinion because abstract concepts could mean different things to different men. Solutions to political questions should be realistic proposals, not theoretical ideas or legalistic notions. It was not the way of man to 'follow up practically any speculative principle, either of government or of freedom, as far as it will go in argument or logical illation'. [*sic*][5] On the contrary: 'The question with me is, not whether you have a right to render your people miserable; but whether it is not your interest to make them happy. It is not what a lawyer tells me I *may* do; but what humanity, reason, and justice tell me I ought to do.'[6] Towards this end government must direct itself. He admitted without hesitation that:

All government, indeed, every human benefit and enjoyment, every virtue, and every prudent act, is founded on compromise and barter. We balance inconvenience; we give and take; we remit some rights

[2] *Works*, III, 26 (Speech on Conciliation with America, 22 March 1775).
[3] Ibid., 160 (Letter to the Sheriffs).
[4] Ibid., 74 (Speech on Conciliation). [5] Ibid., 110. [6] Ibid., 75.

that we may enjoy others; and we choose rather to be happy citizens than subtle disputants.[7]

Not for Burke, then, the inflexible stand upon an absolute right. Every situation must be treated on its own merits. Furthermore, the statesman must not lose sight of the fact that men inevitably pursue their self-interest, 'Man acts from adequate motives relative to his interest; and not on metaphysical speculations.'[8] Men should not, however, be granted complete liberty to pursue their interests. As he put it: 'we must give away some natural liberty, to enjoy civil advantages'.[9]

Burke's approach to imperial questions, then, was exactly in line with his approach to political problems elsewhere. His philosophy proceeded from an acute perception of the realities of numan nature and the significance of history. It was with grim self-righteousness that Burke lectured his fellow members of parliament after the shattering news had reached Britain that the last army had surrendered in America. Parliament's blind enforcement of its imperial rights had almost ruined the country and now actually lost part of the empire.

Oh, wonderful rights that are likely to take from us all that yet remains. What were those rights? Can any man describe them, can any man give them a body and soul answerable to all these mighty costs? We did all this because we had a right to do it: that was exactly the fact.[10]

We should pause here, however, to examine further Burke's undoubtedly sincere distaste for discussing abstract rights and his opposition to parliament's attempts to assert its rights. Viewed against the background of his party loyalties, Burke emerges less as the pragmatic statesman of empire than as the spokesman of the Rockingham Whig party. The leaders of the Rockingham party had been just as keen as the king and his supporters to maintain the rights of parliament over the colonies. The only difference between them had been that the Rockinghams had been more timid than other political groups in parliament in enforcing these rights. Here, then, was one powerful reason for Burke to avoid the discussion of such rights, for such a discussion would only have embarrassed the leaders of the Rockingham party. The Marquis of Rockingham himself had no intention of becoming embroiled in such discussions, and it was he who laid down the basic lines that not only Burke but the other Rockinghamite spokesmen such as Dowdesdell and Fox followed: that parliament had

[7] *Works*, III, 110–11.   [8] Ibid., 112.   [9] Ibid., 111.
[10] Speech at the Opening of the Session, 27 November 1781, *Speeches*, II, 288.

a customary right to tax the colonists 'but that such a right was irrelevant unless the Americans chose to acknowledge it'.[11]

Nevertheless Burke *did* uphold parliament's 'unimpaired and undiminished just, wise, and necessary constitutional superiority' and believed it to be 'consistent with all the liberties a sober and spirited America ought to desire'.[12] He had to accept that in law parliament had 'an unlimited legislative power over the colonies' which he wished to preserve 'perfect and entire'.[13] His objective, therefore, was 'To reconcile British superiority with American liberty.'[14] What Burke objected to was not so much parliament's right to tax but the extent to which parliament was prepared to go in enforcing its rights. He and his party differed from the North ministry over the question of coercing the colonies, a policy which was enforced with disastrous results in 1774. Thereafter it was Burke's intention to *restore* the traditional relationship which had hitherto existed between the Americans and the mother country: 'I propose, by removing the ground of the difference, and by restoring the *former unsuspecting confidence of the colonies in the mother country*'[15] to reconcile them to British rule. Burke continued to believe until the end of 1775 that a change of heart in London would be sufficient to revive the imperial relationship which had suffered such a profound shock on the field of Lexington[16] and hoped that a few concessions would satisfy men who had come to doubt the *raison d'être* of the British empire in North America (a popular contemporary fallacy). Such a fallacy probably had its origin in a tendency widespread amongst those in opposition to the North Ministry, to identify the Americans with the Whigs of 1688, the victims of oppression whose liberties were threatened by parliament's rigid insistence upon its rights. Their refusal to pay taxes to which they had not consented seemed reminiscent of the Whig resistance to James II. The Americans would return to their imperial allegiance as soon as the unjust taxes of which they complained were removed.

To some extent Burke understood this. Although he clung to his

[11] The Marquis of Rockingham to William Dowdeswell, 13 September 1774, Wentworth Woodhouse MSSRI-1504, Rockingham Papers, Sheffield Public Library. I wish to express my thanks to Earl Fitzwilliam and the Trustees of the Wentworth Woodhouse Estates for permission to quote from the Wentworth Woodhouse MSS.

[12] *Works*, III, 7 (Speech on Arrival at Bristol, 1774).

[13] Ibid., 177–8 (Letter to Sheriffs).

[14] Ibid., 7 (Speech on Arrival at Bristol).

[15] Ibid., 31 (Speech on Conciliation).

[16] In April 1775 an unimportant skirmish near Boston became the symbolic inauguration of the American struggle for independence.

belief in the supremacy of parliament and its right to tax the colonies, he believed that the levying of internal taxes might be undertaken by the Americans themselves, 'To mark the legal *competency* of the colony assemblies [*sic*] for the support of their givernment in peace, and for public aids in time of war.'[17] But what if the colonists refused to tax themselves ? This was no difficulty for Burke. Taxation must be founded upon consent, otherwise the empire would become a military dictatorship. The Americans should not be taxed at all if they chose not to be. Their only connection with the mother country would then be the laws of trade, including the Navigation Acts, the commercial foundation of the empire. Burke's American thought, then led to his abandonment of the traditional concept of empire and its replacement by something approaching the modern idea of a free commonwealth of nations. He declared that the policy of taxing the colonists begun by George Grenville to be not only unprecedented but unwise and unnecessary.[18] The prosperity of the colonists in settled times would yield, in Burke's view, considerably more from external taxation than from internal dues such as the hated Stamp Tax. Such dues must be abandoned and the traditional bonds of imperial loyalty must be permitted to reassert themselves. Burke hoped for a voluntary, cultural attachment of the Americans to the mother country:

My hold of the colonies is in the close affection which grows from common names, from kindred blood, from similar privileges, and equal protection. These are ties, which, though light as air, are as strong as links of iron. Let the colonies always keep the idea of their civil rights associated with your government, – they will cling and grapple to you; and no force under heaven will be of power to tear them from their allegiance.[19]

Burke did not believe that a policy of reconciliation would weaken the imperial authority of the British parliament. Such a policy was, indeed, necessary to *restore* that authority and to maintain the empire.

Burke's conception of the integrity of the empire arose from his conviction that the imperial relationship must be voluntary. Between 1775 and 1777 his American thought developed rapidly as he sought constantly to relate it to a changing political and military situation. By the end of 1775 he was prepared to concede to the American congress the right of legislating for the colonies. Thereafter, he was

---

[17] *Works*, III, 92 (Speech on Conciliation).
[18] Ibid., 100–3.   [19] Ibid., 123–4.

prepared to concede almost anything so long as there remained the possibility, however remote, that some form (or even fiction) of imperial unity could be maintained. In the following year he had perforce to take into account the Declaration of Independence. Rejoicing in America's defiant struggle to maintain her liberties against the oppression of the British parliament, Burke lent his blessing to what he had been dreading for years – the separation of the colonies from the mother country. Burke justified this seeming inconsistency by extolling the beauties of liberty and freedom in the state which the Americans were striving to build for themselves.

The Declaration of Independence came as a blow for Burke for it had always been his primary objective to maintain the integrity of the empire. It came as an unwelcome surprise to him. He had underestimated the will of the colonists to resist the British. He said in his speech on conciliation: 'We thought . . . that the utmost which the discontented colonists could do, was to disturb authority; we never dreamt they could of themselves supply it.'[20] The outbreak of hostilities ended, he knew, 'all our prospects of American reconciliation'.[21] He was puzzled and wrote to Richard Shackleton: 'I do not know how to wish success to those whose Victory is to separate from us a large and noble part of our Empire. Still less do I wish success to injustice, oppression and absurdity.'[22] Burke did not expect the Americans to resist the British armies for long. In the interim, he feared the destruction of the system of government which had existed since the Glorious Revolution. He feared that 'other maxims of government and other grounds of obedience than those which have prevailed at and since the Glorious Revolution' were being propagated among the people.[23] By 1777 he was already convinced that the liberties of the country were in great danger. Burke believed that the imperial parliament had become a 'fund of despotism through which prerogative is extended by occasional powers, whenever an arbitrary will finds itself straitened by the restrictions of law'.[24] As late as 1777 in his Letter to the Sheriffs of Bristol Burke continued to cling to the pious hope that an acknowledged but unexercised right of taxation might satisfy the colonists. Clearly however, this was no longer possible and, in his heart, Burke knew it. In the 'Letter' he asserted that for parliament to concede American independence peacefully would damage the constitution less

---

[20] *Works*, III, 59.
[21] Burke to Charles O'Hara, 28 May 1775, *Correspondence*, III, 160–2.
[22] Burke to Richard Shackleton, 11 August 1776, ibid., 286–7.
[23] *Works*, IX, 193 (Address to the King, 1777).
[24] Ibid.

than would a war.[25] Thereafter Burke's advocacy of peace was closely connected to his support of American independence. Any hesitation Burke may have felt in supporting the Americans was dissipated when one of the British armies in America was defeated at Saratoga at the end of 1777. The struggle for the British constitution was being waged on the fields of America. Burke had not given up hope that the Americans might be tempted to return to the imperial fold. But he was no longer concerned to preserve imperial unity for its own sake. For Burke, the imperial conflict had become a struggle for liberty.

Burke believed passionately that the cause of liberty throughout the empire was at stake in the War of American Independence. If the Americans were to be defeated then the principles of Whiggism, those of the British constitution itself, would be overthrown. Liberty throughout the empire was indivisible. If it died in America it would not be long before it would be extinguished in Britain: 'you cannot have different rights and a different security in different parts of your dominions'.[26] Not only was the cause of liberty at stake on the battlefields of America, it was directly threatened at home by the war itself. Like many of his contemporaries opposed to the war, Burke clung to the double fear that if the British armies were victorious they might proceed to turn upon those who had opposed the war but that even if they were unsuccessful the military burdens under which the country was groaning would cause permanent damage to the body politic. The large number of military, naval and supply offices which had sprung up during the war was, for Burke, merely another example of the rising influence of the crown. Even when allowance has been made for rhetorical exaggeration, there can be little doubt that Burke was deeply afraid that the liberties of the empire would be cut off at their source and that there existed a threat to liberty in Britain greater in the 1770s than at any other time since the Glorious Revolution: 'Liberty is in danger of being made unpopular to Englishmen', he said. It was easy for Burke, in this vein, to interpret the coercive acts of 1774 as the symptoms of a new and sinister Toryism. He dismissed them as an attempt 'to dispose of the property of a whole people without their consent'.[27] Thus the suspension of Habeas Corpus appeared less as the erratic and ill judged response of a weak ministry to a crisis than as part of a deep laid plan. In short, the whole American crisis seemed to Burke to be reinforcing and strengthening the court system which had already been the object of his denunciation:

[25] *Works*, III, 147–54 (Letter to the Sheriffs).
[26] Ibid., IX, 194 (Address to the King). [27] Ibid., 176 (Letter to the Sheriffs).

73

War suspends the rules of moral obligation, and what is long suspended is in danger of being totally abrogated. Civil wars strike deepest of all into the manners of the people. They vitiate their politics; they corrupt their morals; they pervert even the natural taste and relish of equity and justice.[28]

Burke hated the war not merely because it threatened to extinguish liberty in the empire. He was alarmed at the Franco-American treaty of 1778. In the event of an American defeat, the French would be gravely weakened in Europe. Nothing could then stop the power of the crown from rising to uncontrollable proportions. On the other hand, if the Americans were victorious over the British then the power of France would be unrivalled in Europe, and then British security would be endangered, as happened in 1778 when a French invasion was nearly launched against British shores. National security and independence, as well as liberty, then, were threatened by the War of American Independence, a further substantial reason why Burke constantly championed the cause of peace and reconciliation.

Burke's American thought was thus less an imperial theory than a renewed plea for party. The Rockingham Whigs thought they were fighting not only the war but the court cabal as well. After the failure of their exertions to avert the war, many members of the party seceded from parliament in the winter of 1776–7. Rockingham wanted the 'infinite Comfort of not feeling – self accused – as having *ever abetted* the System in this Reign, which have brought on all the External Calamities, and which perhaps too, have laid the Foundations for endangering the Internal Felicities of the Constitution of this Country'.[29] Party had once more become a term of public abuse, associated as it was, with opposition to the war. Burke gloried in the controversy, 'For this rule of conduct I may be called in reproach a *party man*; but I am little affected with such aspersions. In the way which they call party, I worship the constitution of your fathers; and I shall never blush for my political company.'[30] Thus in opposing the ministry of Lord North over the American war, in using the kind of political language and in adopting the concepts that he did Burke was effectively extending his earlier political theory and applying it to imperial problems.

In his American attitudes, therefore, Burke was more of a party politician than a philosopher. Mistrusting philosophical speculation he

[28] *Works*, III, 152 (Letter to the Sheriffs).
[29] Rockingham to an unidentified recipient, early December 1776, Rockingham Papers, RI-1095a, Sheffield Public Library.
[30] *Works*, III, 197 (Letter to the Sheriffs).

did not think that political theory could resolve problems of imperial government. He asserted that:

> In the comprehensive dominion which the Divine Providence had put into our hands, instead of troubling our understandings with speculations concerning the unity of empire, and the identity of distinction of legislative powers, and inflaming our passions with the heat and pride of controversy, it was our duty, in all soberness, to conform our government to the character and circumstances of the several people who composed this mighty and strangely diversified mass.[31]

Such bluff Johnsonian common sense, such anti-philosophical philosophy, concealed, in fact, the extent to which Burke's American thinking rested upon three distinct yet related concepts. These were history, expediency and environment.

The lessons of history were never far from Burke's mind. He deplored the fact that ministers ignored history and introduced novel imperial practices which threatened popular liberties. He advocated an attitude towards the Americans consonant with 'the ancient policy and practice of the empire'[32] to which the Americans had lent their agreement. 'Recover your old ground, and your old tranquility' he told the Commons[33] and he went on to warn them:

> Be content to bind America by Laws of trade, you have always done it. Let this be your reason for binding their trade. Do not burthen them by taxes; you were not used to do so from the beginning. Let this be your reason for not taxing.[34]

Burke frequently comes close to asserting that political actions were justified, and only justified, if historical precedents existed for them. There is no doubt that he was just as historically minded in his imperial as in his domestic concerns. He sought to restore old practices. With his party, he looked into the past for his inspiration and for his principles. The past was a storehouse of practical wisdom of ever-present relevance. For example, to revive old practices would win the loyalty of the Americans. To innovate further would serve to alienate them even more. For Burke did not believe that there was anything radically wrong with the political or economic organization of the empire. For example, the colonists derived undeniable benefits from them because 'Their monopolist happened to be one of the richest men in the world' and thus they profited from British capital.[35] But, in Burke's view,

---

[31] *Works*, III, 182.   [32] Ibid., II, 430 (Speech on American Taxation).
[33] Ibid., 431.   [34] Ibid., 433.   [35] Ibid., 384.

in the 1760s parliament began to heap novel and crippling economic restrictions upon America for penny-pinching reasons. The economic policy of the Grenville and Chatham and North administrations struck at the very heart of the principle of 'no taxation without representation'. Burke placed his political opinions in a historical framework. Indeed his imperial attitudes are nothing less than a well-meaning endeavour to restore an imperial world which Burke fondly imagined to have existed in the good old days, before the court system corrupted and distorted political relationships of all kinds.

Closely connected with Burke's view of history was his concept of expedience. This operated at different levels of intellectual sophistication. Perhaps the most subtle of these was Burke's awareness of the uniqueness of historical situations, their complexity, their internal interconnections and external ramifications. Politics ought to take fully into account the peculiar idiosyncrasies of every historical artefact. But such a mentality bred a thorough timidity of undertaking drastic action. He was instinctively fond of supporting established institutions and rights established by history and by custom. Not for Burke the lavish gestures and the large-scale reforms. It was enough to preserve the heritage of the past. This was, in fact, the best means of planning for the future. He asserted that the repeal of the Stamp Act and the Declaratory Act had been decided,

> on principles, not of constitutional right, but on those of expedience, of equity, of lenity and of the true interests present and future of that great object for which alone the colonies were founded, navigation and commerce.[36]

Right political judgement must always relate to the practical rather than the theoretical features of the case, and, in particular, take note of the interests of men and institutions. But Burke's notion of expedience operated at the political level too. He was fond of making the distinction between a right and its enforcement. He insisted not only that the military enforcement of a right was liable to lead to evil consequences but that 'we have no sort of *experience* in favour of force as an instrument in the rule of our colonies'.[37] It was thus unprecedented and did not enjoy the presumption of history.

The extent to which Burke related expedience and history will already be apparent, yet his awareness of the importance of environmental issues throws both into relief. Burke strongly reinforced his argument against the use of force by his discussion of the nature of

[36] *Works*, II, 168–9 (*Observations on a . . . State of the Nation*).
[37] Ibid., III, 48 (Speech on Conciliation).

American society and the factors which conditioned the spirit of its people. Burke took account of the rising population in the colonies, the booming commerce and the thriving agriculture. Such considerations ruled out what Burke described as a 'partial, narrow, contracted, pinched, occasional system for dealing with America'.[38] Burke displayed considerable insight into the spirit of the American people and the conditions which had formed it including traditions of protestantism, free thought, free education and self-government. His understanding of the critically important relationship between circumstances and policy was to be a common element in his political philosophy. But it does not appear to have occurred to Burke that the old mercantilist framework of empire was no longer sufficient to contain these dynamic social forces. Although he was able to utilize his familiarity with American history and society to demonstrate the irrelevance of a military solution to the colonial question, he was unable to advance a more realistic solution himself. Even if it had been possible to restore the imperial situation which existed before 1763, it is extremely doubtful if the Americans would have been satisfied. Burke was willing to go to almost any lengths to restore the old empire. Indeed, he was willing to go so far that he stumbled almost by accident, upon a new concept of the empire.

Burke always maintained that the imperial sovereignty of Britain should be recognized by the colonists, otherwise 'the presiding authority of Great Britain as the head, the arbiter, and director of the whole empire, would vanish into an empty name, without operation or energy'.[39] Nevertheless, he was loath to advocate measures to enforce the supremacy of the imperial government:

> The very idea of subordination of parts, excludes this notion of simple and undivided unity. England is the head; but she is not the head and members too. Ireland has ever had from the beginning a separate, but not an independent, legislature; which far from distracting, promoted the union of whole.[40]

For Burke the empire was a collection of diverse political units under the general and paternal supremacy of the mother parliament. He went, perhaps, as far as anyone could, towards reconciling local separation with imperial unity given the limitations of contemporary thinking about the imperial question, especially the preoccupation with rights. Burke summarized his ideal of the empire thus:

> We have a great empire to rule, composed of a vast mass of hetero-

[38] *Works*, III, 36.   [39] Ibid., II, 169–70 (*Observations*).   [40] Ibid., 113.

geneous governments, all more or less free and popular in their forms, all to be kept in peace, and kept out of conspiracy with one another, all to be kept in subordination to this country; while the spirit of an extensive and intricate and trading interest pervades the whole, always qualifying and often controlling, every general idea of constitution or government. It is a great and difficult object; and I wish we may possess wisdom and temper enough to manage it as we ought. Its importance is infinite.[41]

The role of parliament in the empire was two-fold. The first arose from its function as the local legislature of Great Britain itself

The other, and I think her nobler capacity, is what I call her *imperial character*; in which, as from the throne of heaven, she superintends all the several inferior legislatures, and guides and controls them all, without annihilating any. As all these provincial legislatures are only co-ordinate to each other, they ought to be subordinate to her, else they can neither preserve mutual peace, nor hope for mutual justice, nor effectually afford mutual assistance.[42]

Burke considered that the provincial legislatures should be independent of the mother parliament unless they proved themselves unequal 'to the common ends of their institution'.[43] Parliament must therefore supply these occasional deficiencies from her boundless reserve of sovereignty. Burke well understood that the spheres of authority of the central and local legislatures were difficult to define but he assumed that wise policy operating in accordance with circumstances would establish a viable relationship between mother country and colony. Burke was fond of observing that the real cement of empire was not the laws, still less was it physical coercion or economic subordination: it was more subtle but far more powerful. We quote again Burke's apparent anticipation of the ideal of the modern commonwealth:

My hold of the colonies is in the close affection which grows from common names, from kindred blood, from similar priveleges, and equal protection. These are ties, which, though light as air, are as strong as links of iron. Let the colonies always keep the idea of their civil rights associated with your government; they will cling and grapple to you; and no force under heaven will be of power to tear them from their allegiance. But let it be once understood, that your government may be one thing, and their privileges another; that these two things may exist without any mutual relation; the

[41] *Works*, II, 167.   [42] Ibid., II, 436 (Speech on American Taxation).
[43] Ibid.

cement is gone; the cohesion is loosened; and everything hastens to decay and dissolution.

As he put it 'Magnanimity in politics is not seldom the truest wisdom; and a great empire and little minds go ill together.'[44]

Burke's American thought was the series of public utterances of a party politician, a collection of speeches and addresses and plans whose purpose it was to cope with urgent problems. He viewed the American problem through the eyes of a British parliamentarian – indeed, he could do no other – and although he came nearer than many of his contemporaries to understanding the problem of empire, he could not separate in his own mind the threat to American liberties posed by parliamentary taxation from the threat to the British constitution posed by the court system. This is the essential link between Burke's domestic and imperial thinking. The fact that parliament acquiesced in the taxation of Americans lent a conspiratorial air to the imperial question, in which the sinister cabal around George III was equally intent upon destroying the liberties of Americans as of Englishmen. Burke's imperial thinking embraced the ideal of returning to a 'golden age' of imperial relationships; this ideal of restoring a former age rather than anticipating a new one, characterized Burke's imperial as well as his domestic thought. In the same way that Burke was not and could not be the prophet of the two party system, or the modern system of responsible government, so he cannot be truly described as the prophet of the modern commonwealth of nations.

[44] *Works*, II, III, 126 (Speech on Conciliation).

Chapter IV

The Imperial Problem: Ireland

We saw in our examination of Burke's American thought that his ideas were called forth by political circumstances over which he had no control. The second of the imperial questions with which he had to deal – that of Ireland – was more complex than that of America. It was, in fact, much more than an imperial situation. Social and economic realities lay at the root of the problem. The mass of the native peasantry were Catholic. They resented restrictions placed both upon their religion and their political activities by the Protestant minority, many of them absentee English landlords, who ruled the country and its people. Catholics had no prospect of acquiring education or political power. They had neither the vote nor the right to sit in parliament. The Irish parliament at Dublin had little independent authority and tamely followed the policy of the imperial legislature. The government of Ireland was in the hands of the Lord-Lieutenant who was appointed by the British government. The parliament of Ireland was managed by undertakers who wielded a pro-English majority. In short, a corrupt minority exercised a Protestant Ascendancy over the country. After 1760 the native Irish slowly began to stir and to manifest their discontent with the situation. They came up against the power not only of the Protestant Ascendancy but also that of the British government. For long the Ascendancy and the imperial authorities had presented a united front to the Catholic Irish but conflict between them gradually came to the surface. In this political minefield Burke had to tread with care.

Burke, of course, was an Irishman and his solicitousness for his native country was one of the motivating aspects of his early thought. He admitted in 1780 that it had always been one of his political aims 'to be somewhat useful to the place of my Birth and education'[1] and to

[1] For his detailed vindication of his conduct with respect to Ireland in 1778

attempt to manifest what he described as 'an utter abhorrence of all kinds of public injustice and oppression' which led him, as he said, to take up the crusade of Ireland.[2] He was pleased to go with Hamilton to Ireland in the early 1760s but he was undoubtedly moved by the wretched condition of his fellow countrymen, and nauseated by the horrible violence with which the agrarian disturbances (attributed to the so-called Whiteboys) of these years were put down.

It was about this time that Burke wrote his *Tracts on the Popery Laws*, from which much of our knowledge of his early Irish attitudes can be gleaned. The *Tracts* were a polemic against the injustice and inhumanity of the penal laws against the Irish Catholics, laws which appeared to Burke to aim at the destruction of Catholic property and weaken the institution of Catholic marriage and promote the division of Ireland into two hostile groups. Yet, although the language of the *Tracts* was extravagant their substance was less extreme. He demanded better treatment for the Catholics but neither the dissolution of the Protestant establishment nor any substantial change in the structure of Irish society. Even when he was most radical Burke remained profoundly conservative by temperament and inclination.

Burke's first public stand on Irish questions as a party politican was made in opposition – pretty factious opposition, at that – to a ministerial proposal in 1773 to lay a tax upon the property of absentee Irish landowners. Now Burke, in his nationalistic youth, had advocated just such a tax but he found political objections to it in 1773. Not only was Lord Rockingham one of the greatest of the absentee land-lords but many others in the party held land in Ireland too. Burke, then, had to toe the party line and join in the party's opposition to the tax. He proclaimed that if the tax passed then many of the absentees would be forced by economic reasons to take up residence in Ireland. Burke sincerely believed that if they did so the natural bonds between England and Ireland would be weakened and the fabric of the empire loosened. But Burke knew as well as anyone how much harm the absentee landlords did Ireland. His blind obedience to the party line over this matter does his reputation little credit. In view of the lifetime of devoted service which he gave to his country his attitude requires explanation. What may be said in his defence is that Irish affairs were still relatively peaceful and that the world situation had not invested her with the critically important geographical and strategic role which she acquired later in the decade. And furthermore there was nothing

and 1779, see his letter to Thomas Burgh, dated 1 January 1780, printed in *The Works of Edmund Burke* (2 vols 1834), II, 407–14.

[2] Burke to J. Curry, 14 August 1779, *Correspondence*, IV, 118–20.

inconsistent in Burke, the protagonist of the Declaratory Act, defending the powers of the imperial parliament against a narrowly nationalistic bill.

Burke was an Irish patriot, but, more than that, he was an imperialist. When the American War of Independence had broken out, Ireland could have taken advantage of England's embarrassments to seek local advantage. Burke took a wider view, however, asserting the identity of interests between the two countries within the empire. He saw the importance of Ireland's geographical position in relation to France and England. To keep Ireland in safe hands, Burke saw that the Irish must be made happy, their connection with Britain entirely voluntary. As the crisis of the empire developed in the late 1770s Burke saw the Irish problem in an imperial framework. Indeed, he was convinced that Ireland had an important part to play in the current crisis. 'Ireland was never in the situation of real honour and real consequence in which she now stands. She has the Ballance of the Empire and perhaps its fate for ever, in her hands.' What Burke wanted was for the Irish parliament to address both the king and the English parliament against pursuing a coercive policy in America. If it did 'It was impossible that they should not succeed.'[3] Burke was wrong. It was, in fact, not only possible, but perhaps inevitable! No such address was forthcoming. Burke complained 'Ireland has missed the most glorious opportunity ever indulged by heaven to a subordinate State, that of being the safe and certain mediatour in the quarrels of a great Empire'.[4] What worried Burke and many of his contemporaries was that Ireland, far from being impartial in the struggle between Britain and her colonies, might try to emulate the Americans. This was something against which Burke constantly struggled by seeking to improve the domestic situation of the Irish themselves.

Burke had no illusions about his native land. He knew that its political system was rotten, that the mass of the Catholic peasantry were unwilling to take part in constructive political action and that the ruling Protestants, including both the landed and the monied interests, were unwilling for selfish reasons to assist England in her struggle against the Americans.[5] Burke was right to have reservations about his fellow countrymen. The American Revolution, and especially the Declaration of Independence, had made an impact upon Ireland, where the ruling class – but especially the Presbyterians – began to demand a greater measure of independence of the mother country, a

---

[3] Burke to Richmond, 26 September, 1775, *Correspondence*, III, 217–20.
[4] Burke to Lord Charlemont, 4 June 1776, ibid., 270–1.
[5] Burke to Charles James Fox, 8 October 1777, ibid., 380–8.

demand which England was hardly in a position to refuse especially when the Irish leaders began to acquire popular support for their attempts to widen the sphere of toleration for Roman Catholics.

Considering both the seriousness of the Irish situation and the degree of Burke's concern for his country, he was surprisingly slow to take any initiative on this topic. He supported silently a measure proposed by one of the most independent and talented men of his party, Sir George Savile, to extend toleration for English Catholics. This passed in 1778 and allowed them to lease and sell land. This was merely a prelude to a similar measure for Ireland. Burke now took it upon himself to advise the Irish Catholics to remain loyal to the throne and to petition peacefully for some relaxation of the penal laws which he had condemned in the *Tracts* a decade and a half earlier.[6] Burke believed that religious and civil toleration must proceed together. One was useless without the other. He even opposed a relief bill in 1782 because it excluded Catholics from the franchise and from holding offices. For Burke, the price of religious toleration should not be civil slavery. Civil freedom should precede religious toleration and provide a foundation for its development. Burke had, therefore, a secular view of toleration. He viewed it as a civic as much as a religious question. Thus, in his view, the act of 1782, extended religious toleration 'but it puts a new bolt on civil rights, and rivets it to the old one'.[7]

Toleration was, perhaps, less important an issue in Irish politics in the age of the American Revolution than the commercial relationship of the mother-country with its dependency. Burke believed that some easing of Ireland's restrictive trade laws was urgent, especially when the American war began to cause serious dislocations in Irish trade. Burke clung courageously to his opinions, even at the cost of alienating his Bristol constituents, who bitterly recognized that they would be among the first victims of Burke's generosity towards the Irish.

Burke's courage and selflessness in advocating far-reaching changes in the economic structure of the empire are however less interesting than the arguments he used to support his proposal. Yet again he rested his case upon an appeal to history, arguing that his proposals merely restored the economic arrangements of the empire to what they had been in the later seventeenth century. The Navigation Act of 1672

[6] Burke to J. Perry, 12 July 1778, ibid., IV, 5–10. For details of these proceedings see A. P. Levack, 'Edmund Burke, his Friends and the Dawn of Irish Catholic Emancipation', *Catholic Historical Review*, XXXVII (1951); T. H. D. Mahoney, 'Edmund Burke and Rome', ibid., XL (1953). Professor Mahoney's *Edmund Burke and Ireland* (Harvard University Press, 1960) is the most detailed and authoritative account of its subject.

[7] Burke to Lord Kenmare, 21 February 1782, *Correspondence*, IV, 405–18.

and its benefits applied to Ireland as well as to England.[8] It was only since the Williamite oppression that Ireland had lost her commercial freedom. History and justice were thus both on the side of the Irish. Ireland had demonstrated her loyalty to England on several occasions and furnished her with troops. It was in Britain's own interest, therefore, to reward such fidelity at least with an opportunity for the Irish to compete equally with the English on the home market. Burke was also conscious of another, more ominous, argument that the Irish would force the English to grant such a concession unless it were granted voluntarily.[9] For Burke, the interests of Bristol, the interests of England and of Ireland were subordinate to the interests of the empire as a whole. He regarded himself not merely as a member of parliament but also as a member of an imperial parliament. Only by adopting an imperial attitude could Ireland be saved from going the way of America.[10]

Events completely justified the wisdom of Burke's magnanimity. 1779 was remarkable in Ireland for the sudden growth of the Volunteer Movement. The Volunteers were a body of militia. They had sprung up as a defensive reaction against the incursions of American privateers. They could easily be directed, however, against the British and used to extract concessions from the North administration. The Volunteers were contemptuous of the scanty religious and commercial concessions which the British government was offering in 1779. As the year wore on, Catholics were admitted into the Volunteers and by the autumn of 1779 Ireland seemed poised to go the way of America. Not only was the Irish parliament demanding freer trade. Forty thousand Volunteers pressed home its demand. The American pattern was clearly being repeated when, in the autumn of 1779, non-importation agreements levelled against English goods proliferated in Ireland. Burke of course was deeply alarmed by these symptoms of an impending Irish separatism. He was a British imperialist before he was an Irish nationalist. He approved warmly therefore of the measures that North

---

[8] The Rockingham–Shelburne ministry was agreed on few things. A solution to the Irish problem, however, was one of them. The ministry repealed an act of 1719 which applied the legislation of the English parliament directly and automatically to Ireland. Other detailed measures passed by the ministry limited the authority of the British Privy Council to amend Irish laws.

[9] See Burke's speech of 5 May 1778, *The Parliamentary History*, XIX, 1119–24. It is Burke's Letter to Sir Hercules Langrishe (1792) which contains his most detailed discussion of the Glorious Revolution and its effects upon Ireland, *Works*, VI, 334–6.

[10] See Burke's speech of 15 February 1779, *The Parliamentary History*, XX, 133.

rushed through parliament at the turn of the year.[11] Burke supported free trade in the empire not only because it would be beneficial to the whole empire, not just because it would benefit Ireland but also because it was clearly in the interests of the mother country herself to relax her mercantilist stranglehold upon Ireland.[12] Burke was, therefore, just as uninterested in the traditional *rights* of the British parliament over Ireland as he was in its *rights* over America. He believed that inequalities and grievances ought to be redressed irrespective of rights. Events were soon to demonstrate how wise Burke's indifference to legislative sovereignty really was. 'Our late misfortunes have taught us the danger and mischief of a restrictive coercive and partial policy.' He had believed for some time that 'The prosperity, arising from an enlarged and liberal system improved all its objects and the participation of a trade with flourishing countries is much better than the monopoly of want and penury.'[13] And he ridiculed the prospect that 'America was to be conquered, in order that Ireland should *not* trade thither; whilst the miserable Trade, which she is permitted to carry on to other places, has been torn to pieces in the struggle'. He did not believe trade between England and Ireland was limited, 'as if the objects of mutual demand and consumption, could not stretch beyond the bounds of our Jealousies'.[14] One other argument in favour of free trade appealed to him. It would further the prosperity of the urban middle class (among which was numbered a small but significant Catholic minority) and weaken the power of the Protestant Ascendancy.

The next objective of the Irish was to prevent the British government from retracting the commercial concessions which it had so reluctantly granted. This could only be attained by the Irish being granted some measure of legislative independence. In 1780 and 1781 this prospect became increasingly attractive to the Irish; after Britain's defeat by the Americans at Yorktown towards the end of 1781 it became irresistible. The Rockingham – Shelburne ministry of 1782 which succeeded the ministry of North could do no other than grant legislative independence to Ireland. By this time, indeed, the Volunteers and the 'Patriot' party led by Ireland's liberal statesman, Henry Grattan[15]

[11] These included the removal of restrictions upon the import of Irish wool and glass into England and the opening to the Irish of markets in America, the West Indies and Africa.

[12] Burke to T. Burgh, 1 January 1780, loc. cit.

[13] Burke to Samuel Span, 9 April 1778, *Correspondence*, III, 426.

[14] Burke to Hartford, Cowles & Co., 2 May 1778, ibid., 440–1.

[15] The greatest Irish politician of his generation and the architect of Irish legislative independence. Indeed, in Irish history, the Irish assembly of 1782–1801 is referred to as 'Grattan's Parliament'.

had become the allies of the Rockingham Whigs and the counter-
weights to the Protestant Ascendancy. Burke took little active part in
Irish affairs, excluded as he was from cabinet discussions. Not that
he was uninterested. He went clean against the wishes of his party
colleagues in criticizing the grant of legislative independence. Burke's
disapproval was founded upon his fear that it tended towards the
complete separation of Ireland from the mother country and the
disintegration of the empire. Legislative independence would undermine the position of the Lord Lieutenant and weaken the position of
the Irish Catholics. (The imperial parliament had always existed as a
final court of appeal for them but after 1782 it would no longer be
able to inquire into the actions of the Protestant Ascendancy.) Another
aspect of Burke's imperial conservatism becomes evident. Burke wished
to maintain the traditional structure of the empire by restoring traditional usages in each constituent part, and with traditional usages,
traditional loyalties.

In an attempt to establish greater security for the Irish Catholics,
however, Burke now reversed his earlier position and conceded the
right of Catholics to hold office. This reversal of his earlier attitude
also contradicts his attitude towards the English Dissenters but it
followed logically enough from the new situation in which Irish
Catholics found themselves after 1782. Those Catholics who managed
to attain office would be able to some extent to protect those who did
not. As usual, this was a political rather than a philosophical reason;
for Burke's attitude to Irish legislative independence anticipated his
controversial opposition to Pitt's proposals of 1785 for free trade with
Ireland. No doubt Burke followed his party in its factious opposition
to Pitt's scheme.[16] No doubt, too, his wish to acquire popularity in
Ireland played some part in persuading him to resist the proposals.
Yet his fear that Pitt's proposals might lead in time to the economic
separation of Ireland from England was, at least, consistent with his
earlier and frequently expressed concern to maintain the integrity of
the empire.

The French Revolution caused further changes in Burke's developing
and sometimes complex attitude towards Ireland. The origin of Burke's
new concern was his fear that the depressed Catholic peasantry might
attempt to emulate the French, to destroy the Protestant Ascendancy
and establish a Jacobin revolutionary power, allied to France, in
Ireland. In the last years of his life, therefore, Burke toiled increasingly

[16] Pitt wished to promote the commercial prosperity of Ireland in an attempt
to lower the political tension. This he proposed to do by liberalizing trade
between the two countries.

to safeguard Ireland from revolution. Towards this end he lent his aid to the powerful Catholic Association, tried to restrain it from violence and excesses and encouraged it to aim for the amelioration of the lot of the Catholics and a complete revision of the penal laws. He supported its attempts to admit Catholics into the professions, into the magistracy and to the franchise.[17] In his attempts to safeguard the unity of the empire and to maintain the loyalty of the Catholic population of Ireland, Burke was forced into a thoroughgoing re-examination of his earlier ideas. He continued to work, but now with renewed vigour, for the repeal of the penal laws. Reflecting his attitude towards America in the 1770s (when he had scorned the idea of indicting a whole people) Burke reasserted his belief that the penal laws formed no part of the ancient constitution of the empire and that if Ireland were to be kept within the folds of the empire they must be done away with. This attitude was typical of Burke, both in his concern for the integrity of the empire and his concern for popular liberties. Yet surely Burke was guilty of inconsistency in at least one part of his proposed treatment of the Irish Catholics: his willingness to admit them to the franchise when he was so vehemently opposed to its extension in England.

For Burke, of course, the situation of the two countries was different. In Ireland the Catholics had no representation at all. They were not even 'virtually' represented in the Irish parliament whose representative character had been strangled by the Ascendancy. Therefore, even if the result of admitting the Catholics to the franchise were the increased corruption which Burke anticipated he nevertheless thought it a price worth paying for keeping Ireland in the British empire. There was a further argument in favour of parliamentary reform in Ireland. It might save the country from an Irish Catholic revolution. Burke opposed violent revolution in Ireland for many reasons. Fundamentally, he could not see that violence was necessary when political channels for reform still remained open. Burke did not believe that the British constitution established between 1688 and 1714 forbade Catholic enfranchisement; to enfranchise them, therefore, would not be a violation of the constitution, rather the contrary.

As every one knows, that a great part of the Constitution of the Irish House of Commons was founded about the year 1614, expressly

[17] Edmund sent his son, Richard to Ireland in 1792 to act as the agent of the Catholic Association in an attempt to reform the administration of that country. In this he was unsuccessful. In the following year, after the outbreak of war between England and France, Pitt relented and extended the vote to the Irish Catholics upon the same basis as that already enjoyed by the Protestants.

for bringing that House into a state of dependance, and that the new Representative was at that time seated and installed by force and violence, nothing can be more impolitic than for those who wish the House to stand on its present basis, (as for one I most sincerely do) to make it appear to have kept too much the principle of its first institution, and to continue to be as little a virtual, as it is an actual representative of the Commons. It is the degeneracy of such an institution so vicious in its principle, that is to be wished for. If Men have the real Benefit of a Sympathetic Representation, none but those who are heated and intoxicated with Theory will look for any other. This sort of Representation, my dear Sir, must wholly depend not on the force with which it is upheld, but upon the prudence of those who have influence upon it. Indeed without some such prudence in the use of Authority, I do not know, at least in the present time, how any power can long continue.[18]

Burke did not believe that a Catholic franchise would amount to anything like an attack upon property by numbers. Since 1778 the Catholics had enjoyed the right to acquire property. They had thus acquired an interest to uphold and defend. They, or at least the propertied Catholics, deserved the vote. Burke, then, in admitting Catholics to the vote was extending, not contradicting his own principles. Finally, we may note that Burke never stated that the franchise was a right. Its extension was a matter of expediency. The danger that numbers would be set against property would be reduced by admitting 'settled, permanent substance in lieu of the numbers'.[19] Thus Burke strengthened property against numbers. After a century of discrimination it was a matter of urgent necessity for the British government to conciliate the Irish Catholics. Burke well knew that to enfranchise Catholic property would only affect the outcome of a handful of elections. He wanted not electoral change but a symbolic public act to win the trust of the Catholics. And, in any case, the enfranchisement of the Catholics said Burke was 'not an innovation in the constitution but a restoration of it, the removal of an innovation'.[20]

Yet the swirling and dangerous cross currents of the Irish problem led Burke to discard some of his optimistic ideas. By the end of 1792 the Irish situation was seriously and rapidly deteriorating. The hitherto moderate Catholic Association had fallen into the hands of Wolf Tone,

[18] Burke to an unidentified recipient, February 1797, *Correspondence*, IX, 253–63.
[19] *Works*, VI, 311, 368–73 (Letter to Langrishe, 1792).
[20] Speech on the Address to the Throne, 13 December 1792, *Speeches*, IV, 80.

who supported and propagated the principles of the French Revolution. The outbreak of war between France and Britain in February 1793 ignited a critical situation. At once, the British government adopted the policy of relief which Burke had been advocating for some time. The Relief Act of 1793 admitted the Irish Catholics to both the parliamentary and to the municipal franchises, to the magistracy, and allowed them to sit on juries and to hold commissions. These substantial concessions did not effectively quieten the Irish scene. The tide of revolutionary enthusiasm rose so high that Burke became thoroughly alarmed. He proclaimed that all men whatever their politics or religion must unite against the atheistic anarchy of Jacobinism. In the way of achieving this national inter-denominational crusade against Jacobinism, however, stood the almost insuperable obstacle of the Protestant Ascendancy.

Burke had always hated the Ascendancy. He regarded it as a selfish and sectional attempt by a part only of the Protestants to arrogate to themselves exclusively the privileges of citizenship. They perpetuated their oligarchic dominion by wholesale bribery and corruption. The envy, jealousy and suspicion which resulted were fatal to Burke's hope for national unity in the 1790s. The Relief Act of 1793 had not weakened the power of the Ascendancy: rather it had served to entrench it more strongly.

> That the late change in the Laws has not made any alteration in their Tempers; except that of aggravating their habitual pride by resentment and vexation. They have resolved, to make one, among the many unhappy discoveries of our times. It is this; that neither the Laws, nor the dispositions of the chief executive Magistrate are able to give security to the people, whenever certain leading men in the Country, and in office are against them. They have actually made the discovery; and a dreadful one it is, for Kings, Laws and Subjects: This is what makes all Ideas of Ascendancy in particular factions, whether distinguished by party names taken from Theology or from Politicks so mischievous as they have been. Wherever such Factions, predominate in such a manner, that they come to link (which without loss of time they are sure to do) a pecuniary and personal Interest with the licentiousness of a party domination, nothing can secure those that are under it. If this was not clear enough, upon a consideration of the nature of things, and the nature of Man, the late proceedings in Ireland, subsequent to the repeal of the penal laws would leave no doubt of it.[21]

[21] Burke to Thomas Hussey, 4 February 1795, *Correspondence*, VIII, 138.

It should not be thought that Burke was encouraging an attack upon the Irish aristocracy. Rather he was trying to establish one. As early as 1792 he had proclaimed that he would like to replace the Ascendancy by 'an aristocratick interest . . . an interest of property and education . . . and to strengthen by every prudent means, the authority and influence of men of that description.'[22] He was not thus arguing for a more democratic form of government but for a more aristocratic one, 'provided that the personal authority of individual nobles be kept in due bounds, that their cabals and factions are guarded against with a severe vigilance'.[23] There is some danger that we may mistake and misunderstand Burke's ultimate objectives in Ireland. His sense of nationalism, his conception of the role of Ireland in the empire, his wish to extend toleration and civic rights to the Catholics and, most of all, his passionate desire to break the power of the Ascendancy— tend to conceal the fact that he wished, after all, to establish a society in Ireland dominated by the aristocracy, not by the Ascendancy of the Protestants. Government, for Burke, ought to be aristocratic: 'Our constitution is not made for great, general, and prescriptive exclusions, sooner or later it will destroy them, or they will destroy the constitution.'[24] The purpose of politics was to promote reconciliation. A 'prudent and enlarged' policy ought to be pursued by governments, especially the imperial government in Ireland in the 1790s. If they did not then it would be all too easy for the Jacobins to promote attacks upon religion, property, and 'old traditionary institutions.'[25]

Burke, therefore, opposed the persecution of the Catholics because the stability of Irish society was at stake, and, with it, the security of the empire. His hatred of persecution did not arise from a purely philosophical scruple but from the harsh realities of politics in the tempestuous decade of the 1790s. Besides, it was not so much the case that the persecution was wrong; it was futile. Two centuries of persecution had only strengthened the cohesion of the Catholics and their loyalty to their religion. Events in the last few years of Burke's life appeared to justify his humanitarianism. The British government ignored Burke's advice and relied increasingly upon the use of force and government by the Ascendancy to maintain its rule in Ireland. Although Burke did not live to see the rebellion of 1798, he lived long enough to deplore the growing extremism of the Catholics as well as the blind obduracy of the Protestants. At all costs he was determined to fight the forces of Irish nationalism. Any talk, or any hint, of Irish home rule horrified him:

[22] *Works*, VI, 344-5 (Letter to Sir Hercules Langrishe, 1792).
[23] Ibid., 304.   [24] Ibid.   [25] Ibid., 310.

For, in the name of God, what Grievance had Ireland, as Ireland, to complain of with regard to Great Britain? Unless the protection of the most powerful Country upon earth, giving all her privileges without exception in common to Ireland, and reserving to herself only the painful pre-eminence of tenfold Burthens to be a matter of complaint. The Subject, as a subject is as free in Ireland as he is in England—as a member of the Empire, an Irishman has every privilege of a natural born Englishman, in every part of it, in every occupation, and in every branch of Commerce.[26]

He wished, therefore, to maintain the imperial relationship for the sake of Ireland as much as for the sake of England. Lying beneath the varying and complex elements of Burke's Irish thought, therefore, can be discerned an imperial mentality which renders coherent the divergent aspects of his thinking and makes intelligible the fanatical tone of his later writings.

The sense of apocalyptic despair which Burke felt towards the end of his life over Irish affairs was far more than a senile dread of disorder. He feared the consequences of Irish independence: instant subjugation at the hands of the French. If England did not dominate Ireland then France surely would. 'Ireland *constitutionally* is independent – *Politically* she never can be so.'[27] France would destroy Catholicism and Protestantism as well; everything, therefore, must be subordinated to keeping Ireland free of French influences. In particular, Ireland must be saved from the naivete of her Jacobin sons who fondly believed that the only way to save themselves from the Ascendancy was to go the way of the French.[28] At the same time, he thoroughly understood the almost universal hatred among Catholics for the Ascendancy. He well knew that further emancipation would not reconcile them to the empire. Nothing short of universal suffrage would satisfy them. But any concession would be regarded by the Catholics as a show of weakness.[29] Nevertheless, he was determined to save his country. In his last months Burke would have made any sacrifice, including the concession of universal suffrage, even the destruction of the Ascendancy, to conciliate the Catholics. He died on 9 July 1797 in the unhappy belief that the Ascendancy was hardening its grip on the country and that revolution was now inevitable.

It was well that he died before the rebellion of 1798 for that event

---

[26] Burke to Thomas Hussey, 18 May 1795, *Correspondence*, VIII, 246–7.
[27] Burke to an unidentified recipient, February 1797, loc. cit.
[28] Burke to Thomas Hussey, 18 May 1795, loc. cit.
[29] Burke to Lord Fitzwilliam, 7 May 1797, *Correspondence*, IX, 330–1.

marked the complete disappointment of his hopes. Like many of his contemporaries, Burke could scarcely keep pace with the rapid changes in the British empire in the later eighteenth century. Like many of his contemporaries, he failed to think out a satisfactory solution to the tragic Irish problem. Yet his Irish thought well illustrates the constant pragmatism and undogmatic realism which inform so much of his political philosophy. He did not attempt to force an interpretation of events into conformity with an arbitrary view of the empire. There is, however, a consistency in his overall view of Irish society and Irish history, which ensures that his flexibility does not become a superficial expediency. His humanitarianism, manifested in his anxiety to extend a greater degree of toleration to the Irish Catholics, shines through every aspect of his long career of concern for the Irish. His distaste for the corruption and exclusiveness of the Ascendancy was always with him. Finally, his conviction that the destiny of Ireland was indissolubly linked with that of England provided yet another plank of consistency in the history of his Irish thought. For here, as in his American thought, Burke was the great conciliator, trying to restore the imperial links between Irishmen and Englishmen on the one hand, and between Irishmen and Irishmen on the other.

Chapter V

The Imperial Problem: India

Burke's ideas on British rule in India were consistent in their general outline with other aspects of his imperial thinking. On America he had objected to parliament's *right* to tax the colonies arbitrarily. On Indian affairs he opposed the *right* of the East India Company to govern India arbitrarily. On neither issue did he deny the status of the legislative right involved. For Burke there existed profound humanitarian and moral issues which transcended legislative custom. Similarly, his later works attacked the French revolutionaries for destroying the *ancien régime* in France and in Europe. This attitude was consonant with his attacks upon the East India Company for its destruction of an *ancien régime* in India, for its tampering with chartered rights, for its destruction of an ancient ruling class. His solicitousness for the Irish Catholics was matched by his concern for the welfare of the mass of the Indian people. Further, the awareness of environmental and socializing factors which he had displayed on American affairs was reflected in a similar understanding of Indian society. In a debate in 1781 he asserted that 'we must now be guided, as we ought to have been with respect to India, by studying the genius, the temper, and the manner of the people, and adapting to them the laws that we establish'.[1] In this way, different aspects of Burke's thought complement each other, develop comparable themes and reflect similar attitudes. Burke was always ready to expand his vision and to incorporate into his thought new circumstances and new situations. This is one reason why his thought is not dull and uniform but vibrant and variable. Burke was not impressed by the 'right' of the East India Company to misgovern India. Such a right constituted a monopoly and therefore a trust, over which parliament should exercise vigilance. The Company's

[1] Speech of 27 June 1781, *The Parliamentary History*, XXII, 555.

rights were not unlimited. If it violated the trust which parliament reposed in it then parliament could and should revoke it. It was not to be, however, before the 1780s that he expounded fully his doctrine of the trust owed by the imperial parliament to the people of India. The company's 'right', therefore, was restricted by the necessity for it to govern in accordance with the habits of the people themselves, with their history and character, rather than in accordance with the paper precedents of legislative custom.

The nature of Burke's involvement in Indian politics can only be appreciated and its intensity understood by realizing how far he felt himself to be personally involved in the affairs of the company and of Warren Hastings. His crusades to reform the government of India coincided with the decline of Burke's party fervour, when his active and restless intellect was hungry for new challenges and starved of political idealism. His persecution of Hastings began during the dark days of Burke's career, when his public reputation was at its lowest and when he felt the need to justify his career to posterity. To this end, the impeachment of Hastings would be his monument.[2] He pored over partisan accounts of the Company's rule in India – and of Hastings' part in it – and read into them a conflict of principles, a conflict in which he, Burke, was on the side of right and Hastings the side of wrong. For Burke, the impeachment was to be like a medieval morality play, acted out in public, bristling with salutary moral and political lessons for Britain. There can be no disputing the fact that Burke considered his Indian activities to be the most important events of his career. Towards the end of his life he wrote:

> Let everything I have done, said or written be forgotten but this. I have struggled with the great and the little on this point during the greater part of my active Life; and I wish after death, to have my Defiance of the Judgements of those, who consider the dominion of the glorious Empire given by an incomprehensible dispensation of the Divine providence into our hands as nothing more than an opportunity of gratifying for the lowest of their purposes, the lowest of their passions and that for such poor rewards, and for the most part, indirect and silly Bribes, as indicate even more the folly than the corruption of these infamous and contemptible wretches.[3]

[2] Burke to Sir Philip Francis, 10 December 1785, *Correspondence*, V, 241–4. (Hastings had been Governor-General of Bengal between 1772 and 1785.)

[3] Burke to French Laurence, *circa* 27 February 1796, *Correspondence*, VIII, 397–9.

Burke was determined to refute the charge that he had been moved merely by personal antagonism against Warren Hastings.

> In reality, you know that I am no enthusiast, but (according to the powers that God has given me) a sober and reflecting man. I have not even the other very bad excuse, of acting from personal resentment, or from the sense of private injury – never having received any; nor can I plead ignorance, no man ever having taken more pains to be informed. Therefore, *I* say, Remember.[4]

It is important to understand how *symbolic* the impeachment was for Burke. He did not seriously expect to convict Hastings. What he aimed to do through the theatrical drama of the impeachment was to assert certain general principles which should be observed in the government of India. It is not too much to say that he was less concerned with the truth about Hastings' rule than with the morality of imperial responsibilities in the sub-continent. His attack on Hastings became less a search for truth than a personal and political vendetta, a propaganda campaign thinly coated with philosophical generalities. If Burke cannot be shown to have been guilty of deliberate distortion and falsification of the evidence then he can be shown to have indulged his passion against Hastings over and above the requirements of judicial deliberation. Burke was pleading a case and a cause before a public audience; although he stated that 'my motives are clear from private interest, and public malice',[5] his attitude towards the evidence was little short of cavalier: 'I know that the country (India) under his care is sacked and pillaged and I know he is the Government and I know a great deal more.'[6] But this conviction did not rest upon an empirical basis, 'We ought to be very careful not to charge what we are unable to prove.'[7] Burke declared that he was out to prove merely *a general evil intention.*[8] In stating the case for the impeachment before the House of Commons Burke was fully aware of tactical considerations:

> in order to bring about the great primary object of a strong case, I wish that the substance of the Charge should be either left to my own discretion, or, what I should like much better, that we should find some way of previously settling our plan of Conduct.[9]

---

[4] Burke to French Laurence, 10, 12 February 1797, *Correspondence*, IX, 238.
[5] Burke to Lord Thurlow, 4 December 1784, ibid., V, 198.
[6] Burke to Lord Thurlow, 14 December 1784, ibid., 204.
[7] Burke to Sir Philip Francis, 10 December 1785, loc. cit.
[8] Ibid.
[9] Burke to Henry Dundas, 25 March 1787, ibid., 312.

Furthermore, Burke was certainly aware of the value of ministerial help. He was prepared to abstain from much of his systematic opposition to Pitt's ministry for the sake of obtaining the help of the government.

> I shall therefore beg leave to add, that if ever there was a common National Cause totally seperated from Party it is this. A body of men, unlimited in a close connexion of common guilt and common apprehension of danger in the moment, with a strong and just confidence of future power if they escape it, and possessed of a measure of wealth and influence which perhaps you yourself have not calculated at any thing like its just magnitude, is not forming, but actually formed in this Country. This faction is at present ranged under Hastings as an Indian leader; and it will have very soon, if it has not already, an English Leader of considerable enterprise and no contemptible influence. If this faction should now obtain a Triumph it will be very quickly too strong for your Ministry. I will go further, and assert without the least shadow of hesitation, that they will turn out too strong for any one description of national interest that exists, or, on any probable speculation that can exist in our time. Nothing can rescue the Country out of their hands, but our vigorous use of the present fortunate moment, which if once lost is never to be recovered, of effectually breaking up this corrupt combination by effectually crushing the Leader and principal Members of the Corps.[10]

He naturally wanted to have his evidence presented to the Commons in the most favourable light. On one occasion he remarked to Dundas that 'Those Witnesses, upon whom we can personally prevail, must immediately come to Town to have their Evidence methodized.'[11]

In general, then, on matters pertaining to the impeachment Burke was prepared to seize every tactical advantage he could, losing no opportunity of blackening Hastings' character and expounding the enormity of his crimes. Much of Burke's Indian 'thought' then was expressed for motives of propaganda; it did not arise from philosophical considerations at all. Nevertheless, it is less the truth or falsehood of Burke's facts which needs to concern the present discussion than the ethical objectives towards which his Indian work was directed.

When this has been said, there is much in Burke's Indian thought

---

[10] Burke to Henry Dundas, 25 March 1787, *Correspondence*, 314.
[11] Ibid., 1 November 1787, ibid., 356.

that redounds to his credit. If he did not attain the highest standards of political honesty during the impeachment of Hastings then it remains true that Burke's motives were never self-interested. If he hated Warren Hastings, he hated not the man but the corruption Burke thought him to represent. A propagandist by his own admission, at least he sought to do his public duty, to awaken his fellow countrymen to the plight of the Indians. Burke was no crank, no alarmist. He was giving expression to fears and anxieties which had become increasingly common since the 1760s, especially the anxiety that the riches to be derived from the plunder of India might be directed towards the corruption of the British constitution. Although he exaggerated, he exaggerated in the best of causes, the cause of humanity and his exaggerations always had *some* basis in fact. He spent many long and weary hours preparing committee reports for the Commons on Indian affairs. (Burke was consequently one of the leading experts on Indian affairs of his political generation.)

What distinguished Burke from so many of his contemporaries was less his expert knowledge, however, than his consuming interest in Indian affairs. What accounts for the intensity of Burke's feelings for India? To some extent he was fascinated by the ancient order of Indian civilization and alarmed at what he took to be its desecration at the hands of the East India Company. He idealized Indian society and admired its law, its hierarchy and its religion. He argued that in spite of its turbulent history of invasion and war, India remained a Hindu polity in which the government behaved in accordance with the spirit and institutions of the people. Hastings threatened to destroy this Hindu polity and to innovate by introducing into India alien customs. Burke hated the idea of trying to anglicize India. It was the duty of the British to extend their oriental horizons, tolerate alien practices and promote their growth. Most important of all, the system of Indian law must not be destroyed. In India religious and civil laws were not separate systems, as in England, but part of one uniform system. It was to destroy the trust which parliament had vested in them for the company's servants to destroy that sensitive and delicate system. It was with this above all that Burke was fascinated, this above all he wished to preserve sound and entire.

Burke's early attitude towards India was determined largely by party considerations. In 1767 and 1773 he *defended* the East India Company from *ministerial* supervision. This was not the same as rejecting the notion of *parliamentary* supervision; for the moment, it appeared to Burke to be necessary to defend the independence of the company and to prevent its revenues falling into the hands of the crown. He attacked the Regulating Act[12] as 'contrary to the eternal laws of right and wrong – laws that ought to bind men, and above all men legislative assemblies'.[13] (We may be forgiven for not taking too seriously either on this occasion or later, during the impeachment, Burke's invocations of the Natural Law, preferring to recognize them as the rhetorical devices which Burke used to support his arguments whenever they needed reinforcement.)

Between 1773 and 1783 Burke completely shifted his ground on India. Growing familiarity with the subject brought him to fear the corrupting effects of Indian money upon the British constitution.[14] When the time came for parliament to renew the Regulating Act of 1773 (which had passed only for a duration of seven years) parliamentary discussion of the company's rule was inevitable. When the ministry of Lord North came out in support of the East India Company – and of Warren Hastings – the Rockinghamite opposition smelled a rat. Spurred on by the tales of Sir Philip Francis[15] who had his own personal axe to grind against Hastings, they dominated the deliberations of the Select Committee of 1780–1. At the same time as the Select Committee was sitting, a Secret Committee was also investigating Hastings' Governor Generalship of Bengal. By 1783 Burke had completely reversed his former role as defender of the East India Company. Burke was the driving force in the Select Committee which proceeded to publish no fewer than eleven reports. These were enough to remove any lingering doubts in his mind of Hastings' guilt. By 1783, therefore, Burke was prepared completely to reverse his earlier opinions. His India bills of 1783 proposed to do what he had criticized the North ministry for doing in 1773, namely, restraining the activities of the Company by bringing them under parliamentary surveillance. Burke had recourse to the argument that since 1773 the Company had broken the trust which parliament had entrusted to it and that therefore its charter ought to be revoked. We should be clear that Burke was perfectly prepared to rest the case for ministerial intervention upon a

[12] Lord North's Regulating Act of 1773 allowed the East India Company to continue to govern India for trading purposes, provided for a substantial loan to keep the Company solvent, reorganized the government of India and made it answerable to the British parliament.

[13] For Burke's early position on India see P. J. Marshall, *The Impeachment of Warren Hastings* (Oxford, 1965), 1–9.

[14] Burke to Rockingham, 27 April 1782, *Correspondence*, IV, 448–50.

[15] Francis became a committed member of Burke's party through his own personal vendetta against Hastings. His influence upon Burke, however, has been shown by Dr Marshall to have been exaggerated in the past, *The Impeachment of Warren Hastings*, 2–21, *passim*.

detailed scrutiny of the Company's record, not upon any abstract right. Burke thus proposed to bring the government of India under the control of a commission appointed by the ministry, not by the crown. His great speech on 1 December 1783 defended the measures and the philosophy behind them. Burke looked to his bills to cure the ills in the government of India. Of the two bills, the first vested the administration of the East India Company in seven commissioners and nine assistant commissioners, removable only by parliament. The second bill laid down regulations for the Company's servants to observe. The charge that the Indian policy of the coalition ministry was directed wholly towards maintaining Fox and his friends in office, suggested by a cursory glance at the first bill is, in fact, refuted by the details of the second.[16] Nevertheless, there is no escaping the fact that the coalition ministry was attacking chartered rights ostensibly in the party interest. The notorious overthrow of the ministry in the House of Lords[17] left Burke in no doubt that Hastings and the Company had directly interfered in British politics on this occasion. This conjecture became a certainty in Burke's mind after the defeat of his party at the 1784 election. He refused to accept the decision of the people as final and in 1786 he persuaded both the ministry of Pitt and the House of Commons to impeach Hastings, a significant achievement and a remarkable success for one man. Burke's lonely Indian crusade had begun.

The major theme of the impeachment was Burke's affirmation of the right of parliament not only to inquire into the affairs of the East India Company but also to exercise surveillance over the government of India. As we have seen, immediate political considerations together with a passionate humanitarianism inspired Burke's concern. There was one further motive: his belief that the British control of India might be endangered if the Company's arbitrary rule were allowed to continue. He said in December 1783 'that if we are not able to contrive some method of governing India *well*, which will not of necessity become the means of governing Great Britain *ill*, a ground is laid for their eternal separation'.[18] Misgovernment of India might, therefore, provoke a movement for Indian independence. All of this amounted to an overwhelming case for parliamentary surveillance. There was one critical difficulty with Burke's position. How could a good Rockingham Whig possibly profess any opinion which contravened the

[16] See the authoritative account in J. Cannon, *The Fox-North Coalition* (Cambridge, 1969), 106–23.
[17] Ibid., 124–44.
[18] *Works*, IV, 7 (Speech on the India Bill, 1 December 1783).

traditional Whig principle of the sanctity of chartered rights. Burke surmounted this difficulty by distinguishing between the *fundamental laws of the land* (such as Magna Carta) which were unalterable, and documents (like the charter of the East India Company) which were not. The former was a charter 'to restrain power and to destroy monopoly', the latter was a charter 'to establish monopoly and to create power'.[19] Burke did not question the rights of the Company as far as they went:

Those who carry the rights and claims of the company the furthest, do not contend for more than this; and all this I freely grant. But granting all this, they must grant me in my turn, that all political power which is set over men, and that all privilege claimed or exercised in exclusion of them, being wholly artificial, and for so much a derogation from the natural quality of mankind at large, ought to be some way or other exercised ultimately for their benefit.[20]

In short, these rights were a trust. They were neither unlimited nor unrestricted. Burke laid it down that 'it is of the very essence of every trust to be rendered *accountable*; and even totally to *cease* when it substantially varies from the purposes for which alone it could have a lawful existence'.[21] And he went on to assert 'that if the abuse is proved, the contract is broken; and we re-enter into all our rights: that is, into the exercise of all our duties'. That is, Burke was out to promulgate, as he put it, 'the *magna charta* of Hindostan'.[22]

Burke thought it to be unsatisfactory to proceed upon a theoretical and arbitrary presumption about the rights and wrongs of the Company's rule. 'I feel an insuperable reluctance in giving my hand to destroy any established institution of government, upon a theory, however plausible it may be.'[23] Therefore to justify his taking the administration of India out of the hands of the Company Burke needed to prove that the evils perpetrated by the Company were of such a magnitude as to warrant any infringement of the charter.

The abuse affecting this great object ought to be a great abuse. It ought to be habitual, and not accidental. It ought to be utterly incurable in the body as it now stands constituted. All this ought to be made as visible to me as the light of the sun, before I should strike off an atom of their charter.[24]

The first was self-evident in view of the extent of the Indian dominions

[19] *Works*, IV, 9. [20] Ibid., 11. [21] Ibid., 12.
[22] Ibid., 13. [23] Ibid., 14. [24] Ibid., I, 15.

and the size of the population. Burke sought to demonstrate the second proposition by proving firstly:

> that there is not a single prince, state, or potentate, great or small in India, with whom they have come into contact, whom they have not sold. I say sold, though sometimes they have not been able to deliver according to their bargain – Secondly I say, that there is not a single treaty, they have ever made, which they have not broken – Thirdly, I say, that there is not a single prince or state, who ever put any trust in the company, who is not utterly ruined; and that none are in any degree secure or flourishing, but in the exact proportion to their settled distrust an irreconcilable enmity to this nation.[25]

Burke demonstrated the validity of his propositions with a mass of evidence, most of it carefully chosen to fit his case, as indeed, such evidence had to be. He developed this theme further by showing that political disaster had been compounded by the commercial havoc which had been wreaked upon the natives of Bengal by the Company. Burke concluded in high dudgeon:

> In effect, Sir, every legal, regular authority in matters of revenue, of political administration, of criminal law, of civil law, in many of the most essential parts of military discipline, is laid level with the ground, and an oppressive, irregular, capricious, unsteady, rapacious, and peculating despotism without a direct disavowal of obedience to any authority at home, and without any fixed maxim, principle, or rule of proceeding, to guide them in India, is at present the state of your charter-government over great kingdoms.[26]

Long before the Coalition Ministry of 1783, therefore, Burke had made up his mind about the Company. In 1781, for example, he had declared that 'we find the Country infinitely injured, & the Treasures & revenues both of the Company & the subordinate powers wasted & decayed'.[27] Burke however, did not allow his party activities to prevent him from attending to the 'real wants of the people' of India.[28] In any case, as we have noticed on several occasions, his party favour was declining in the 1780s as his interest in India quickened. This did not prevent him from opposing Pitt's India Bill of 1784[29] on the

[25] *Works*, I, 21.   [26] Ibid., 93.

[27] Burke to Sir Thomas Rumbold, 23 March 1781, *Correspondence*, IV, 343–7.

[28] *Works*, IV, 122 (Speech on the India Bill, 1 December 1783).

[29] Pitt's India bill was similar to Burke's in many ways but left patronage in the hands of the Company subject only to a royal veto on appointments.

grounds that it 'put the whole East India Company into the hands of the Crown'.[30] Like many of his party colleagues, Burke came to believe a new myth after 1784 which in many ways was similar to the old Bute myth. Burke and others believed that after 1784 Pitt's government was using the influence of the crown to build up a new aristocracy in Britain, a new aristocracy which would replace the traditional elite of Britain, a new aristocracy based upon corruption and service in India. Burke confessed that the new court plan was more successful than ever the old one had been. The first victims of its corrupt and tyrannical success were the Indians. The only possible remedy was to reassert the function of parliament in exercising vigilance over the constituent parts of the constitution.

> It is difficult for the most wise and upright government to correct the abuses of remote, delegated power, productive of unmeasured wealth, and protected by the boldness and strength of the same ill-got riches. These abuses, full of their own wild native vigour, will grow and flourish under mere neglect. But where the supreme authority, not content with winking at the rapacity of its inferior instruments, is so shameless and corrupt as openly to give bounties and premiums for disobedience to its laws, when it will not trust to the activity of avarice in the pursuit of its own gains, when it secures public robbery by all the careful jealousy and attention with which it ought to protect property from such violence, the commonwealth then becomes totally perverted from its purposes; neither God nor man will long endure it, nor will it long endure itself. In that case, there is an unnatural infection, a pestilential taint fermenting in the constitution of society, which fever and convulsions of some kind or other must throw off.[31]

Burke's condemnation of Indian administration was, therefore, many-sided. The rule of the Company, in general, and of Hastings, in particular, was the very antithesis of what government ought to be because it did not consult the happiness of the governed. They did not govern the Indians with a due concern for their own experience and character. As he said of British politicians, 'We had not steadily before our eyes a general, comprehensive, well connected, and well-proportioned view of the whole of our dominions, and a just sense of their true bearings and relations.'[32] In 1781 he urged the Ministry of North to establish justice as the principle of all its proceedings as

[30] Speech on Pitt's India Bill, 16 January 1784, *Speeches*, II, 493.
[31] *Works*, IV, 318 (Speech on the Nabob of Arcot's Debts, 28 February 1785).
[32] Ibid.

the best method of ensuring the abiding loyalty of the Indians. As it was, government persecuted instead of protected the Indians. Parliament, the only recourse open to the Indians, was under the control of their oppressors after 1784. These oppressors were not the political agents of Great Britain at all.

> It is not the English nation in India, it is nothing but a seminary for the occupation of offices. It is a nation of placemen, it is a republic, a body of people, a state, made up of magistrates, there is no one to watch the powers of office . . . being a kingdom of merchants, they are actuated by the spirit of the body – in other words, they consider themselves as having a common interest separate from that of the country in which they are, where there is no control of the persons that understand the language, and manners, and customs of the country.[33]

Hastings, of course, was the epitome of this avaricious separatism, this negation of government and of empire.

No account of his imperial philosophy can ignore the importance of the intense moral concern displayed by Burke on Indian affairs. His moral starting point was the proposition taken by Burke wittingly and directly from Montesquieu, unwittingly and indirectly from Grotius, that conquest does not permit arbitrary rule but rather carries with it moral duties and moral obligations 'to preserve the people in all their rights, laws and liberties' and 'to preserve and protect the people the same as if the Mogul's empire had existed, to observe the laws, rights, usages and customs of the natives, and to pursue their benefit in all things'.[34] Burke totally rejected Hastings' argument that the actions of Englishmen committed in India had to be judged according to local standards because 'the laws of morality are the same everywhere'.[35] Morality, for Burke, was not a question of geographical location. Furthermore, he brushed aside Hastings' further argument: that he had to govern as he found things. Burke saw no need for Hastings to capitalize on all manner of prevalent corruption.[36] The fact of conquest imposed considerable moral obligations upon the conqueror. Although conquest gave him considerable arbitrary discretion in matters of government, the greater the discretion, the greater the compulsion to deal justly. Burke denied that it had ever been part of the legitimate policy of the Company to wield arbitrary power. Not only *had* it never been, it *never could be*. The Company had never had

[33] Speech on Opening the Articles of Impeachment, 15 February 1788, *Speeches*, IV, 312–13.
[34] Ibid., 308–9.   [35] Ibid., 305.   [36] Ibid., 375 (18 February 1788).

such powers to wield. It had never had them because parliament had never given them and never could.

> My Lords, the East India Company have not arbitrary power to give him; the king has no arbitrary power to give him; your Lordships have not; nor the Commons, nor the whole legislature. We have no arbitrary power to give, because arbitrary power is a thing which neither any man can hold nor any man can give. No man can lawfully govern himself according to his own will; much less can one person be governed by the will of another. We are all born in subjection, – all born equally, high and low, governors and governed, in subjection to one great, immutable, pre-existent law, prior to all our devices and prior to all our contrivances, paramount to all our ideas and all our sensations, antecedent to our very existence, by which we are knit and connected in the eternal frame of the universe, out of which we cannot stir. This great law does not arise from our conventions or compacts; on the contrary, it gives to our conventions and compacts all the force and sanction they can have. It does not arise from our vain institutions. Every good gift of God; all power is of God; and He who has given the power, and from whom alone it originates, will never suffer the exercise of it to be practised upon any less solid foundation than the power itself. If, then, all dominion of man over man is the effect of the Divine disposition, it is bound by the eternal laws of Him that gave it.[37]

Nobody can deny the sincerity and the moral force of passages such as this. To acknowledge these characteristics does not, however, itself clarify the status of the moral argument that Burke used and, in particular, it does not reveal the significance which attaches to his appeals to the Natural Law.

It is worth repeating what we said earlier: that Burke's appeals to the Natural Law ought not to be 'lifted' from their place in a speech or even in the impeachment as a whole. Their rhetorical impact is completely lost if they are treated as 'quotations' or as academic data which, taken together 'prove' Burke's attachment to the Natural Law. It is worth repeating that Burke never believed that he could convince the court of the illegality of Hastings' actions. His intention was to persuade the world that those same actions, while not illegal, were both immoral and illegitimate. To effect such a persuasion was the function of Burke's invocations of the Natural Law during the trial. The Natural Law was needed – increasingly – as the trial wore on, as

[37] Speech on Opening the Articles of Impeachment, 15 February 1788, *Speeches*, IV, 308–9.

a rhetorical device because the managers found that more and more of their evidence was ruled to be inadmissible by the judges according to precedent. It was convenient – perhaps necessary – for Burke to establish another standard by which his evidence would not be dismissed. Sincere, Burke undoubtedly was in his condemnation of Hastings but that there was an element of calculation in his rhetoric will be denied only by his most unthinking admirers.[38] The theatrical impact of his Natural Law perorations was just as important as their logical precision. Indeed, it was probably far more important. It was all very well for Burke to tell the judges that Hastings' crimes were 'not against morals, but against those eternal laws of justice which you are assembled here to assert'.[39] But what were 'those eternal laws of justice'? The judges did not know and they cannot have been much enlightened by Burke's explanation:

> There is one thing, and one thing only, which defies all mutation that which existed before the world, and will survive the fabric of the world itself; I mean justice; that justice, which, emanating from the Divinity, has a place in the breast of every one of us, gives us for our guide with regard to ourselves and with regard to others, and which will stand after this globe is burned to ashes, our advocate or our accuser before the great Judge, when He comes to call upon us for the tenor of a well-spent life.[40]

Until – and unless – such passages are endowed with some meaning, Burke's appeals to the Natural Law must be treated with considerable reserve.

In fact, none of the great 'moral' themes of the impeachment of Warren Hastings rested upon a Natural Law basis. The idea that the government of the empire ought to be conducted in the interests of the governed, that government should act within the law, that conquest carried with it responsibilities, that government ought to be carried on in accordance with the spirit and traditions of the governed – these commonplaces of the British (and European) constitutional tradition were taken over by Burke and applied to the problems of India.

Too much can be – and has been – claimed for Burke's Indian crusade. Morley, for example, asserted that Burke won a new status for Indians in the empire and overthrew a corrupt system of government. Burke did nothing of the kind. The abuses in the government of India against which Burke raised his voice were already well known

[38] Speech on Opening the Articles of Impeachment, 18 February 1788, *Speeches*, IV, 374.

[39] Ibid., 303–4 (15 February 1788).

[40] *Works*, XVI, 417 (Speech at the Close of the Impeachment, 16 June 1794).

to the public; even while the impeachment was dragging on, steps were being taken to ameliorate them. Pitt's India Bill of 1784 permanently established parliamentary control of the East India Company and the beginning of Cornwallis' regime in the following year marked the inauguration of a new phase in the life of 'John Company'. We should be prepared to place Burke's Indian crusade in its proper perspective in both British and Indian history. We should be prepared to acknowledge, and thus to try to understand, the personal and political motives which prompted Burke's inexhaustible industry. We should, moreover, attempt to relate his Indian thought to other aspects of his imperial philosophy. And if that philosophy reflected the variations in the nature of the imperial problem in different parts of the empire then no more can be expected from the 'philosopher in action'.

Chapter VI

The French Revolution

In Burke's French revolutionary thought political philosophy became incidental to a generalized view of man and society. Although his French thought was, to a large extent, consistent with his earlier constitutional and imperial theories, it is much too facile a view to contend that Burke's later thought 'arose out of' his earlier ideas or that it was in some way 'an extension of' them. For Burke now had a new objective: to defend the *ancien régime* in France and in Europe. To achieve this objective it was necessary for him to demonstrate that radical political change was not only unworkable but, in the context of the *ancien régime*, positively undesirable. He therefore underlined the danger of innovation and disruption which might be thrust upon a social system by introducing new and alien elements into an old social and political fabric. In one sense, Burke's historical perspective was limited. Although he was aware of the great developments of history and the variations of culture and society between one continent and another he could neither see that the England of Pitt and Rockingham was dying nor that a new commercial and industrial society was already emerging. The central feature of Burke's French revolutionary thought was his concern to preserve the old society.

In this role, his thinking was just as abstract and as speculative as that of the writers whom he attacked. He hated the radical authors because their works weakened the old prejudices and habits which formed the psychological foundations of the *ancien régime*. Burke's assumptions that the life of the individual is rooted in the life of the state and that the life of the state is rooted in its history were just as arbitrary as comparable assumptions made by the 'Jacobin' theorists whom he so vehemently denounced. Abstract and speculative his philosophy might be, Burke deliberately, however, chose to sustain the role of critic of contemporary thought. His revolutionary thought was his reaction to the current enlightenment philosophy of religion, of society and of man. The Enlightenment elicited deep intellectual anxieties in Burke's mind to which he gave expression in an anti-revolutionary philosophy. This proceeded from an anti-rationalist position. Liberty, for example, was not an abstract proposition but a social reality. Property was not to be regarded as a mental construct. It was, in practical terms, the bulwark of the social order. Inevitably, then, Burke's anti-rationalism strengthened his enduring presumption in favour of any established government or existing institution. The state thus became a vehicle for maintaining and for transmitting the structure and traditions of a society irrespective of popular sentiment. He proclaimed that in his French writings 'He proposed to convey to a foreign people, not his own ideas, but the prevalent opinions and sentiments of a nation, renowned for wisdom, and celebrated in all ages for a well understood and well regulated love of freedom.'[1] But he was speaking only for the propertied class of his country. He did not speak to and he did not write for the man who read Paine's *Rights of Man*. Indeed, it was man's duties rather than his rights which impressed him during the 1790s. In a very real sense, then, Burke was the spokesman of the *ancien régime* in Europe during the revolutionary crisis.

The French Revolution occurred when Burke's career – and his morale – were at their very nadir, and when the impeachment of Warren Hastings, upon which he had pinned all his hopes, was dragging along tediously. Even worse, the king's illness of the winter of 1788–9 had found Burke's party divided and utterly incapable of taking political advantage of the situation. It was less his party's failure which distressed Burke – he had grown accustomed to failure during the past twenty years – than the failure of his party colleagues to uphold the traditional Whig doctrine of hereditary succession during the Regency crisis of 1788–9.[2]

As to the Prince, I found him deeply concerned that the Ideas of an elective Crown should not prevail. He had experienced, and you had all of you fully experienced the Peril of these doctrines on the question of the Regency. . . . I supported the Princes Title to the

---

[1] *Works*, VI, 76 (Appeal from the New to the Old Whigs, 1791).

[2] The king's illness during the winter of 1788–9 threatened to create a vacancy upon the throne. The natural candidate for the Regency, the Prince of Wales, was closely associated with the opposition and there is little doubt that a Regency would have resulted in Pitt's resignation and the formation of a ministry under the Duke of Portland, Rockingham's successor, and led, in the Commons, by Fox. There is a good account of the crisis in J. W. Derry, *The Regency Crisis, and the Whigs, 1788–9* (Cambridge, 1963).

Regency upon the Principle of his Hereditary Right to the Crown: and I endeavoured to explode the false Notions, drawn from what has been stated as the Revolution Maxims. . . . I endeavoured to shew, that the Hereditary succession could not be supported, whilst a person who had the Interest in it, was, during a virtual interregnum, excluded from the Government; and that the direct tendency of the measure, as well as the grounds upon which it was argued, went to make the Crown itself elective contrary (as I contended) to the fundamental Settlement made after the Revolution.[3]

Burke bitterly resented his party's inability to support the basic principles upon which it had been founded. He had become irascible, tetchy and resentful, an object of ridicule and a figure of fun in the House of Commons. Apparently he had outlived his political usefulness. An embarrassment to his colleagues, isolated and with no political future, Burke had sunk to the lowest point in his career. The revolution transformed that reputation and saved it from the relative obscurity to which Burke appeared to be destined.

More than any other aspect of his thought, Burke's French ideas need to be related to the political circumstances of the time if they are to be understood. For all its generalizations and its defence of the *ancien régime* in France, the *Reflections on the Revolution in France* (1790) were indisputably directed towards a *British* rather than a French or European audience and to a particular domestic situation. Burke was worried about the growth of radicalism in his own party and in writing the *Reflections* he was attempting to alert the party leaders, and, indirectly, the Prince of Wales, to the dangers to which radical opinions, however innocent and however sincerely held, could run. Indeed, Burke was mainly concerned with the French Revolution as a practical example and a timely illustration of the dangers of radicalism to Englishmen. He was, at first, more concerned with the practical *effects* of revolution than with its causes or its ideological motivations. His earliest, serious reservation about the revolution was his fear that the National Assembly would not be strong enough to function as a government. This was the rock upon which the ship of the *ancien régime* had foundered: 'I very much question, whether they are in a condition to exercise any function of decided authority'.[4] The Assembly would be too weak to assert itself against mob rule. Burke's earliest doubts about the revolution, therefore, sprang from his belief

[3] Edmund Burke to William Weddell, 31 January 1792, *Correspondence*, VII, 58.

[4] Burke to William Weddell, 27 September 1789, ibid., VI, 25.

that democracy in France would not give rise to stability. This caution ripened into a conviction that the organs of the revolutionary state would become subjected by degrees to the pressures of mob rule and military dictatorship. Hence Burke condemned the French Revolution because it had destroyed liberty ('the birthright of our species'[5]), because it had failed to maintain the conditions in which a free man could exist 'in a perfect state of legal security, with regard to his life, to his property, to the uncontrolled disposal of his Person, to the free use of his Industry and his faculties.'[6] Yet he made neither a constructive suggestion nor proposal to assist the French to overcome their fortuitous inability as a nation to establish liberty. The reason for their failure was not hard to find: Burke believed that the revolution *must* fail because it derived its inspiration from a false and abstract philosophy. 'It is with man in the concrete, it is with common human life and human Actions you are to be concerned. . . . Never wholly separate in your Mind the merits of any Political Question from the Men who are concerned in it.'[7]

Up to this point, his intention was to dissuade his fellow-countrymen from imitating the French. Then, in January 1790, Burke stumbled across what he could regard as nothing but definite proof that a plot existed. For none other than Thomas Paine chose to confide in Burke his thorough approval of the revolution and his sincere wish that 'The Revolution in France is certainly a Forerunner to other Revolutions in Europe.' He expressed the wish that future alliances in Europe should be alliances of the peoples of Europe against the courts of Europe.[8] This removed any lingering doubts that Burke might still have entertained about the revolution.

> In all appearance, the new system is a most bungling, and unworkmanlike performance, I confess I see no principle of coherence, co-operation, or just subordination of parts in this whole project, nor any the least aptitude to the condition and wants of the state to which it is applied, nor any thing well imagined for the formation, provision, or direction of a common force. The direct contrary appears to me.[9]

What most concerned Burke, however, was the possibility that there existed in Britain a faction dedicated to emulating the French. A few

[5] Burke to Charles-Jean Francois Depont, November 1789, *Correspondence* VI, 39–50.
[6] Ibid.   [7] Ibid.
[8] Thomas Paine to Burke, 17 January 1790, ibid., 67–75.
[9] Burke to an unidentified recipient, January 1790, ibid., 78–81.

weeks later, on 9 February, Burke announced to a surprised House of Commons – and an even more astonished opposition party – his hostility to the French faction in England who wished to level the state. He concluded by warning the Whig party that if it professed support for democratic principles then he would break with it. Edmund Burke's counter-revolution had begun.[10]

Towards the end of the same year he published his *Reflections*. His purpose in giving the tract to the world was to confirm his fellow-countrymen in their belief in the aristocratic, hereditary nature of the British constitution and to demonstrate its incompatibility with the revolutionary principles of France. In August 1791 he issued his *Appeal from the New to the Old Whigs* in which he exposed the principles of the radical wing in the opposition party, demonstrating their inconsistency with those of the old 'Revolution' Whigs. Burke warned one of his readers against taking the 'Appeal' too philosophically, however: 'But surely you forget, that I was throwing out reflexions upon a political event, and not reading a lecture upon theories and principles of Government.'[11] The outbreak of war between France, on the one hand, and Austria and Prussia, on the other, in the spring of 1792 confirmed the prediction which he had already made: that the revolution could only be saved by a foreign war. Yet the war introduced a novel and dangerous factor into the situation. It raised the political temperature and quickened the speed of developments inside France. The imprisonment of the French king in August 1792 touched a chord of hysteria in Burke. By then, he had noted ominously, the French had begun to regard the war as a messianic crusade to spread revolution throughout Europe and to destroy its christian, feudal foundations. Burke viewed the war as an attack upon the ideal of a mixed, aristocratic government. Without the aristocratic principle, Burke believed, 'every Dominion must become a mere despotism of the Prince, or the brutal Tyranny of a ferocious and atheistic populace'.[12] He was horrified at the imprisonment of Louis XVI in August 1792.

This last Revolution, whatever name it may assume, at present bears no one Character of a National Act. It is the Act only of some desperate Persons, Inhabitants of one City only, instigating and hiring at an enormous Expence, the lowest of the people, to destroy the Monarch and Monarchy, with whatever else is respectable in Society. Not one Officer of the National Guards of Paris, which

[10] 9 February 1790, *The Parliamentary History*, XXVIII, 337–73.
[11] Burke to W. C. Smith, 22 July 1791, *Correspondence*, VI, 303–4.
[12] Burke to Richard Burke Junior, 29 July 1792, ibid., VII, 160.

Officers are composed of nothing higher than good Tradesmen, has
appeared in this business. It is not yet adopted throughout France
by any one Class of People. No regular Government of any Country
has yet an Object with which they can decently treat in France, or
to which they can rationally make any official Declaration whatsoever.[13]

Burke openly proclaimed the doctrine that Britain ought to intervene
militarily in France. If she did so, she would be merely following
precedents which had saved the constitution in the past.

But an abstract principle of public law, forbidding such interference,
is not supported by the reason of that law, nor by the Authorities
on the Subject nor by the practice of this Kingdom, nor by that of
any civilized Nation in the World. This Nation owes its Laws and
Liberties, his Majesty owes the Throne on which he sits, to the
contrary principle. The several Treaties of Guarantee to the protestant
Succession, more than once reclaimed, affirm the principle of
interference which in a manner forms the basis of the public Law of
Europe.[14]

Britain's failure to intervene would only fill the Jacobins with fresh hope
and renewed enthusiasm.

Burke rested his case and waited for events to justify his warnings.
The September Massacres, the trial and execution of the French king
and French threats against England led gruadually but inevitably to
the outbreak of war between the two countries early in 1793. Burke
was keen to impress upon the government of William Pitt that the
war ought neither to be a war for trade nor merely a war of national
independence but a crusade against the principle of Jacobinism itself.
The government would pursue a short-sighted policy of national
aggrandizement at its peril. The world must be made safe for the
ancien régime. It would not be safe until Jacobinism had been uprooted
in France itself. Thus in 1795, when war weariness led the British
to negotiate with the French, Burke was nearly beside himself at the
prospect of negotiating peace with a regicide republic. Peace with
France could not be permanent because it was the intention of the
Jacobins to destroy Britain. Peace was in the interests of the Jacobins
only in so far as it would give them time to regroup and rest before
renewing their assault upon property and hierarchy throughout
Europe. Until his death in 1797, Burke never ceased to advocate

[13] Burke to Lord Grenville, 18 August 1792, *Correspondence*, VII, 174.
[14] Ibid., 176.

bloody war upon the armies of Jacobinism. His counter-revolution had in effect become a crusade.

The motivation for and the context of Burke's French thought were overtly propagandist. Burke's French revolutionary thought, it should be remembered, was intended to be a refutation of the radical theories of radicals, such as the unfortunate Dr Richard Price, of whom Burke made such an example in *The Reflections*. Burke reacted instinctively against what he took to be their superficial commitment to the idea of the inexorable progress of society and the inevitable perfectibility of man. The historical method which he adopted in many of his writings was curiously circular. It is difficult to disentangle his historical method from his political theory. Burke found the vindication of his appeals to history in history itself and the historical conclusions which he reached affected his method. For he derived from his study of history the conclusion that rational speculation about the destiny of states was a fruitless and unprofitable undertaking; schemes by abstract thinkers to plan a utopian society must come to naught because they rest on the assumption that the life of states can be ordered, predicted and arranged, that the beneficial effect of a reform, or group of reforms, can be guaranteed. As he had been saying for years, not only the institutions and the customs but also the 'spirit' of a people are the products of the ages. Burke thus tied the present closely to the past and drew a discreet veil over the future. His philosophy, because of its historical orientation, was profoundly conservative. Burke's reforming impulses were directed towards restoring the legacy of the past and freeing it of corruption. His stress upon history, tradition and prescription inclined him to fear the consequences of abstract philosophy: 'The triumph of philosophy is the universal conflagration of Europe',[15] thundered Burke.

The cardinal error of the Jacobins was to ignore history and to apply the principles of science to the unquantifiable matter of social life. They stressed the physical and material side of man's nature to the exclusion of those intangible aspects of the personality which render men human. Furthermore, Burke professed to distrust 'reason' because it was nothing more than the speculations of particular men and he saw no reason to endow their ponderings with an infallible status. Burke was familiar with the view that the reason affected only a small part of man's nature, that instinct and emotion impinged upon the rest and that the kingdom of reason touched only a small part of human action. 'Politics ought to be adjusted, not to human reasonings, but to human

[15] *Works*, VII, 324 (Preface to William Burke's Translation of Brissot's Address to his Constituents).

nature: of which the reason is but a part, and by no means the greatest part', he had stated as early as 1769.[16] This meant that apparently 'irrational' aspects of men's behaviour had their importance. For example, customs and traditions, for Burke, were not simply medieval relics to be retained for the sake of nostalgia or antiquarianism. They acquired their own raison d'etre through their existence time out of mind. The cumulative wisdom of successive generations had recognized their value and they had, consequently, survived.[17]

We must be extremely careful, however, of regarding Burke as an 'anti-rationalist' philosopher. Although he would, no doubt, have been glad to be regarded in this manner by posterity we should notice that his anti-rationalism does not stretch very far. Certain aspects of the political philosophy which Burke expounded in the 1790s arose from a 'rationalist' style of argument. To some extent, this tactic was forced upon him because he had to meet and refute the contract theories of radical writers, the starting point of their (not his) philosophy. Burke adopted the view that in the matter of the contract man has no choice, that the nature of the contract arises from the nature of man himself and thus it lasts for ever. Burke's contract theory freezes social relationships in their 'original' state.

> Once social relations had been settled upon some compact, tacit or expressed, there is no power existing of force to alter it, without the breach of the covenant, or the consent of all the parties. Such is the nature of a contract. And the votes of a majority of the people, whatever their infamous flatterers may teach in order to corrupt their minds, cannot alter the moral any more than they can alter the physical essence of things. The people are not to be taught to think lightly of their engagements to their governours; else they teach governours to think lightly of their engagements towards them. In that kind of game in the end the people are sure to be losers.[18]

For Burke these propositions were unchangeable; men have power to alter neither their duties nor the morality which dictates them. The obligations of the contract are thus timeless.

> Society is indeed a contract. Subordinate contracts for objects of mere occasional interest may be dissolved at pleasure – but the state ought not to be considered as nothing better than a partnership

[16] R. R. Fennessy, *Burke, Paine and the Rights of Man* (The Hague, 1963), 62.
[17] Ibid., 62–75 *passim.*, for a detailed critique of Burke's idea of rights.
[18] *Works*, VI, 201–2 (*Appeal*).

agreement in a trade of pepper and coffee, calico or tobacco, or some other such low concern, to be taken up for a little temporary interest, and to be dissolved by the fancy of the parties. It is to be looked on with other reverence; because it is not a partnership in things subservient only to the gross animal existence of a temporary and perishable nature. It is a partnership in all science; a partnership in all art; a partnership in every virtue, and in all perfection. As the ends of such a partnership cannot be obtained in many generations, it becomes a partnership not only between those who are living, but between those who are living, those who are dead, and those who are to be born. Each contract of each particular state is but a clause in the great primaeval contract of eternal society, linking the lower with the higher natures, connecting the visible and invisible world, according to a fixed compact sanctioned by the inviolable oath which holds all physical and all moral natures, each in their appointed place. This law is not subject to the will of those, who by an obligation above them, and infinitely superior, are bound to submit their will to that law.[19]

Burke's contract, then, is quite different to the logical construct of other writers. It is permanent, binding and unchangeable. It also has a moral sanction, since duties, arising from the contract 'arise from the relation of man to man, and the relation of man to God, which relations are not matters of choice'.[20]

The 'state of nature', for Burke, was therefore a state of inhuman anarchy to which man *must* not choose to return. He asserted that human institutions, far from imposing artificial restraints upon man, as many enlightenment writers declared, liberated him from the anarchy of the state of nature and enabled him in an orderly freedom to develop his faculties. Burke thus freed himself from what had been one of the traditional concerns of political philosophy: speculation concerning the origins of society derived from abstract notions of the state of nature. Burke was content to draw certain general principles from his discussion of the state of nature. His idea of contract and his idea of the state of nature led him to the conclusion that government and its obligations were not determined by its origins but by the nature of man and his moral duties. Indeed, he considered discussion of the origins of government futile. In a well known passage, Burke declared: 'The foundations, on which obedience to governments is

[19] *Works*, V, 183–4 (*Reflections on the Revolution in France, 1790*).
[20] Ibid., VI, 204–5 (*Appeal*).

founded, are not to be constantly discussed. That we are here, supposes the discussion already made and the dispute settled.'[21] Thus he would give a presumption in favour of established institutions to govern the individual 'until some intolerable grievance shall make us know that it does not answer its end, and will submit neither to reformation nor restraint'.[22]

These characteristic conceptions of contract and the state of nature were almost certainly intended by Burke to be a rebuttal of the fashionable ideas of the enlightenment. In departing, as it were, from the Age of Reason, Burke opened up the field of political science and began to penetrate its depths. His state of nature was not the pre-contractual situation of anarchic man but the post-contractual state of civil society. Burke shifted philosophy away from the logical and legal manner of thinking which had traditionally characterized its discussions. This he did because he regarded such questions as problems not of logic or of law but of practice, that is, of politics. Burke, therefore, rejected entirely the fashionable concept of nature. In the sense that Burke's 'nature' was somewhat more realistic and historical than many contemporary versions of nature then he may be regarded as less speculative than his radical opponents. At least, he succeeded in conforming nature to man and exploded the enlightenment's attempt to force a mythical man to conform to a non-existent nature. It is hardly surprising that his version of 'natural rights' did not even mention the typical 'pre-social' rights of rebellion and resistance to authority. On the contrary, men were bound to obey legitimate, i.e. prescriptive, authority. Burke's natural rights amounted to the normal benefits of social living, those of order, security, justice and peaceful possession of property and labour.[23] The purpose of the state was to preserve those rights. These were social rights. They did not include political power. Rights to political power were not 'natural'. Such rights were acquired not through the contract but through experience (i.e. history) and according to circumstances. Rights do not exist apart from society. They evolved through time with customary obligation, traditional morality and established institutions. Burke had no time for those theorists who were for ever stressing the rights of the individual at the expense of the power of the state. Natural rights could only exist in society; they are not anterior to it. For Edmund Burke, then, rights

---

[21] Speech on the Unitarians' Petition, 11 May 1792, *Works*, X, 51–2.
[22] Ibid., 52–3.
[23] This idea of natural rights owes much to Montesquieu. See F. T. M. Fletcher, *Montesquieu and English Politics, 1750–1800* (1939), 109–13.

were not legal or personal matters, but the residue of experience and time, enshrined in the institutional apparatus of society.

The totality of a society existed in time through prescription and inheritance. But since rights depended upon society, Burke believed that society had to be preserved if natural rights were to survive. Because European society was traditionally elitist, Burke, in defending that society, was, inevitably, defending the prescriptive ownership of property and the prescriptive title to political authority of a few hundred aristocratic families. For example, one of the most important of Burke's natural rights was the right to own property. In the context of Europe at the end of the eighteenth century, the right to property, and the right to transmit property by inheritance and by prescription, meant that those who already enjoyed the ownership of property would be the chief beneficiaries of Burke's crusade. The events of the 1790s, of course, reinforced Burke's elitism. The lynch-pin of this elitism was his belief that immemorial possession legitimized both the ownership of property and titles to political authority, no matter how that property or that authority had originally been acquired.[24] Prescription served for Burke the purpose which natural rights served for the radicals. It legitimized authority. This is the crucially important function of his conception of prescription in his philosophy:

> It is not calling the landed estates, possessed by old *prescriptive rights*, the 'accumulations of ignorance and superstition', that can support me in shaking that grand title, which supersedes all other titles, and which all my studies of general jurisprudence have taught me to consider as one principal cause of the formation of states; I mean the ascertaining and securing *prescription*. But these are donations made in the 'ages of ignorance and superstition'. Be it so. It proves that these donations were made long ago; and this is *prescription*; and this gives right and title. It is possible that many estates about you were originally obtained by arms, that is, by violence, a thing almost as bad as superstition, and not much short of ignorance but it is *old violence*; and that which might be wrong in the beginning, is consecrated by time, and becomes lawful. This may be superstition in me, and ignorance; but I had rather remain in ignorance and superstition than be enlightened and purified out of the first principles of law and natural justice. I never will suffer you, if I can help it, to be deprived of the well-earned fruits of your industry, because others may want your fortune more than you do,

[24] P. Lucas, 'Edmund Burke's Doctrine of Prescription or an Appeal from the New to the Old Lawyers', *Historical Journal*, XI (1968), 35–9.

and may have laboured, and do now labour, in vain, to acquire even a subsistence. Nor on the contrary, if success had less smiled on your endeavours, and you had come home insolvent, would I take from any 'pampered and luxurious lord' in your neighbourhood one acre of his land, or one spoon from his sideboard, to compensate your losses, though incurred (as they would have been incurred) in the course of a well-spent, virtuous and industrious life. God is the distributor of his own blessings. I will not impiously attempt to usurp his throne, but will keep according to the subordinate place and trust in which he has stationed me, to secure the order of property which I find established in my country.[25]

Burke's view of the historical process, his conception of nature and his scepticism of 'reason' determine his idea of the state. His prescriptive conception of the state did not permit him to express anything like an 'idea of progress', or even an evolutionary or linear view of history. His idea of the state is 'organic' in the sense that he appealed to experience and recognized that states and institutions can and must change but it remains true that this change was not to be directed to a future ideal. Political change, for Burke then, operated correctly when it restored the state to its original nature. In short, Burke had no vision of a different political or social order. Not only that. His very instincts tended towards restoration and conservation: his philosophy was so solidly based upon prescription that his idea of the state acquired a tremendous inertia.

His idea of the state was also something of a curiosity in European thought. It is different to the customary 'state' inhabited by eighteenth-century philosophers. It is even different to the 'state' inhabited by Burke himself earlier in his life. In his later writings he stressed the powers of the state; in his earlier writings he had emphasized the rights of the individual against those of the state. Burke's 'state' of the 1790s was a very different thing from the 'state' of Locke, Montesquieu and most of the radicals (who contented themselves with a state in which the central government exercised very little authority; little more, in fact, than the regulation of diplomatic affairs and the currency). In the 1790s he strongly reaffirmed his belief that the state was a trust based upon heredity, property and law. As the role of the state in his political thought loomed larger, his conception grew of its delicacy and complexity. 'Government is a contrivance of human wisdom to provide for human wants', he wrote.[26] The organization of a state and

[25] Burke to Captain Thomas Mercer, 26 February 1790, *Correspondence*, VI, 95.　　　　　　　　　　　　　　[26] *Works*, V, 122 (*Reflections*).

its government was 'a matter of the most delicate and complicated skill'.[27] It followed, then, that one man, or one group of men, ought not lightly to pull down what the centuries had fashioned, in accordance with the wants and needs of a people.

Burke emphatically did not believe that government ought to be conducted according to the wishes of the majority. When the people demanded change such change must be pursued in accordance with the political and social context of the country concerned, its history, traditions and customs. Institutions must be reformed in accordance with their original principles, spirit and purposes. Reform should preserve rather than destroy. There was another reason why Burke closed his ears to the voice of the majority. Political wisdom was not a matter of collecting voices and counting heads. In 1791 he wrote: 'Political problems do not primarily concern truth or falsehood. They relate to good or evil.'[28] All of this did not mean that Burke was opposed to reform. For much of his career, indeed, he was far in advance of public opinion. What he would not allow was radical change based upon the will of the multitude whose effects could not be foreseen and which might introduce alien principles and damaging innovations in ancient polities. The art of the reformer was a fine and delicate art which required a leader of profound wisdom to decide what needed reform, when and how it should be accomplished, what priorities should be observed and how to apply the principles of equity and justice. Reform should proceed less from will than from necessity, less from theory than from experience. Burke, clearly, left little room for reform in his later political theory, although he by no means ruled it out altogether. At a time when established institutions throughout Europe were under assault he had, no doubt, little enthusiasm for encouraging further attacks upon them.

Consequently, Burke left little room in his doctrines for rebellion. He conceded that if the existence of society itself were threatened by its leaders and if means of effecting peaceful political change had been exhausted, then, and only then, rebellion was permissible. This was scarcely more than acknowledging that a society ought to be allowed to survive. In practice, and in the case of France, Burke appeared to rule out rebellion if a constitution existed which could be reformed and, ultimately, become the vehicle for political change. In his Letter to a Member of the National Assembly (January 1791) Burke stated that 'the attempt to oppress, degrade, impoverish, confiscate, and extinguish the original gentlemen, and landed property of a whole

[27] *Works*, VI, 210 (*Appeal*).
[28] Ibid., V, 125 (*Reflections*).

nation cannot be justified under any form it may assume'.[29] But presumably the abuses of the *ancien régime* could! It is difficult to escape the conclusion that, in his fear of revolution, Burke overlooked just those aspects of the society of the *ancien régime* which had made revolution or the danger of revolution possible. In particular, he was quite unwilling to concede the legitimacy of changes in the distribution of wealth and changes in the socio-economic structure of Europe.

Burke's French thought was an even more vigorous defence of elitism than his earlier thought had been. Yet he did all that he could to conceal the fact. He denied that he wished to 'confine power, authority, and distinction to blood and names, and titles. . . . There is no qualification for government but virtue and wisdom, actual or presumptive.'[30] Nevertheless, he insisted that the road to power ought not to be paved too smoothly. Although he made a few gestures in the direction of merit, Burke was quite content to preserve the system of privilege in Europe and to tolerate its class distinctions and its other inequalities. Indeed, he thought it a characteristic feature of property to be unevenly distributed. 'Its defensive power is weakened as it is diffused'[31] for the greater the diffusion of property the greater will be the envy it creates among men jealous of their neighbour's portion. Burke not only tolerated this inequality but thought its perpetuation through inheritance 'one of the most valuable and interesting circumstances belonging to it'.[32] We should be clear why Burke defended the rule of a small, propertied class. It was not because the rule of that class acted as a barrier against totalitarianism – the eighteenth-century state was too weak to establish a centralized, totalitarian structure – but because it acted as a barrier against mob rule and anarchy. He contemplated France with horror, where the multitude had succeeded in destroying the rule of a propertied minority, but the French people had not received one square metre of the estates of the aristocracy, church and monarchy.[33] The old society had been succeeded not by democracy or equality but by slavery, famine and war.

Burke's defence of a 'natural aristocracy', therefore, is integral to his conception of social stability, 'To be honoured and even privileged by the laws, opinions, and inveterate usages of our country, growing out of the prejudice of ages, has nothing to provoke horror and indignation in any man.'[34] Burke saw order and hierarchy, privilege and inequality, in all social systems and thus in all governments. The mass

[29] *Works*, VI, 4–5 (Letter to a Member of the National Assembly, 1791).
[30] Ibid., V, 106 (*Reflections*).   [31] Ibid., 108.   [32] Ibid., 108.
[33] Speech at the Opening of the Session, 13 December 1792, *Speeches*, IV, 76.
[34] *Works*, V, 254 (*Reflections*).

of the people should rest content in their position of natural sub-ordination. 'They must respect that property of which they cannot partake.'[35] Burke's famous defence of the 'natural aristocracy' is perhaps one of the most open admissions of elitism in the whole of British philosophy.

> A true natural aristocracy is not a separate interest in the state, or separable from it. It is an essential integrant part of any large body rightly constituted. It is formed out of a class of legitimate presump-tions, which, taken as generalities, must be admitted for actual truths. To be bred in a place of estimation; to see nothing low and sordid from one's infancy; to be taught to respect one's self; to be habituated to the censorial inspection of the publick eye, to look early to publick opinion; to stand upon such elevated ground as to be enabled to take a large view of the wide-spread and infinitely diversified combinations of men and affairs in a large society; to have leisure to read, to reflect, to converse; to be enabled to draw the court and attention of the wise and learned wherever they are to be found; – to be habituated in armies to command and to obey; to be taught to despise danger in the pursuit of honour and duty, to be formed to the greatest degree of vigilance, foresight, and circumspection, in a state of things in which no fault is committed with impunity, and the slightest mistakes draw on the most ruinous consequences – to be led to a guarded and regulated conduct, from a sense that you are considered as an instructor of your fellow-citizens in their highest concerns, and that you act as a reconciler between God and man – to be employed as an administrator of law and justice, and to be thereby amongst the first benefactors to mankind – to be a professor of high science, or of liberal and in-genuous art – to be amongst rich traders, who from their success are presumed to have sharp and vigorous understandings, and to possess the virtues of diligence, order, constancy, and regularity, and to have cultivated an habitual regard to commutative justice – these are the circumstances of men, that form what I should call a *natural* aristocracy, without which there is no nation.[36]

The French Revolution was nothing less than an attack upon the natural aristocracy in France. The Jacobin movement throughout Europe had for its objective the destruction of the natural aristocracy throughout Europe. The leaders of revolution were 'men of no rank, of no consideration, of wild, savage minds, full of levity, arrogance &

[35] *Works*, V, 432 (*Reflections*).   [36] Ibid., VI, 217–18 (*Appeal*).

presumption, without morals, without probity, without prudence'.[37]
These revolutionaries had no stake in any country. They were motivated
by envy and by greed. Burke tried to explain how such men had
managed to acquire the influence and power which they had:

In the long series of ages which have furnished the matter of history,
never was so beautiful and so august a spectacle presented to the
moral eye, as Europe afforded the day before the Revolution in
France. I knew indeed that this prosperity contained in itself the
seeds of its own danger. In one part of the society it caused laxity
and debility; in the other it produced bold spirits and dark designs.
A False philosophy passed from academies into courts, and the great
themselves were infected with the theories which conducted to their
ruin. Knowledge, which in the two last centuries either did not
exist at all, or existed solidly on right principles and in chosen hands,
was now diffused, weakened, and perverted. General wealth loosened
morals, relaxed vigilance, and encreased presumption. Men of
talent began to compare, in the partition of the common stock of
publick prosperity, the proportions of the dividends with the merits
of the claimants. As usual, they found their portion not equal to
their estimate (or perhaps to the publick estimate) of their own
worth. When it was once discovered by the Revolution in France,
that a struggle between establishment and rapacity could be maintained, though but for one year, and in one place, I was sure that a
practicable breach was made in the whole order of things and in
every country. Religion, that held the materials of the fabric together,
was first systematically loosened. All other opinions, under the name
of prejudices, must fall along with it, and property, left undefended
by principles, became a repository of spoils to tempt cupidity, and
not a magazine to furnish arms for defence. I knew, that, attacked
on all sides by the infernal energies of talents set in action by vice
and disorder, authority could not stand upon authority alone. It
wanted some other support than the poise of its own gravity.
Situations formerly supported persons. It now became necessary
that personal qualities should support situations. Formerly, where
authority was found, wisdom and virtue were presumed. But now
the veil was torn, and, to keep off sacrilegious intrusion, it was
necessary that in the sanctuary of government something should be
disclosed not only venerable, but dreadful. Government was at
once to shew itself full of virtue and full of force. It was to invite

[37] *Works*, VII, 165 (Remarks on the Policy of the Allies, 1793).

partisans, by making it appear to the world that a generous cause was to be asserted, one fit for a generous people to engage in.[38]

We should not underestimate the extent to which Edmund Burke carefully distinguished the French Revolution from other and earlier revolutions: 'It is a revolt of *innovation,* and thereby the very elements of Society have been confounded and dissipated.'[39] The revolution was an attack upon the basic foundations of European civilization. ('Its spirit lies deep in the corruption of our common nature'.)[40] Burke grimly perceived that Europe stood on the brink of another Dark Age. The false philosophy of the revolution was spreading throughout Europe, sapping its will to resist, undermining the pillars of the old society, releasing the lowest instincts in men. The essence of this disease of Jacobinism was the release of man's basest energies and, unrestrained by religion or by civilization, their harnessing to the Jacobin cause. For Burke, one of the fundamental strengths of Jacobinism was its dangerous appeal to the envy of man.

It is the contempt of Property, and the setting up against its Principle, certain pretended advantages of the State, (which by the way exists only for its conservation) that has led to all the other Evils which have ruined France, and brought all Europe into the most imminent danger. The beginning of the whole mischief was a false Idea, that there is a difference in property according to the description of the persons who hold it under the laws, and the despoiling a Minister of Religion is not the same Robbery with the Pillage of other Men. They, who thro' weakness gave way to the ill designs of bad men in that confiscation, were not long before they practically found their Error. The spoil of the Royal Domaine soon followed the seizure of the Estates of the Church. The appenages of the Kings brothers immediately came on the heels of the usurpation of the Royal Domaine; The Property of the Nobility survived but a short time the appenages of the Princes of the Blood Royal.[41]

Burke took revolutionary France as the prototype Jacobin state founded upon the ending of inequality and the destruction of the natural aristocracy. He did not find its early history attractive, 'Laws overturned; tribunals subverted; industry without vigour; commerce

---

[38] *Works*, VII, 362–4 (Letter to William Elliot, 1795).
[39] Burke to le Chevalier de Rivarol, 1 June 1791, *Correspondence*, VI, 268.
[40] *Works*, VIII, 389 (Second Letter on a Regicide Peace, 1796).
[41] Burke to Comte Mercy-Argentau, *circa* 6 August 1793, *Correspondence*, VI, 389.

expiring; the revenue unpaid, yet the people impoverished; a church pillaged, and a state not relieved; civil and military anarchy make the constitution of the kingdom.'[42] In spite of the considerable amount of rhetorical exaggeration in passages such as this, of one thing Burke was in no doubt: through their insistence upon the philosophy of the rights of man, the Jacobins wished to restructure Europe upon a new basis, rank and heredity counting for nothing, property separated from power, rank from dignity. Jacobinism introduced *'other interests into all countries than those which arose from their locality and natural circumstances'*[43] Power was taken by the Jacobins out of the hands of the natural aristocracy and placed in the hands of 'tradesmen, bankers, and voluntary clubs of bold, presuming young persons; advocates, attornies, notaries, managers of newspapers, and those cabals of literary young men called academics'.[44] This reversal of the natural order of things was typical of Jacobinism. For Jacobinism itself was the reverse of all the customs and norms of civilized life. In particular, Burke thought it a novelty, in all the governments that the world had ever known, for prescription to be regarded as a bar and not as a claim to possession.[45]

In short, then, Jacobinism was a European movement that threatened to reverse the natural order of things and to plunge Europe once more into a Dark Age of anarchy and turbulence. From the historical point of view Burke saw the revolutionary era as the disintegration of Christian Europe. The common, feudal and Christian foundations of European society were the very objects of Jacobinism. Authority and institutions of all kinds were the objects of its attack. Jacobinism weakened authority by constantly assaulting it. The resulting instability was essential to the success of its attack. For Jacobinism itself was the state of social and political instability in which no tie was secure, no authority safe and no order strong enough to prevail.[46] In a Jacobin state like France, Burke saw instability erected into a system. In such a state nothing was constant, nothing was certain. Man's political principles no longer derived from his interests. Political power no longer arose from the ownership of permanent (landed) property. Immediate self-interest was the only public standard for the men who ran the revolution:

'the agitators in corporations . . . societies in the towns formed of directors of assignats, and trustees for the sale of church lands,

[42] *Works*, V, 87–8 (*Reflections*).   [43] Ibid., 80.
[44] Ibid., VII, 14, 19 (*Thoughts on French Affairs, 1791*).
[45] Ibid., IX, 64–5 (Fourth Letter on a Regicide Peace, 1797).
[46] Ibid., 58–9.

attornies, agents, money-jobbers, speculators, and adventurers, composing an ignoble oligarchy founded on the destruction of the crown, the nobility and the People'.[47]

The central issue in the struggle, for Burke, was that of religion· The laws and institutions of society stood upon a Christian foundation· The Jacobins' first objective was to weaken and destroy the church; that done, the other institutions of society would collapse in turn.[48] He viewed the war which broke out in Europe in 1792 as nothing less than a war for the survival of religion. Jacobinism was not merely another ideology thrown up by another sect. The French Jacobins had declared 'a war against all sects and all religions'.[49] They were a new species of man, a new breed of political animal, incompatible with the Christian brotherhood of Europe. Their principles represented an attempt to regenerate the moral constitution of man and to condition him in the ideals of the rights of man.[50]

Burke contended, therefore, that the war against the Jacobins must be a crusade on the part of Christian Europe to preserve the independence of nations and the property, liberty and religion of individuals from universal havoc and atheism.[51]

We are in a war of a *peculiar* nature. It is not with an ordinary community, which is hostile or friendly as passion or as interest may veer about, not with a state which makes war through wantonness, and abandons it through lassitude. We are at war with a system, which, by its essence is inimical to all other governments, and which makes peace or war, as peace and war may best contribute to their subversion. It is with an *armed doctrine* that we are at war. It has, by its essence, a faction of opinion, and of interest, and of enthusiasm, in every country. To us it is a Colossus which bestrides our channel. It has one foot on a foreign shore, the other upon the British soil. Thus advantaged, if it can at all exist, it must finally prevail. Nothing can so completely ruin any of the old governments, ours in particular, as the acknowledgement, directly, or by implication, of any kind of superiority in this new power. This acknowledgement we make, if, in a bad or doubtful situation of our affairs, we solicit peace, or if we yield to the modes of new humiliation, in which alone she is content to give us a hearing. By that means the terms cannot be of our choosing, no, not in any part.[52]

[47] *Works*, V, 349 (*Reflections*).   [48] Ibid., 176–82.
[49] Ibid., VII, 175 (Remarks on the Policy of the Allies).
[50] Ibid., VI, 34 (Letter to a Member of the National Assembly).
[51] Ibid., VIII, 236–41 (Second Letter on a Regicide Peace).
[52] Ibid., 98 (First Letter on a Regicide Peace, 1796).

It was, in any case, impossible to make peace with revolutionary France. She considered herself to be outside the public law of Europe, at liberty to pursue her own interests by disrupting the balance of power in Germany and Italy as well as in Europe as a whole.[53] She was determined to destroy the old states of Europe and erect in their place a series of client-states which, through their instability and weakness, would be dependent upon the revolutionary mother-country. 'It is not the Cause of Nation against Nation but . . . the cause of mankind against those who have projected the subversion of that order of things under which our part of the world has so long flourished.'[54] There could, therefore, be no peace with an armed ideology. Every reverse and every setback which the allies suffered in the war confirmed Burke in his belief that to negotiate peace with the regicide republic would be dangerous. Britain should pursue the war with as much vigour as possible. He was never satisfied that a defensive war would be adequate to contain and to destroy Jacobinism.

> . . . we ought, first of all, to be sure, that it is a species of danger, against which any defensive measures, that can be adopted, will be sufficient. Next we ought to know, that the spirit of our laws or that our own dispositions, which are stronger than laws, are susceptible of all those defensive measures, which the occasion may require. A third consideration is, whether these measures will not bring more odium than strength to government; and the last; whether the authority that makes them, in a general corruption of manners and principles, can ensure their execution.[55]

Burke constantly advocated a military strike at Paris and the destruction of Jacobinism once and for all but, as the above quotation suggests, he was, if anything, most of all concerned to safeguard England from revolution. He saw with alarm the proliferation of radical societies and the growing support for French principles even within his own party.[56] He found great cause for concern in 'the irresolution and timidity of the middle sort of men in the country who did nothing to restrain demagogues from their attempts to whip up a popular frenzy and thus things proceed, by a sort of activity of inertness'. Burke gloomily anticipated that the constant proselytizing of the Jacobins at home, together with military reverses abroad, would unsettle the people and

[53] *Works*, VIII, 337–9 (Third Letter on a Regicide Peace, 1797).
[54] Burke to Comte Mercy-Argentau, *circa* 6 August 1793, *Correspondence*, VI, 387.
[55] *Works*, IX, 11 (Fourth Letter on a Regicide Peace).
[56] Ibid., VI, 80–5 (*Appeal*).

drain their confidence in the leaders of the country. Popular clamouring for peace would erode the authority of the government, the strength of the legal system and magistracy, and, in turn, allow and encourage the popular spirit to rise even higher. Burke knew that the outcome of the European religious wars against the Jacobins hung upon the survival of England, which in turn depended upon the successful outcome of an aggressive military policy abroad and a united front of the propertied classes at home. Only then could Britain and Europe save themselves from the enemy and launch the counter-revolution against the Jacobins.[57]

Burke saw clearly what the purposes of the counter-revolution should be. He would have nothing to do with the Jacobins. He not only refused to negotiate with them, he would not even allow them to exist. He would not rest until the propertied classes of the *ancien régime* in France had been restored. To that end, the monarchy must be re-established and its property entirely restored, and with it 'the whole fabrick of its ancient laws and usages, political, civil, and religious'. Clearly, the purpose of Burke's counter-revolution was to restore the hereditary, natural aristocracy of the *ancien régime*. In other words, Burke would not allow the Jacobins' seizure of property to start another prescriptive cycle. He wrote on 6 August 1793:

> The people at large in all countries ought to be made sensible that the Symbols of publick Robbery never can have the Sanction and the currency that belong exclusively to the Symbols of publick faith. If any Government should be settled in France upon any other Idea than that of the faithful restitution of all property of all descriptions and that of the rigorous and exemplary punishment of the principal authours and contrivers of its Ruin, I am convinc'd to a certainty, that property, and along with property, Government must fall, (in the same manner in which they have both fallen in France) in every other state in Europe.[58]

'The truth is, that France is out of itself – The moral France is separated from the geographical.'[59] Burke meant that, according to his own principles, the French 'people' no longer existed. For the French to be reconstituted as a people required the re-establishment of her

---

[57] The passionate conviction which lay behind Burke's fears accounts for the many letters and works which he wrote in the period from 1791 to 1797. These he used to attempt to influence his friends but, more importantly, the ministers. In these attempts he was almost invariable unsuccessful.

[58] Burke to Comte Mercy-Argentau, *circa* 6 August 1793, loc. cit.

[59] *Works*, VII, 139 (Remarks on the Policy of the Allies).

natural aristocracy, her traditional leaders, the emigré aristocracy. Only Frenchmen could recivilize Frenchmen, revive old loyalties and re-establish old institutions. For Burke, then, counter-revolution was *not* a means of obtaining military victory over the French. Such a military victory was only a preliminary, a necessary preliminary, to the re-establishment of French society. The contest, in Burke's mind, was not between Britain and France. It was between legitimate and illegitimate government.

These were the general principles of Burke's counter-revolutionary theory: how to implement counter-revolution was, to a large extent, a matter of circumstance and of necessity. Burke judged that counter-revolution could not generate itself spontaneously from within France. Britain must take 'the directing part' in the anti-French alliance and be 'the soul of the whole confederacy'.[60] Yet the allies must act in concert with the emigrés; they should not impose a settlement upon them. What Burke suggested was that the French nobles of the blood should appoint a regent who should be approved by the *parlements*, then recognized by the allies. This would help to re-establish things 'according to nature and to its fundamental laws'.[61] Thereafter France would have to be liberated and organizations of loyalists – to rival those of the Jacobins – set up. In this context, the church could play a vital role in rallying the people around the standard of the legitimate government of France. Burke was indifferent to the details of the restored regime to be erected in France so long as it was a legitimate government, dedicated to preserving the security of property, for property not numbers, was the basis of government. 'First, therefore, restore property, and afterwards let that property find a government for itself.'[62]

In his counter-revolutionary writings Burke was fond of contrasting the British constitution with that of Jacobin France to establish his thesis that the former rather than the latter most nearly accommodated itself to the nature of man.

The states of the Christian world have grown up to their present magnitude in a great length of time, and by a great variety of accidents. . . . Not one of them has been formed upon a regular plan

[60] *Works*, VII, 98–104 for Burke's discussion of the counter-revolution inside France. (Heads for Consideration on the Present State of Affairs, 1792.)
[61] For Burke's survey of Europe and his general discussion of the prospects for counter-revolution, see *Works*, VII, 25–46 (*Thoughts on French Affairs*).
[62] Speech on a bill to enable French subjects to enlist in regiments for continental service, 11 April 1794, *Speeches*, IV, 166.

or with any unity of design. As their constitutions are not systematical, they have not been directed to any peculiar end. . . .

The British state is, without question, that which pursues the greatest variety of ends, and is the least disposed to sacrifice any one of them to another, or to the whole. It aims at taking in the entire circle of human desires, and securing for them their fair enjoyment.[63]

It does not follow that Burke recommended other countries to imitate the British system of government. They had their own traditional constitutions which they ought to utilize to their own advantage. The French constitution of the *ancien régime* was well-suited to the French. The representation of estates was the natural and only just representation of France. 'It grew out of the habitual conditions, relations, and reciprocal claims of men. It grew out of the circumstances of the country, and out of the state of property.'[64] While there was a constitution in existence it was the duty of the rulers of the state to govern in accordance with it. In the case of Britain, for example, the constitution derived from three separate principles. Monarchy, aristocracy and democracy must all be supported 'on grounds that are totally different though practically they may be, and happily with us they are, brought into one harmonious body'. He asserted that if only one of the three members was endangered then he would support it to maintain the harmony of the whole.[65]

Burke believed – quite wrongly – that the nature of the British constitution had been unchangeably settled at the time of the Glorious Revolution. He appeared to believe that the Revolution Settlement precluded the possibility of all future change, assuming that the provisions of the legislation of the period bound future parliaments. Furthermore, Burke believed that it was the function of the eighteenth-century aristocracy to defend that constitution and to preserve its benefits by whatever political means might be appropriate – the activities of party, the passage of economical reform legislation or as in the 1790s, the waging of war on revolutionary France. He found nothing inconsistent in his attacks upon the French Revolution in the last decade of the century and his support of the Americans in the 1770s. This was not an admission that rebellion was permissible.

[63] Burke's historical account of the background to the *ancien régime* can be found in *Works*, VIII, 253–6 (Second Letter on a Regicide Peace).

[64] Burke discusses the relationship of a representative system to the property structure of a state in *Works*, VI, 56–60 (Letter to a Member of the National Assembly).

[65] Ibid.

Burke believed that the Americans stood 'in the same relation to England, as England did to King James II in 1688' and that they had taken up arms to defend their right to tax themselves 'for the purposes of maintaining civil and military establishments'.[66] Burke proclaimed that his theory of the British constitution, outlined in the *Reflections*, was consistent with the Revolution Settlement, and that what he said in the 1790s was directly derived from the ideology of the Rockingham Whigs.

During the party struggles of the early 1790s Burke was particularly anxious to defend himself from the *New Whigs* in his party who believed that not only the Rockinghams' support of the Americans but their defence also of the Glorious Revolution should have led him to support the French Revolution and the cause of radical reform in Britain. Burke, in fact, thoroughly disapproved of the kind of specious logic used by the 'New Whigs' not only to establish the doctrine of the sovereignty of the people but also to demonstrate 'that in the people the same sovereignty constantly and unalienably resides; that the people may lawfully depose kings, not only for misconduct, but without any misconduct at all'.[67] Burke refuted the opinion that the people may set up and maintain any form of government they chose, that magistracy was not 'a proper subject of contract'.[68] How, then, did Burke succeed in explaining away the Glorious Revolution? Burke argued from the Sachaverell impeachment that

. . . a breach of the *original contract*, implied and expressed in the constitution of this country, as a scheme of government fundamentally and inviolably fixed in king, lords and commons. – That the fundamental subversion of this ancient constitution, by one of its parts, having been attempted, and in effect accomplished, justified the Revolution. That it was justified *only* upon the *necessity* of the case; as the *only* means left for the recovery of that *ancient* constitution, formed by the *original contract* of the British state: as well as for the future preservation of the same government.[69]

From another point of view, Burke occasionally argued that the Glorious Revolution was designed to preserve property 'guarded by the sacred rules of prescription'. The Glorious Revolution, then, was a revolution *in accordance with* the principle of prescription. The situation of France was different.

With us it was the case of a legal monarch attempting arbitrary

[66] *Works*, VI, 123 (*Appeal*).   [67] Ibid., 147.
[68] Ibid.   [69] Ibid., 148.

power – in France it is the case of an arbitrary monarch, beginning from whatever cause, to legalise his authority. The one was to be resisted, the other was to be managed and directed; but in neither case was the order of the state to be changed, lest government might be ruined, which ought only to be corrected and legalized.

The Glorious Revolution, for Burke, was a revolution prevented, not effected, a condition restored, not destroyed.

> In the stable fundamental parts of our constitution we made no revolution, no, nor any alteration at all. We did not impair the monarchy. . . . The nation kept the same ranks, the same orders, the same privileges, the same franchises, the same rules for property, the same subordinations, the same order in the law, in the revenue, and in the magistracy; the same lords, the same Commons, the same corporations, the same electors.[70]

As for France, 'It is a *revolt of innovation*, and thereby the very elements of society have been confounded and dissipated.'[71]

Burke was in no doubt that the most important aspect of the Glorious Revolution had been the restoration of the monarchy 'for without monarchy in England, most certainly we never can enjoy either peace or liberty'.[72] He emphasized the hereditary nature of monarchy, rejecting *New Whig* ideas that the people could choose and cashier their kings. This proposition he defended by referring not merely to the hereditary nature of the British monarchy and to the laws of the land but to the functions of monarchy in society:

> *Je mesure mon attachement par l'utilité de leurs fonctions jamais augustes et sacrées. Quelles sont ces fonctions? De garder le peuple contre les entreprises des grands, et les grands contre les invasions des peuples, de tenir tout dans sa place et dans son ordre habituel, de consolider l'assemblée, de tout finir dans un sain Milieu, de tout applanir sous l'égalité de la justice et non celui des chimères folles, insolentes, qu'on prêche et qu'on réalise en France.*
>
> *Conservez l'ordre pour lequel la Monarchie est ordonnée, vous conserverez les Monarques. Permettez la subversion de cet ordre, permettez la magistrature, la prêtrise, la Noblesse, d'être flétries et foulées aux pieds, les monarques et la monarchie périront ensemble.*[73]

[70] *Works*, V, 19–20 (Speech on the Army Estimates, 9 February 1790).
[71] Burke to the Comte de Rivarol, 1 June 1791, *Correspondence*, VI, 268.
[72] *Works*, V, 64 (*Reflections*).
[73] Burke to M. de Sandouville, *post*-13 October 1792, ibid., VII, 263.

But hereditary monarchy could not stand unsupported.

> The support of the permanent orders in their places and the reconciling them all to his government, will be his best security, either for governing quietly in his own person, or for leaving any sure succession to his posterity. Corporations which have a perpetual succession, and hereditary nobles who themselves exist by Succession are the true guardians of Monarchical succession. On such orders and institutions alone an hereditary monarch can stand.[74]

The relationship between monarchy and aristocracy was particularly important. 'In a monarchy the aristocracy must ever be nearer to the crown than to the democracy, because it originated in the crown as the fountain of honour'.[75] The aristocracy, he had learned from the French experience, was the first line of defence for the monarchy. Early in 1792 he wrote:

> The name of the Monarchy, and of the hereditary monarchy too, they preserve in France, and they feed the person whom they call King, with such a Revenue, given to mere luxury and extravagance, totally separated from all provision for the State, as, I believe, no people ever before dreamed of granting for such purposes. But against the Nobility and Gentry they have waged inexpiable War. There are, at this day, no fewer than ten thousand heads of respectable families driven out of France; and those who remain at home, remain in depression, penury, and continual alarm for their Lives.[76]

All of these crimes had been undertaken by and on behalf of 'the people'. Running through all of Burke's revolutionary thought is the assumption that the people have no right to political power. This is a strain of thought which went back to the earliest days of his political career. He never tired of making the point that government, far from being a matter of arithmetic, was a delicate and sophisticated proceeding, requiring the understanding of the total political situation in its many aspects and their prudential management, not blind subservience to public opinion. The politician must listen to the popular voice but he must not be led by it. His duty was to maintain the constitution and the establishments of the state. The principle that political power should be exercised on behalf of the people and in the public interest was not at all the same thing as slavishly following the cries of the mob. The politician had his responsibilities to the people but he also

[74] Burke to Rivarol, 1 June 1791, loc. cit.
[75] Speech on the Quebec Act, 11 May 1791, *Speeches*, IV, 32.
[76] Burke to William Weddell, 31 January 1792, loc. cit.

had his responsibilities to God.[77] Burke did not rule out the possibility that 'There may be situations in which the purely democratic form will become necessary', but there is little doubt that these cases he regarded as exceptional. Of those who, parrot-like, chanted the contemporary catch phrases about popular power, Burke asked:

Have they never heard of a monarchy, directed by laws, controlled and balanced by the great hereditary wealth and hereditary dignity of a nation, and both again controlled by a judicious check from the reason and feeling of the people at large acting by a suitable and permanent organ?[78]

Burke had a clear conception of the deferential attitudes of the people in his ideal polity: 'They must respect that property of which they cannot partake. They must labour to obtain what by labour can be obtained.'[79] For Burke, 'The tyranny of a multitude is a multiplied tyranny', as the French Revolution illustrated perfectly clearly.[80] For in France the people were not their own masters. They were, therefore, easily corruptible and easily controllable, through flattery, through lavish promises and through demagoguery. As he wrote in *The Appeal*: 'The pretended *rights of men* . . . cannot be the rights of the people. For to be a people, and to have these rights, are things incompatible. The one supposes the presence, the other the absence, of a state of civil society.'[81] In many of the later works, Burke argued directly against proposals to extend the franchise. His most famous argument against it was his computation that only about 400,000 people at the most should enjoy the franchise, 'those of adult age, not declining in life, of tolerable leisure for such discussions, & of some means of information'.[82] If men did not deserve the vote, their opinions on the issues of the day could safely be neglected. In any case, in constitutional theory, the problem did not arise. For parliament was infallible when it came to collecting the sentiments of the people.

In legal construction, the sense of the people of England is to be collected from the house of Commons, and, though I do not deny the possibility of an abuse of this trust as well as any other, yet I

---

[77] Burke discusses the moral duties of political leaders in *Works*, V, 176–8 (*Reflections*).
[78] Ibid., 229.   [79] Ibid., 429.
[80] Burke to Captain Thomas Mercer, 26 February 1790, *Correspondence*, VI, 96.
[81] Burke's principal discussion of natural rights is in *Works*, VI, 208–15, passim (*Appeal*).
[82] Ibid., VIII, 140–1 (First Letter on a Regicide Peace).

think, that without the most weighty reasons, and in the most urgent exigencies, it is highly dangerous to suppose that the house speaks any thing contrary to the sense of the people, or that the representative is silent when the sense of the constituent, strongly, decidely, and upon long deliberation, speaks audibly upon any topick of moment. If there is a doubt, whether the house of commons represents perfectly the whole commons of Great Britain, (I think there is none) there can be no question but that the lords and the commons together represent the sense of the whole people to the Crown, and to the world. Thus it is, when we speak legally and constitutionally. In a great measure, it is equally true, when we speak prudentially; but I do not pretend to assert, that there are no other principles to guide discretion than those which are or can be fixed by some law, or some constitution; yet before the legally presumed sense of the people should be superseded by a supposition of one more real, (as in all cases, where a legal presumption is to be ascertained,) some strong proofs ought to exist of a contrary disposition in the people at large, and some decisive indications of their desire upon this subject.[83]

His suspicion of popular sovereignty did not mean that Burke was in any way opposed to popular liberty. As we have seen, he rejected the French version: 'It was a liberty without property, without honour, without morals, without order, without government, without security of life. In order to gain liberty they had forfeited order, and had thus forfeited every degree of freedom.'[84] Burke contrasted French liberty with the defence of liberty undertaken in England at the Glorious Revolution. As in the 1770s, Burke understood liberty to be a consequence of civil order and personal restraint. It was not to be taken as the theoretical foundation of government, 'The Revolution was made to preserve our *antient* indisputable laws and liberties, and that *antient* constitution of government which is our only security for law and liberty.'[85] He had no faith in unrestricted liberty: 'But what is liberty without wisdom, and without virtue? It is the greatest of all possible evils; for it is folly, vice, and madness, without tuition or restraint.' It was the easiest thing in the world to remove restraint but it was much more difficult to establish free government, 'that is, to temper together these opposite elements of liberty and restraint in one consistent work'.[86] Not that liberty was only for a few:

I certainly think that all Men who desire it, deserve it. It is not the

[83] *Works*, VIII, 323–4 (Third Letter on a Regicide Peace).
[84] See above, p. 110.　　　[85] *Works*, V, 74 (*Reflections*).　　　[86] Ibid., 434.

Reward of our Merit or the acquisition of our Industry. It is our Inheritance. It is the birthright of our Species. We cannot forfeit our right to it, but by what forfeits our title to the privileges of our kind; I mean the abuse or oblivion of our rational faculties, and a ferocious indocility.[87]

Burke's liberty has nothing to do with political power or with economic equality. Burke's ordered liberty is the freedom of every man to enjoy the natural rights of social, civilized life.

No account of Burke's later philosophy is complete without some discussion of the place occupied by religion in the corpus of his revolutionary thought. That place is by no means as straightforward as some modern commentators have maintained. Burke himself confessed that the workings of Divine Providence in history were beyond man's understanding and he admitted that he saw no discernible patterns in the history of civilizations.

It is often impossible, in these political enquiries, to find any proportion between the apparent force of any moral causes we may assign and their known operation. We are therefore obliged to deliver up that operation to mere chance, or, more piously, (perhaps more rationally,) to the occasional interposition and irresistible hand of the Great Disposer. We have seen states of considerable duration, which for ages have remained nearly as they have begun, and could hardly be said to ebb or flow. Some appear to have spent their vigour at their commencement. Some have blazed out in their glory a little before their extinction. The meridian of some has been the most splendid. Others, and they the greatest number, have fluctuated, and experienced at different periods of their existence a great variety of fortune. At the very moment when some of them seemed plunged in unfathomable abysses of disgrace and disaster, they have suddenly emerged. They have begun a new course and opened a new reckoning; and, even in the depths of their calamity, and on the very ruins of their country, have laid the foundations of a towering and durable greatness. All this has happened without any apparent previous change in the general circumstances which had brought on their distress. The death of a man at a critical juncture, his disgust, his retreat, his disgrace, have brought innumerable calamities on a whole nation. A common soldier, a child, a girl at the door of an inn, have changed the face of fortune, and almost of nature.[88]

[87] Burke to Depont, November 1789, loc. cit.
[88] *Works*, VIII, 79–80 (First Letter on a Regicide Peace).

Furthermore, in spite of his strong religious convictions and his frequent appeals to the Divine Providence, towards the end of his life Burke began to despair of the future of European culture, civilization and Christianity. Burke could not begin to understand the cosmic reasons why God was prepared to leave man to the mercy of the Jacobins. If the French Revolution was an atheistic attack upon Christianity, then why did God allow it to succeed? Burke did not have satisfactory answers to these questions and went to his grave a bewildered and demoralized man, believing that the curfew of European civilization had been sounded. From the very beginning, he had regarded the French Revolution as a profanity, an atheistic assault upon the sacred principles of Christianity, an infection of the moral order by the rationalistic individualism of the Enlightenment which attacked the basic units of society, the family, the church, the community and the corporate institutions of the nation. How Burke's God could permit the disruption of society and the destruction of the church of Christ, his means of maintaining virtue, morality and order in the world of man, is a question which takes us to the very limits of our knowledge of Burke's philosophy.

Only on rare occasions did Burke allow such insoluble problems to distract him from more practical considerations. His primary concern with religion was with its social and political manifestations. Burke always believed that politics could never be separated from morality and that political rights and duties required a moral justification. Furthermore Burke was aware of the 'benefits which society in general derived from the morality founded upon the belief of the existence of a God, and the comforts which individuals felt in leaving this world, in the hope of enjoying happiness in the next'.[89] It was scarcely surprising if Burke defended strongly the religious establishments then under attack from radical reformers.

Church establishments for Burke fulfilled several important functions in the life of the state. They acted as the vehicle of man's religious awareness, 'the first of our prejudices, not a prejudice destitute of reason, but involved in a profound and extensive reason. It is first, and last, and midst in our minds'.[90] Furthermore, they placed before the governors of a state 'high and worthy notions of their function and destination'.[91] It also operated 'with an wholesome awe upon free citizens' in that it impressed upon them the notion that power was a *trust*.[92] The Church of England was in an anomalous position with respect to the state, attached to it, but in many ways, independent of it. It was not an organ of the state but one of the largest independent

[89] *Works*, VIII, 81–2.   [90] Ibid., V, 176 (*Reflections*).   [91] Ibid.   [92] Ibid.

owners of landed property in the country.[93] Attacks upon the church, therefore, became attacks upon the whole social order. Church and state were inextricably bound up together in their struggle for survival in civil society. The example of France persuaded Burke that under the pretence of reform the whole church could be brought crashing down and after it the civil institutions which buttressed the fabric of the state. Naturally, then, in Burke's later thought, there occurred a gradual but noticeable shift in the direction of strengthening the powers and rights of the state at the expense of the degree of individual dissent which Burke had earlier been prepared to allow. He laid it down that 'government, representing the society, has a general superintending control over all the actions, and over all the publicly propagated doctrines of men'. Therefore, 'A reasonable, prudent, provident and moderate coercion, may be a means of preventing acts of extreme ferocity and rigour.'[94] It would be mistaken to assume that Burke believed in an *alliance* between church and state. He was too Erastian to make such an assumption.

> An alliance is between two things that are in their nature distinct and independent, such as between two sovereign states. But in a Christian commonwealth the church and state are one and the same thing, being different, integral parts of the same whole.

Therefore the Christian magistrate must concern himself with religious affairs and opinions. 'As religion is one of the bonds of society, he ought not to suffer it to be made the pretext of destroying its peace, order, liberty, and its security.'[95] There is no doubt that Burke believed a careless and casual toleration of religious opinions which were fundamentally different to those entertained by most British people to be a dangerous mistake. He warned: 'we have consecrated the state, that no man should approach to look into its defects or corruptions but with due caution; that he should never dream of beginning its reformation by its subversion'.[96] Therefore, 'He who gave our nature to be perfected by our virtue, willed also the necessary means of its perfection – He willed therefore the state – He willed its connexion with the source and original archetype of all perfection.'[97] As the state and its coercive power come to occupy a larger place in his political thinking, then, the

[93] A point which Burke chooses to ignore.
[94] Speech on the Catholic Dissenters' Relief Bill, 1 March 1791, *Speeches*, III, 543.
[95] Speech on the Unitarians' Petition, 11 May 1792, ibid., IV, 55–7.
[96] *Works*, V, 183 (*Reflections*).   [97] Ibid., 186.

emphasis which he had earlier placed upon individual rights diminished.

In the 1790s, therefore, Burke perceptibly changed his ground on the question of toleration for Dissenters. He identified their doctrine indiscriminately with the principles of democracy, accusing them of wishing to imitate the French Revolution. Although the Dissenters' view of the state was different to that of Burke (that is, their notion of the voluntary congregation contrasted with his conception of the hereditary corporation in a close relationship with the state) it was ridiculous for him seriously to charge them with plotting the downfall of church and state. Occasionally Burke would make an example of the statements of certain dissenting ministers, only to plunge himself into some terrible logical and theological tangles. On one occasion, in attempting to refute the view that the state had no right of coercion over the beliefs of individuals, his didactical method led him to the remarkable conclusion that the state 'had an uncontrollable superintending power over those opinions, and it was highly necessary for the prosperity, the safety, the good morals, and the happiness of the community, that it should have such a power'.[98] It was tragic that the crisis of the church and state in the 1790s should have made into an unbridgeable chasm of opinion a difference of view which Burke had formerly been well prepared to tolerate. It was with anger and horror that Burke refuted the Dissenters' belief that toleration and relief were rights and not privileges. (The right to hold dissenting opinions was emphatically *not* one of Burke's natural rights.) He regarded the church-state not as a voluntary association but as a corporate entity, imposing uniformity in most essentials. He rejected all thought of further relief for the Dissenters because in the conditions of the 1790s he had come to identify religious dissent with political subversion.

Edmund Burke's state in the 1790s was not an open society. It was an embattled castle with Dissenters swarming at the gates. Burke found it impossible to comply with their demands.

As long as they continue to claim what they desire as a *Right*; so long will they find it difficult to obtain it. Parliament will not hear of an *abstract principle*, which must render it impossible to annexe any qualification Whatsoever to the capacity of exercising a publick Trust; and I am myself much of the same Mind; though I would have these qualifications as few and as moderate as possible. This high claim of *Right*, leaves with Parliament no *discretionary* power whatsoever concerning almost any part of *Legislation*, which is almost all of it, conversant in qualifying and limiting some *Right or*

[98] Speech on the Catholic Dissenters Relief Bill, loc. cit.

other of man's original nature. As long as principal Leading men among the dissenters make *Associations* on this *Subject*; so long will they keep up the general Alarm. As long as they shew, not a cool, temperate, conscientious dissent, but a warm, animated and acrimonious Hostility against the Church establishment, and by all their words and actions manifest a settled design of subverting it, so long will they, in my poor opinion, be met, in any attempt whatsoever of the least consequence, with a decided opposition.[99]

Burke really believed that nine tenths of the Dissenters were 'entirely devoted, some with greater some with less zeal, to the principles of the French Revolution', more dangerous than the Jacobites of the eighteenth or the republicans of the seventeenth century.

For my part, I shall never think that a party, of at least seven hundred thousand souls, with such recruits as they can pick up, in this Kingdom, and with a body united with them in Sentiments and principles, and more susceptible of violent passions, can be in the present state of things, a ground, upon which one can rest in perfect Security. A foreign factious connexion is the very essence of their politicks. Their Object is avowedly to abolish all national distinctions and local interests and prejudices, and to merge them all in one Interest and one Cause, which they call the rights of man. They wish to break down all Barriers which tend to separate them from the Counsels, designs, and assistance, of the republican, atheistical, faction of Fanaticks in France. France, in the very plenitude of any power which she possessed in this Century, would be no Object of serious alarm to England, if she had no connexion with parties in this Kingdom. With a connexion here which considers the predominant power in France as their natural friend and ally, I should think Three of four departments in Normandy more formidable than the whole of that once great Monarchy. At this moment I think, There is no danger from them. But our danger must be from our not looking beyond the moment.[100]

Burke's earlier Whig theories of limited government tended to give way in the 1790s to an emphasis on the powers of state. In 1772, he had considered the will of the majority to be an important consideration in his discussions of toleration. Twenty years later it was of no account at all. He was less concerned with the merits of toleration than with the *consequences* of toleration.

[99] Burke to John Noble, 14 March 1790, *Correspondence*, VI, 100–4.
[100] Burke to Henry Dundas, 30 September 1791, ibid., 418–22.

The Burke who in his early career had admitted only moderate, restorative reform for an immediate purpose and a predictable end threw up his hands in horror when he thought he saw the bastions of European order crumbling. His reaction was emotive and hysterical, his analysis of events superficial and rhetorical. For example, his account of the *ancien régime* in France scarcely mentioned those economic and social aspects of the kingdom of Louis XVI which, in the end, destroyed both him and it. Like all alarmists, Burke ascribed evil events to evil men and evil ideas. There is considerable truth – perhaps more than many of Burke's admirers concede – in the charge that Burke viewed events from above and that he acquired a partisan view of the situation. For example, it never seems to have occurred to him to inquire into the astonishingly widespread *acquiescence* in the revolution in France. Furthermore, his continued support for a bankrupt monarchy was as astonishing as it was pertinacious, his lacrimonious sympathy for the privileged orders who had persistently and selfishly refused to permit any diminution of their enormous privileges astounding. Equally unrealistic was his sublimely peaceful view of British history. He completely ignored the Civil War and skated rapidly over the frequent outbreaks of religious and political instability in Tudor, Stuart and early Hanoverian England. His abandonment of most of the humanitarian reforms which he had previously espoused was regrettable. His earlier, real, if cautious, meliorism degenerated into a superficial fear of the mob. He continued to accept the divine right of the aristocracy to run not only Britain but every part of Europe without pausing for a moment to consider to what extent they had been, were, or would be fit to do so. He had more sympathy for the minor deprivations of a few aristocratic French families than he had for the sufferings of the poor of Europe. His willingness not only to tolerate, approve, but also applaud the existence of inequality was narrow-minded in the age of Rousseau. His willingness to tolerate any abuse in a working political system was curiously dated in the age of the enlightened despots. It is not that Burke's expediency made him short-sighted. Indeed, his expediency has been much exaggerated. The clue to the shortcomings of his political philosophy perhaps follow from his *method*. His style of arguing didactically from one subject to a pre-determined conclusion was essentially that of the politician rather than the philosopher of the state. As a man of affairs, deeply and politically concerned in the issues with which he dealt, Burke was able to take neither a detached and broad view nor adopt a sober, historical assessment in any of his campaigns and crusades. But one further thing may yet be said about

Burke's revolutionary thought. There was room for a critic of the revolution in the Europe of the 1790s. Burke was not that critic. He lacked the detachment to fill that role. Burke rejected the new order entirely, from its supposed ideological origins to its allegedly disastrous consequences. The revolutionary thought of Edmund Burke offered neither an analytical interpretation nor a critical rebuttal of the ideals of the French Revolution. In the last analysis, he was mainly concerned to argue the revolution out of existence.

CONCLUSION

Edmund Burke was a philosopher of an unusual kind. He believed that political philosophy had, at best, a modest function to perform in the life of society. Political philosophy defined questions; it could not solve problems. Nevertheless, Burke saw an inseparable relationship between politics and philosophy. Without the latter, the former would degenerate into a meaningless expediency. His conception of the limited function of political philosophy arose, perhaps, from Burke's view of man. Burke believed in the essential weakness and corruptibility of human nature, in the incapacity of the average man to resolve his problems in a rational manner, in the irrelevance of most 'rational' solutions to political problems, in the dangers inherent in most forms of political activism, especially those radical experiments with existing institutions which might cause unforeseeable damage. Edmund Burke's conservatism arose, therefore, directly from one of the most fundamental assumptions in his thought. Indeed, it was a function of his own political philosophy to defend the established order of things.

Burke's conservatism was also to a considerable extent conditioned by his philosophical method. This can be described in many ways and by many words but perhaps few would incline to dispute the assertion that Burke's method was *practical*. His practical involvement in party politics, his first-hand experience of public life, his familiarity with Ireland, and also, to a point, with France, the energy which he expended in mastering the details of colonial America, revolutionary France and Warren Hastings' India – all these provide an impressive factual and practical basis for his political philosophy. Paradoxically, it was the fact that Burke was such an accomplished expert in many of the affairs of his time which helped to make him so conservative. His detailed knowledge of affairs revealed to him the true complexities of political situations and political problems together with the irrelevance of so many of the nostrums of the right and the left. His political preoccupations served to orientate Burke's interests and to direct his attention to the present and to divert him from the past. To some extent, at least, this was why he was uninterested in origins and precedents. It was characteristic of Burke, for example, to defend the owners of present property and to neglect to inquire into their title to ownership by investigating how they obtained it.

His method is also didactic and rhetorical. Not for Burke the calm, detached 'philosophical' discussion. Burke's political philosophy *is* the philosophy of the politician. It was evolved in the press and on the floor of the House of Commons, in public and in party. His political philosophy is the disputation of a public figure constantly engaged in controversy and conflict. His inquiries, it goes without saying, were not intended to be academic treatises. They were directed towards the solution of certain pressing political problems not towards explaining the workings of society or the operation of the Divine Providence. He is uninterested, therefore, in establishing the truth of general conclusions from his investigations although he occasionally found it useful to buttress his practical suggestions with the fruitful generalizations which he was able to extract from almost any political or historical situation. It is, consequently futile to argue about Burke's consistency. As a practical politician, Burke was consistent or inconsistent depending upon the level at which commentators choose to pitch their inquiries and to define the words they use. It does not seem to be particularly fruitful to demand whether Burke retracted or adhered to his early ideas and opinions. *He moved on.* He moved on to different areas of political conflict and to fresh conflicts of principles. The most consistent thing about Burke's political philosophy, indeed, was not one or other of his 'theories' but his philosophical method.

That method was, perhaps, best displayed in Burke's contribution to the American problem. As we have seen, his thought kept pace with events and his ideas were always directed towards remedying some situation. Burke was well aware of the legacy of the past and its significance in political disputes but he utilized that awareness to assist his understanding of the colonial problem. Characteristically, he assumed that there was nothing basically wrong with existing institutions, consoling himself with the sanguine feeling that new men and fresh attitudes were all that were needed to reduce the political temperature and to solve all problems. Hence he wished to understand the human factor in the American situation and went to some trouble to familiarize himself with those environmental influences which had conditioned the spirit of liberty in America. His characteristic lack of interest in rights and their enforcement reflected his belief that man rather than his institutions was the primary agent in the historical process. In exactly the same way, on Irish affairs he thought it more important to remedy the grievance felt by the Irish people than to assert the legislative sovereignty of the British parliament for its own sake.

As we remarked earlier, Burke's ability to eschew a legalistic approach to politics was one of the most refreshing and most original aspects of his approach to statecraft. Yet, in other ways, his philosophy – even its most basic assumptions – amounted to little more than an unthinking acceptance and reiteration of some of the traditional themes of political and intellectual life which had become embedded in the European consciousness. His horror of corruption he derived, no doubt, from the classical authors whom he read in his youth. To the idea of corruption he closely related the Machiavellian idea of the balance of the three constituent parts of the constitution (monarchy, aristocracy and democracy). Burke, like so many of his contemporaries, believed that if one of the three became too powerful, then, the balance of the constitution would be upset. This unsettling of the constitution could only occur if the 'independence' of any part of it were infringed; such an infringement could only occur through corruption. That was not the end of the matter, for the constitutional dislocation of a state would be followed, gradually but inexorably, by the wholesale corruption of the people which, in turn, would lead to the overthrow of the state. Like many of his contemporaries, Burke blindly accepted assumptions such as these. Essentially, men of his generation were afraid of power. Political philosophy was devoted to discussing how to limit it rather than how to use it. Yet from these simple assumptions of an ancient European tradition so much in Burke's career followed. The conception of party, for example, was connected to Burke's wish to re-establish the independence of the British parliament. Party not only cured 'Discontents'; it also safeguarded the independence of the individual member. Party was thus one of Burke's suggestions for dealing with the eternal problem of corruption.

In the same way, he adopted an idea that was common to practically all thinkers and writers of the eighteenth century. This was the ideal of *restoration*, the notion that the ideal towards which politicians ought to address themselves was not some future utopia but the revival of a Golden Age and the re-application of its principles to a contemporary situation. We have already seen how powerfully this belief moved Burke, not only in his party thought but in his more general theories of the British constitution and also in his attitudes towards the empire, especially Ireland and America. This ideal was, of course, a metaphysical, not an historical assumption. Politics, for Burke's generation in Britain, did not concern 'progress'. It was concerned with an ancient cycle of renewal, restoration, corruption, decay, disintegration and, once more, renewal.

Underpinning Edmund Burke's political philosophy, then, was a mentality which rendered coherent the diverse and seemingly unconnected experiences of his career. The influence of Lord Bute and the spreading of corruption from the British court were no different, when all was said and done, from the corruption exported to India by the East India Company and practised by Warren Hastings. This, in its turn, was merely a manifestation of the same force for evil as the corrupt operations of the Protestant Ascendancy in Ireland. Burke's *remedies* to all these problems differed according to the situation. The *problem*, however, was fundamentally the same in all these cases.

It is within considerations such as these that the interpretation of Burke's thought must proceed. Not that Burke followed the unstated assumptions of his age invariably. As we have observed, he injected new elements into the sterile Whiggism of the mid-eighteenth century. In converting Whiggism into the ideology of opposition he laid particular emphasis upon the popular nature of politics and the public responsibilities of those who govern. He redefined Whiggism in a novel, prescriptive manner which still left room for reform (albeit restorative), the protection of liberty and the extension of toleration. Late in his career, however, Burke found it necessary to lay emphasis not upon the progressive ideas of the day but upon the fundamental units of society whose existence he sincerely believed to be endangered. His thought became directed towards justifying the social purpose of the state, of property, of government, of monarchy, of aristocracy and of the church establishment. The *conclusions* which Burke reached during the 1790s were not in their general direction inconsistent with those he had reached earlier in his career. The events of that decade only served to confirm Burke's belief that political change best operated when it restored the state to its original nature. The 1790s, in short, reinforced strongly the conservatism which was already such a marked feature of his political philosophy and elicited a more substantial, more theoretical and more soundly philosophically based statement of it than Burke had hitherto made.

During his final years the philosopher of restorative Whiggism propounded a philosophy of conservation which many commentators have too hastily identified with Conservatism. It may readily be conceded that Burke's political philosophy both made Conservatism possible and paved the way for its ultimate expression in the decades after his death. Burke's political philosophy, it may be said, acts as a bridge between the restorative Whiggism which dominated the English mind in the middle and later eighteenth century and the Romantic Conservatism of the early nineteenth. There can be no doubt that his attack upon the political philosophies of the Enlightenment and of the English Dissenters challenged the status which 'reason' had enjoyed in European thought for over half a century. His assertion of the importance of custom, of habit and of instinct in the life of man and of society drastically curtailed the realm of reason. For Burke, both men and societies were too complex and too delicate to lend themselves to the sophisticated yet superficial generalizings of the Philosophes. Burke was horrified at the effects upon society of the proliferation of Enlightenment rationalism; in particular, he deplored its subversive effects upon the basic units of civilized, social life, the family, the church and the state. Burke's 'conservatism' consists of far more, however, than the recognition of the importance of 'non-rational' considerations in society. Burke perceived the universality of change in human history and the transience of the present. He trembled on the verge of an organic view of social life which observed societies as living things with a past and a future contained within a historical world of continuity. Yet Burke, while he caught an early glimpse of the organic notion of the state, lacked a perspective on the future which the organic theory, in its fully developed form, demanded. Burke was so anxious to preserve the fruits of the past in the present that he was unable to look to the future. Burke rejected the Enlightenment's characteristic idea of progress because of his pessimism concerning man's capabilities to organize society upon a basis of controlled and progressive reform. In this sense, too, then, Burke's Political Philosophy is a bridge between restorative Whiggery and the Romantic movement.

All such labels are, however, of very limited use. They may help to suggest ideas and to establish relationships between thinkers and schools but they probably do more harm than good. Burke was an idiosyncratic figure in his time. He is impossible to label. It is wiser to understand why this is so than to fail to resist the temptation to apply a label to him. He rejected many aspects of the Whiggism of Locke but even more of the radical thought of men like Burgh, Cartwright and Paine. In some ways Burke was an unusual figure for the eighteenth century for he explicitly and powerfully rejected many of its most fundamental ideas. He detested its intense legalism and its preoccupation with precedent. He almost entirely ignored its idea of the unchanging nature of man. He rejected its simplistic belief in progress. He refuted the existence of its idyllic 'state of nature' in which free men peacefully nodded their assent to the contract. He disagreed with the widespread view that men were rational and independent agents capable of pursuing rational courses of action. He accepted only with severe reservations the opinion that man had 'natural rights' which it was the function of the state to preserve. In spite of his conservatism, then, Burke cast aside several of the fetters which had for long restricted the development of political philosophy. He succeeded in breaking new ground and in opening up new problems for investigation. Edmund Burke not merely made a contribution to the development of political philosophy but, in a very real sense, succeeded in extending its horizons and in enlarging its province.

BIBLIOGRAPHY

During the 'Burke Revival' of the last two decades an enormous amount of material on Burke has been published. Only a small portion of it, however, can be recommended with any enthusiasm.

On Burke's life:

The older biographies are now out of date in their general political interpretation but R. Murray's *Edmund Burke* (1931), and Sir Philip Magnus's *Edmund Burke: A Life* (1939) retain some value as readable and balanced accounts of their subject. Carl B. Cone's *Burke and the Nature of Politics* (2 vols, University of Kentucky Press, 1957, 1964) is a detailed and ambitious work. Although we are fortunate to have a scholarly, modern biography of Burke, Cone is rather uncritical of his subject and somewhat superficial in his treatment of the politics of Burke's times. On certain aspects of his career Burke has been well served. T. H. D. Mahoney's *Edmund Burke and Ireland* (Harvard, 1960) collects together most of the relevant material in a competent manner. N. C. Phillips, 'Edmund Burke and the County Movement', *English Historical Review* (1961), discusses a significant turning point in his career while P. J. Marshall, *The Impeachment of Warren Hastings* (Oxford, 1965), reaches standards of scholarship and impartiality which Burke studies badly need. On many issues, however, the reader can only be advised to read of Burke's day to day involvement in politics in his *Correspondence* (general editor, T. Copeland) and to read his *Works*.

Philosophy

The 'New Conservative' interpretation of Burke's philosophy with its concentration upon the Natural Law has been the most powerful vehicle for Burke studies since the last war. This interpretation has not been accepted in England although in America it continues to colour much that is written on Burke. It owed much to Leo Strauss, *Natural Right and History* (Chicago, 1953), and Russell Kirk, *The Conservative Mind from Burke to Santayana* (New York, 1953). The Introduction to R. Hoffman and P. Levack (eds), *Burke's Politics* (New York, 1949), is an early – and extreme – anticipation of the Natural Law interpretation. For statements of the Natural Law school see Russell Kirk, 'Burke and Natural Rights', *The Review of Politics*, XIII (1951), the more moderate and far more compelling essay by Charles Parkin, *The Moral Basis of Burke's Political Thought* (Cambridge, 1956), and the most complete discussion of the subject by Peter Stanlis, *Edmund Burke and the Natural Law* (Ann Arbor, Michigan, 1958). F. Canavan, *The Political Reason of Edmund Burke* (Durham, North Carolina, 1960) is an influential and interesting discussion. The Natural Law interpretation was qualified rather than criticized by B. T. Wilkins, *The Problem of Burke's Political Philosophy* (Oxford, 1967).

An alternative – and far more convincing – approach to Burke's philosophy is to attempt to understand what Burke really meant and to explain the concepts which he used. This had been patchily done and no 'interpretation' of Burke's philosophy as such exists. What could be done is dazzlingly illustrated by J. G. A. Pocock's masterful 'Burke and the Ancient Constitution', *Historical Journal*, III (1960). Pocock stresses Burke's debt to the Common Law tradition of the previous century but makes no claim that Burke can *only* be understood in these terms. C. P. Courtenay's, *Montesquieu and Burke* (Oxford, 1963), is in many ways a similar reassertion of Burke's traditionalist outlook. (For the beginner, indeed, Courtenay offers perhaps the best brief introduction to Burke's philosophy that exists.)

Particular aspects of Burke's philosophy have been adequately dealt with as follows: A. M. Osborn *Rousseau and Burke* (1940); R. Fennessy, *Burke, Paine and the Rights of Man* (The Hague, 1963); Harvey Mansfield Jnr, *Statesmanship and Party Government* (Chicago, 1965) is a controversial though brilliant example of a philosophical analysis of Burke's thought. Burke's idea of prescription has been perceptively and engagingly dealt with by Paul Lucas, 'On Edmund Burke's Doctrine of Prescription; Or, An Appeal from the New to the Old Lawyers', *Historical Journal*, XI (1968). Lucas breaks new ground in this article and opens the way towards an effective synthesis of Burke's ideas of History, Change and Prescription.

INDEX